Peripheral Retinal Degenerations

Venera A. Shaimova
Editor

Peripheral Retinal Degenerations

Optical Coherence Tomography and Retinal Laser Coagulation

Second Edition

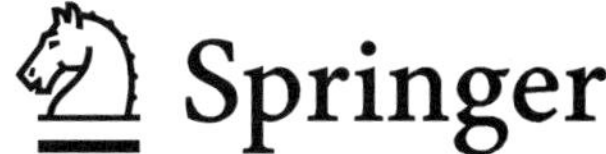

Editor
Venera A. Shaimova
Department of Ophthalmology
Chelyabinsk Laser Surgery Institute
Chelyabinsk
Russia

English text edited by Yana Gorodechnaya

The authors and the editor express deepest appreciation to Prof. Y. Astakhov for his invaluable contribution to writing this atlas

ISBN 978-3-319-48994-0   ISBN 978-3-319-48995-7   (eBook)
DOI 10.1007/978-3-319-48995-7

Library of Congress Control Number: 2017937371

Printed on acid-free paper

This Springer imprint is published by Springer Nature
The registered company is Springer International Publishing AG
The registered company address is: Gewerbestrasse 11, 6330 Cham, Switzerland

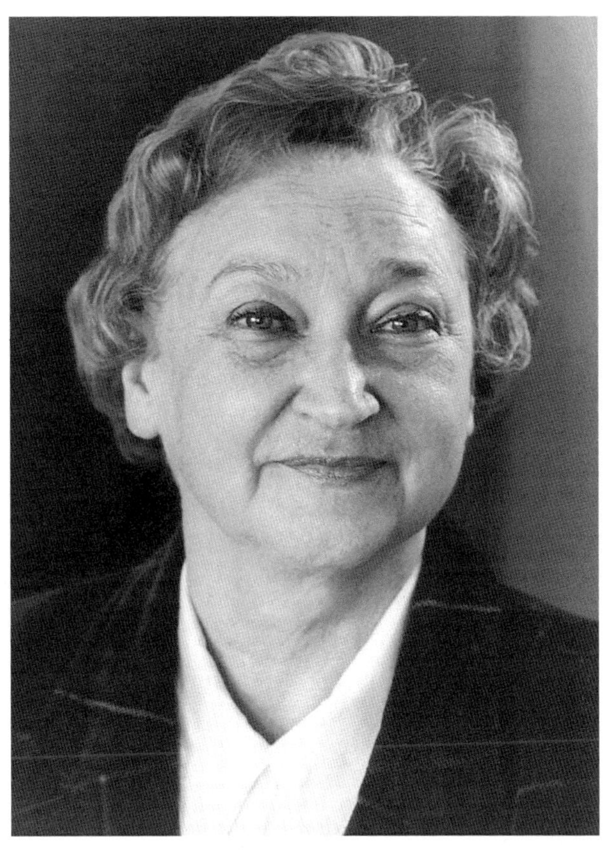

In memory of my Teacher, Honored Scientist of the Russian Federation, Professor Larisa Nikolayevna Tarasova

Foreword

Modern OCT technology generates high-quality images and improves visualization of the retina and choroid. Optical coherence tomography has been adopted by ophthalmologists all over the world, and it is mainly used for the study and treatment of posterior pole and macular diseases.

Venera A. Shaimova and her colleagues brilliantly show here the possibility and the necessity to go beyond the central retina and to also use OCT imaging for the study and treatment of the retinal periphery disorders. OCT assessment and interpretation involves both a technical dimension and an intellectual aspect.

Venera A. Shaimova and the other authors wrote this atlas with these facts in mind, to help and guide the clinician in assessing, classifying, and selecting OCT information. The authors gave all attention and stressed the special importance of the visualization of peripheral retina. Peripheral degeneration features and vitreoretinal traction are technically difficult to highlight, but are of great importance in making appropriate diagnosis and in selecting between laser treatment and surgical treatment strategies.

The authors have done a wonderful work in making outstanding peripheral retina OCT scans that will help ophthalmologists recognize, localize, diagnose, and study lesions in peripheral parts of the retina. I am personally very well aware of the difficulty in focusing and obtaining such beautiful images of the far periphery. The images in this atlas are of the highest quality, showing perfectly vitreal and retinal abnormalities.

The aim of this OCT atlas is to teach OCT users the use and utility of clinical OCT imaging of the retinal periphery. Venera A. Shaimova's atlas guides the general ophthalmologist as well as the retina specialist to obtain the best OCT views and to easily read these OCT images in both typical and atypical aspects of the retinal periphery.

In the first chapters of this book, the authors discuss the principles of OCT, describe the techniques of central retina and retinal periphery scanning, and explain the settings used to obtain such high-quality images. The authors describe the different types of vitreoretinal interface, and the pathologies leading to retinal detachment (tractions and adhesions). Wonderful OCT scanning of the periphery allows for the classification of the vitreoretinal interface into different categories, thereby facilitating the identification of risk factors for rhegmatogenous retinal detachment. Patients can then be classified into three groups: with no risk of rhegmatogenous retinal detachment, with moderate risk requiring follow-up, and lastly a third group at high risk requiring laser photocoagulation.

The following chapters review peripheral retinal degeneration classification and show the mechanisms leading to posterior vitreous detachments and retinal detachments. Other chapters illustrate retinal, vitreoretinal, and chorioretinal degenerations. These disorders are illustrated by black-and-white, color fundus pictures and OCT scans. An in-depth description of retinal and vitreoretinal interface features is given. The last chapter summarizes the place that laser treatment occupies in the management of peripheral retinal pathologies. This chapter reviews the current and sometimes discussed indications for laser therapy, describes its frequent and rare complications, and eventually assesses the results to expect from laser treatment.

OCT imaging of the retinal periphery has a practical and clinical interest for the everyday practice of ophthalmology. This atlas describes how to diagnose diseases and when to plan for laser treatment or surgery in a variety of peripheral retina disorders, and is aimed at quite a vast audience.

I think that this beautiful and up-to-date atlas gives a timely answer to a widely felt clinical need.

Bruno Lumbroso
Former Director of the Rome Eye Hospital
Director of the (Private) Italian Macula Center
General Secretary of the Italian Laser Society

Preface

Dear colleagues,

This is the second edition of the atlas of *Peripheral Retinal Degenerations*, based on a detailed analysis of clinical aspects obtained by SD OCT and fundus photography.

Optical coherence tomography (OCT) allows to acquire high-resolution cross-sectional images of ocular tissue structures that differ in reflectivity. OCT scanning is effective in evaluating retinal structure, interpreting morphological and reflectivity characteristics of retinal layers, and detecting pathological changes and follow-up. This technique is mainly used in analyzing pathologic conditions in macular and optic nerve areas.

We aimed to elaborate a methodology for SD OCT imaging of peripheral retinal degenerations. Our method proved efficient in estimating the layer-by-layer structure of peripheral retinal degenerations, condition of vitreoretinal interface, as well as in keeping clinical records and maintaining the follow-up control. We used OCT to detect retinal degenerations that present the highest risk for rhegmatogenous retinal detachment, and to justify the need for prophylactic laser treatment of peripheral vitreoretinal degenerations.

This atlas is a result of many years of work, and we hope that it will be useful for ophthalmic clinicians.

Our most sincere appreciation is extended to **Professor Yuri Astakhov** for his invaluable help in writing this atlas. We are infinitely grateful to **Professor Bruno Lumbroso** for his attention and his most kind words.

Chelyabinsk, Russia   Venera A. Shaimova

About the Editor

Venera A. Shaimova, MD, Dr. Sc. Med, is a Retina Specialist and Laser Surgery Expert with over 30 years of experience in ophthalmology. She is the author of 3 scientific research works (Ph.D. thesis, Dr. Sc. thesis, Peripheral Retina OCT Study Report) and 97 publications including 1 atlas and 4 patents. Dr. Shaimova and her colleagues at Centre ZRENIYA were the first in Russia to obtain high-quality OCT images of peripheral retina and are now launching an in-depth study of peripheral retinal degenerations.

Dr. Shaimova is a Senior Researcher at Chelyabinsk State Laser Surgery Institute and Chief Physician at Centre ZRENIYA Medical Clinic, Chelyabinsk, Russian Federation. Dr. Shaimova is also a member of EURETINA (European Society of Retina Specialists), Russian Glaucoma Society, and Russian Society of Ophthalmologists.

Contents

Contributors

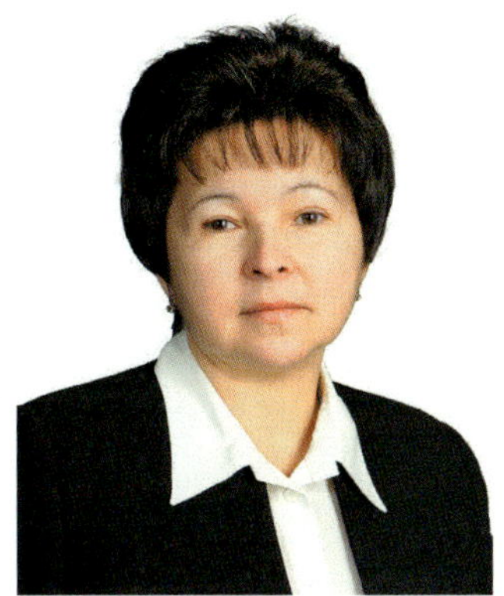

Venera Airatovna Shaimova, MD, Dr. Sci. Med. Senior Researcher, Chelyabinsk State Laser Surgery Institute, Chelyabinsk, Russian Federation

Director, Chief Physician, Retina Specialist, CENTER ZRENIYA Medical Clinic, LLC, Chelyabinsk, Russian Federation

Corresponding author - shaimova.v@mail.ru, 99-d Komsomolski Prospect, CENTER ZRENIYA Medical Clinic, LLC, Chelyabinsk, Russian Federation

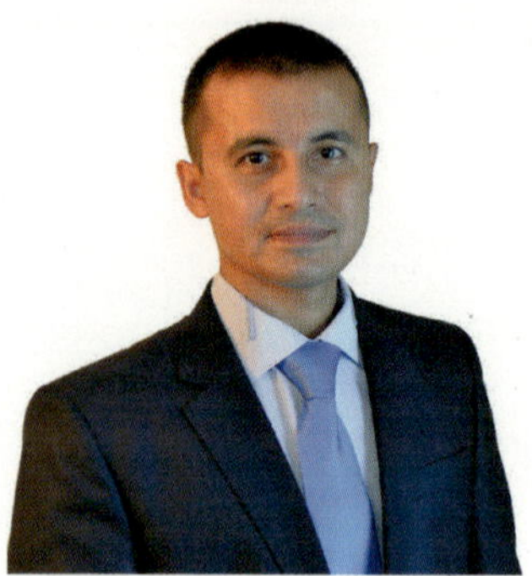

Ruslan Bulatovich Shaimov, MD, PhD General Director, CENTER ZRENIYA Medical Clinic, LLC, Chelyabinsk, Russian Federation

Head of Ophthalmology Department, Municipal Budgetary Healthcare Institution, City Clinical Hospital No 6, Chelyabinsk, Russian Federation

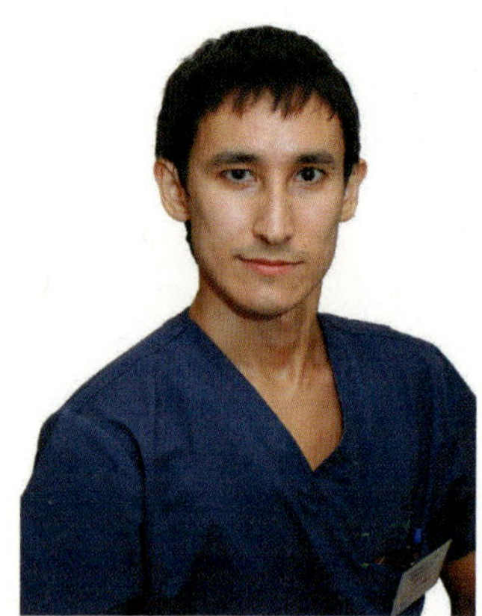

Timur Bulatovich Shaimov, MD Research Student, Ophthalmology Department of Postgraduate Education Faculty, South Ural State Medical University, Chelyabinsk, Russian Federation

Ophthalmologist, CENTER ZRENIYA Medical Clinic, LLC, Chelyabinsk, Russian Federation

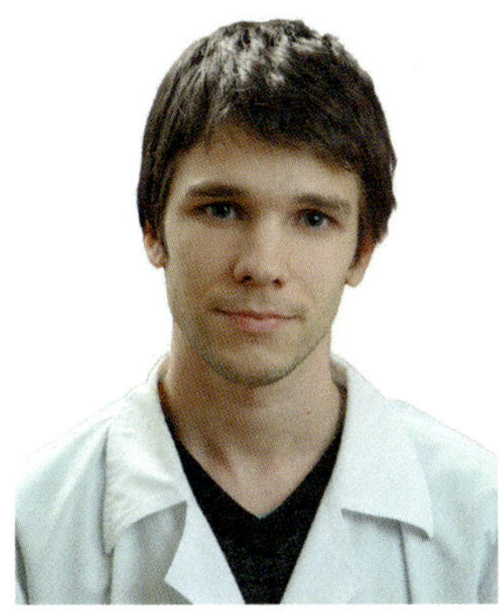

Alexey Yurievich Galin, MD Ophthalmologist, CENTER ZRENIYA Medical Clinic, LLC, Chelyabinsk, Russian Federation

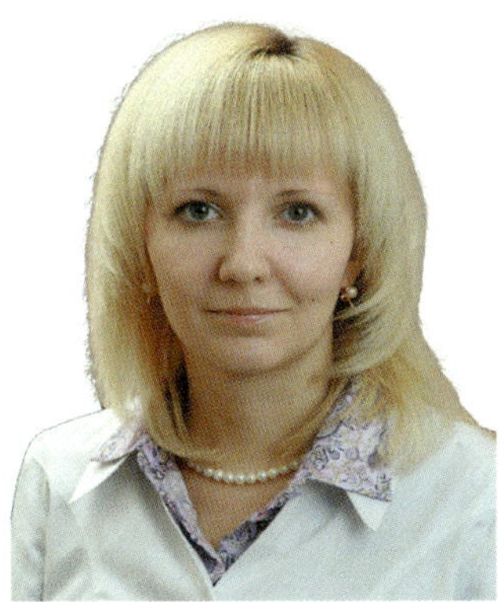

Tatiana Anatolievna Shaimova, MD Ophthalmologist, CENTER ZRENIYA Medical Clinic, LLC, Chelyabinsk, Russian Federation

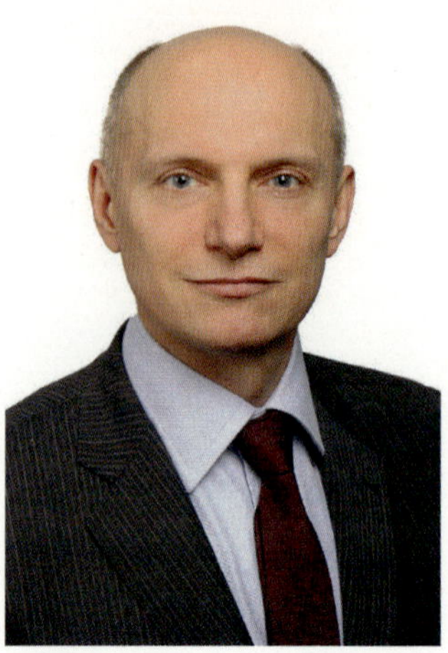

Ernest Vitalievich Boyko, MD, Dr. Sci. Med., Professor, Honored Doctor of Russian Federation Head of St. Petersburg Branch of S. Fyodorov Eye Microsurgery Federal State Institution, St. Petersburg, Russian Federation

Head of Department of Ophthalmology, Mechnikov North-West State Medical University, St. Petersburg, Russian Federation

Professor, Department of Ophthalmology, S.M. Kirov Military Medical Academy, St. Petersburg, Russian Federation

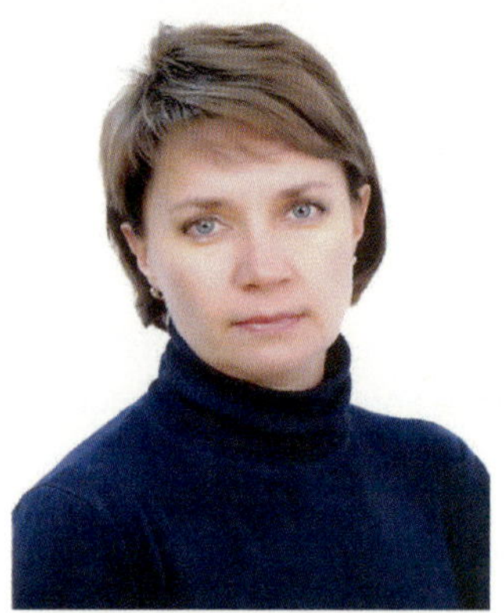

Olga Gennadievna Pozdeeva, MD, Dr. Sci. Med., Professor Chief Physician, Municipal City Clinical Hospital No 2, Chelyabinsk, Russian Federation

Professor, Eye Diseases Department, South Ural State Medical University, Chelyabinsk, Russian Federation

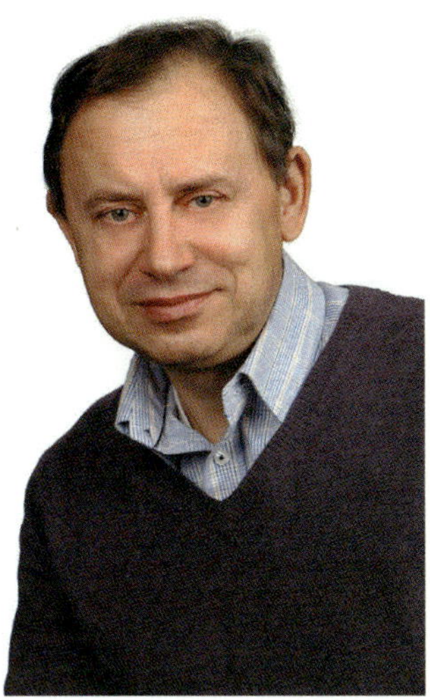

Alexey Valentinovich Fomin Clinical Marketing Director, Tradomed Invest, Moscow, Russian Federation

Methods and Principles of Peripheral Retinal OCT-Scanning

Timur B. Shaimov, Alexey Y. Galin, and Alexey V. Fomin

OCT-Scanning Methods

The eye examination included standard ophthalmic exam and spectral domain optical coherence tomography (SD OCT) with RTVue-100 (Optovue, USA) and RTVue XR Avanti (Optovue, USA). The fundus photography was taken using Nikon NF-505AF (Nikon, Japan) and VISUCAM 500 (Carl Zeiss Medical Technology, Germany) fundus cameras.

It is essential to explain the procedure to the patient before OCT-scanning, so that the patient understands and meets the operator's requirements. The eye pupil was dilated before the procedure.

The method of visualizing peripheral retinal degenerations consists of three steps:

Step 1 The retinal degeneration is localized by means of indirect ophthalmoscopy using +60 D, +78 D, and +90 D lenses and a three-mirror Goldmann lens (Fig. 1.1a, b) and depicted on the retina degenerations scheme (Fig. 1.2a).

Step 2 SD OCT of the retinal periphery is performed (Fig. 1.2b).

Step 3 SD OCT scanning results are analyzed (Fig. 1.3).

While performing the OCT scan, the patient's gaze was oriented in the desired direction with the head slightly rotated towards the area of degeneration (Figs. 1.2 and 1.4). If required, the OCT was calibrated according to the patient's refraction prior to the procedure. We made several scans and selected images with the highest detail. The scanning direction and the axial scan depth were adapted to the location of the retinal lesion. We aimed to standardize the procedure by making the scan in the optimal signal area between the horizontal reference arms and aligning the B-scan edges at the same height to ensure equal image intensification. We used the following scanning protocols: *Line* (axial length 6–12 mm), *Enhanced HD Line* (axial length 12 mm), *3D Macular* (scan area 6×6 mm), and *3D Retina* (scan area 7×7 mm). The maximal scan size was limited by the optimal signal area (see above) and depended on the location of the fundus scanning area and the degree of pupil dilation. The automatic dioptric

T.B. Shaimov (✉)
Ophthalmology Department of Postgraduate Education Faculty, South Ural State Medical University, Chelyabinsk, Russian Federation

Center Zreniya Medical Clinic, LLC, Chelyabinsk, Russian Federation
e-mail: timur-shaimov@mail.ru

A.Y. Galin
Center Zreniya Medical Clinic, LLC, Chelyabinsk, Russian Federation

A.V. Fomin
Tradomed Invest, Moscow, Russian Federation

© Springer International Publishing AG 2017
V.A. Shaimova (ed.), *Peripheral Retinal Degenerations*, DOI 10.1007/978-3-319-48995-7_1

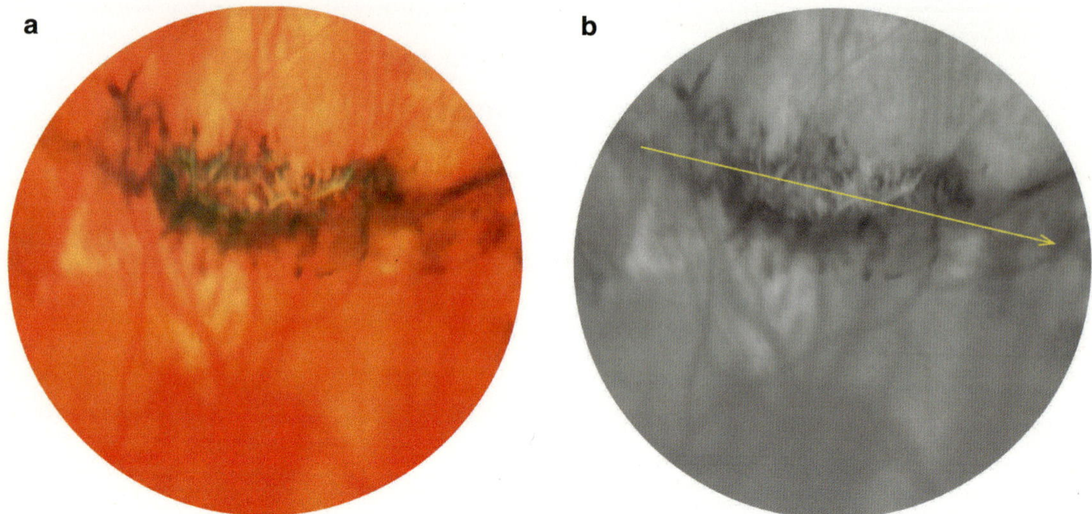

Fig. 1.1 (**a**) Lattice degeneration at the superior retina equator (*right* eye); (**b**) Scanning direction

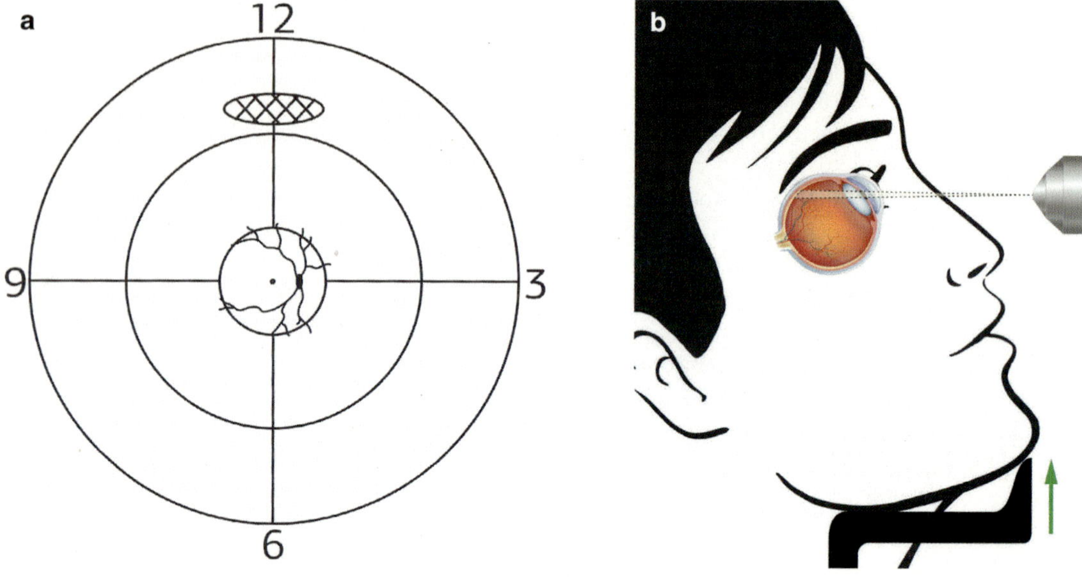

Fig. 1.2 Scanning of the retinal periphery depending on the degeneration's location; (**a**) Schematic location of the degeneration; (**b**) Patient positioning during superior peripheral retina scanning

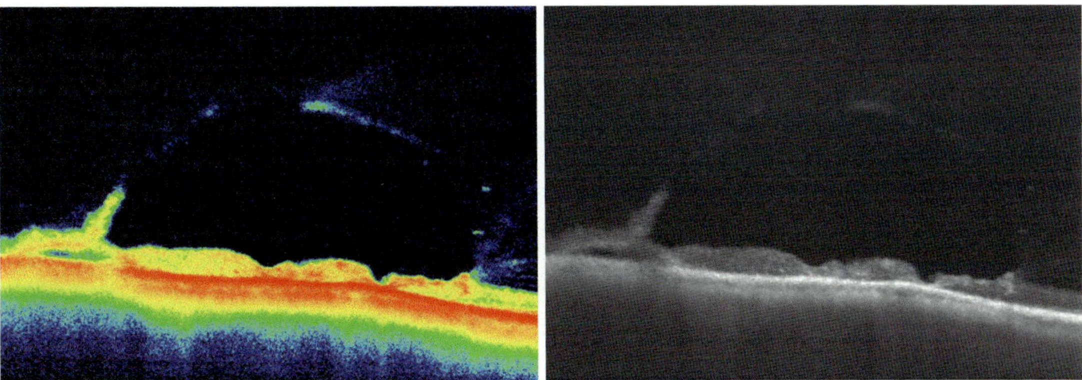

Fig. 1.3 OCT image of lattice degeneration (according to OCT-scanning direction indicated by *line* in Fig. 1.1b) in *Line* protocol. Marked vitreoretinal tractions on the lesion margins, atrophic holes, marked thickening (hyperreflectivity area), and a shallow detachment of the neurosensory retina

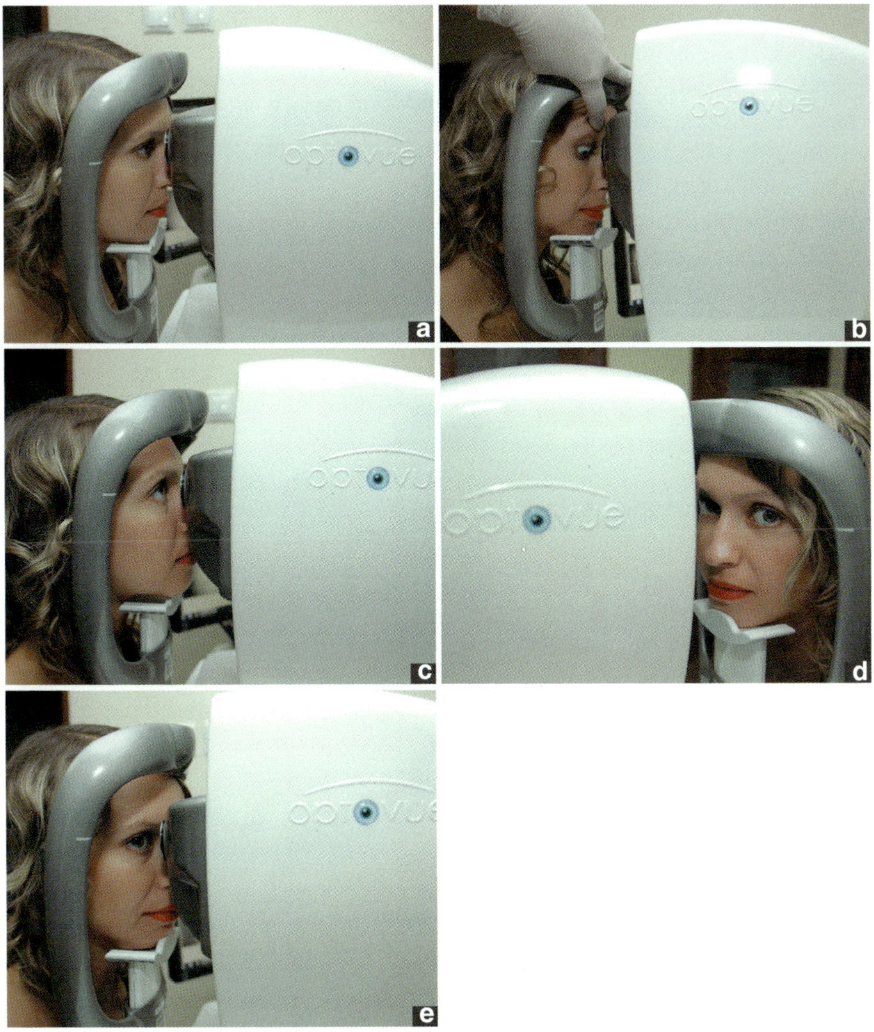

Fig. 1.4 Gaze direction and head positioning for the OCT-scanning (*right* eye): (**a**) Central retina; (**b**) Inferior retina; (**c**) Superior retina; (**d**) Medial (nasal) retina; (**e**) Lateral (temporal) peripheral retina

adjustment (both unifocal and bifocal) and axial adjustment is very important since these parameters change while switching from the central retina to the periphery (Fig. 1.4). The superior and inferior fundus regions are preferably investigated in the horizontal direction, while the temporal and nasal regions are usually investigated in the vertical direction. We shifted the scanning pattern in the viewfinder to ensure a more precise positioning of the line scanner and a successful imaging of the far-peripheral lesions. This also allowed to perform the scanning of any part of the lesion with no change in the patient's gaze direction and head positioning.

The following parameters were used in the linear OCT-scanning:

- RTVue-100 – axial resolution: 5 μm; scanning speed: 26,000 A-scans/s; 1,024 pixels per A-scan; linear scanning speed: 0.038 s; averaging no. of scans: 32
- RTVue XR Avanti – axial resolution: 5 μm; scanning speed: 70,000 A-scans/s; 1,024 pixels per A-scan; linear scanning speed: 0.014 s; average no. of scans: 120

To analyze OCT scans, the following morphometric parameters were measured: thickness of the unaltered retina, depth and length of the lesion, size of the vitreoretinal traction at the site of vitreoretinal adhesion.

It is important to mention several factors that may influence the quality of retinal photography and OCT scanning, such as: media transparency, degree of pupil dilation, deep/shallow setting of the eyes, nystagmus, head tremor, patient compliance and operator's experience.

OCT-Scanning Principles

The basic principle of SD OCT technology is to investigate the target tissue by comparing spectral characteristics of the back-reflected light with those of the reference beam (A-scan).

The coherent light beam (laser beam) passes through the ocular structures and is reflected, scattered and/or absorbed by different tissues depending on their characteristics and depth, which results in the interaction between the back-reflected and scattered light and changes in the spectral characteristics of the back-reflected light. The reflected light with multiple "optical echoes" is detected by the multichannel spectrometer, and the resulting interference patterns are compared to those of the reference beam using Fourier analysis. The spectral differences are used to reconstruct an A-scan, which shows the optical characteristics of the target tissues and their location. A compilation of A-scans represents a B-scan line. Three-dimensional scans are obtained from the array of cross-sectional B-scans; 3D scans have different densities of A-scans compared to B-scans.

The majority of the OCT scans in this Atlas were obtained using the RTVue-100 scan (Optovue, USA). The RTVue-100 scan uses a low-coherent infrared (IR) laser centered at a wavelength of approximately 840 nm with a bandwidth of 50 nm. The axial resolution of the retinal scanning is 5 μm, and the scanning speed is 26,000 A-scans/s. The peripheral retina was usually scanned in the linear and 3D modes. Table 1.1 summarizes the characteristics of the linear and 3D scanning by RTVue-100.

Table 1.1 RTVue-100 scanning protocols

Scan protocol	Scan range (mm)	Number of A-scans in a B-scan	Maximal number of averaged scans	Maximal number of lines in scan
Line	2×12	1,024	32	1
Line HD	2×12	4,096	1	1
Cross line	2×12	2×1,024	16	2
3D Macular	Up to 10×6	513	1	101
3D Reference	7×7	385	1	141

Several scans were obtained with the RTVue XR Avanti (Optovue, USA) (Fig. 1.5). This device incorporates the technological advances of the previous models RTVue-100 and iVue, and offers a scanning speed of 70,000 A-scans/sec, which is three times faster than the RTVue-100 (Table 1.2). The *Line* scan size on the retina is widened to 12 mm, and the axial scan direction in the *Line* protocol is enhanced up to 3 mm (2 mm in the RTVue-100 and other models), which gives more information on the posterior cortical layers of the vitreous adjacent to the retina. It also improves scanning quality in retinal detachment and bullous retinoschisis. The enhanced axial size of the scanning area improves the scanning process by minimizing the impact of suboptimal light direction (e.g., oblique lighting angle) in patients with a high degree of myopia or in peripheral retinal scanning.

To increase the signal-to-noise ratio and the contrast ratio of the B-scan, multiple scanning of the target region is performed (up to 250 scans). The averaging algorithm analyzes the obtained B-scans and removes the noise, resulting in high-contrast, noise-free images. The built-in eye-tracking system prevents blurring of the image caused by eye movement during long scanning sessions. This eye-tracking system uses the IR camera, which recognizes the eye movements of the patient at 30 Hz, and the

Table 1.2 RTVue XR Avanti scanning protocols

Scan protocol	Scan range (mm)	Number of A-scans in a B-scan	Maximal number of averaged scans	Maximal number of lines in scan
Line	2×12	1,024	250	1
Cross line	2×12	2×1,024	2×160	2
3D Retina	7×7	385	1	141
3D Widefield MCT	12×9	320	4	320

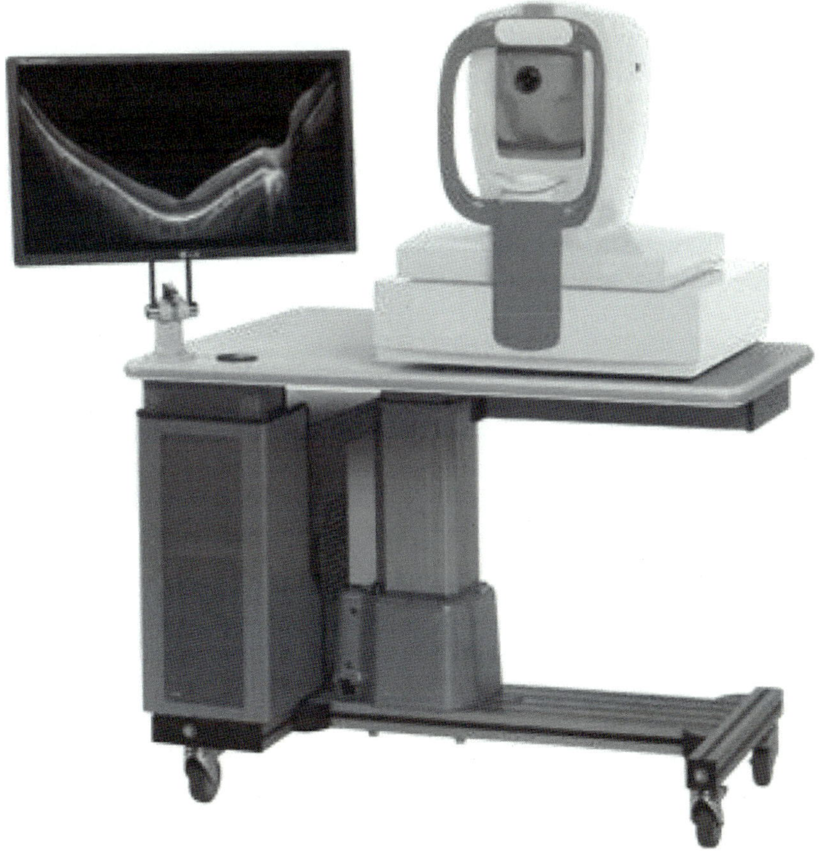

Fig. 1.5 Optovue RTVue XR Avanti

optomechanical system, which scans the target retinal region. This eye-tracking system also increases the B-scan quality (Fig. 1.6).

The RTVue XR Avanti enables detailed assessment of the vitreous using linear scanning in the *Enhanced HD Line* protocol (Fig. 1.7). *Enhanced HD Line* imaging offers the possibility to change the point of signal enhancement and can thus register minimal differences in tissue density (e.g., in the vitreous). The operator uses the "Vitreous" slider bar (Fig. 1.7 bottom right) to obtain high-contrast vitreous images and to localize vitreoretinal adhesions and vitreoretinal traction. Vitreous imaging requires a certain level of experience in manual Z-axis (dioptric) adjustment and polarization adjustment. *Enhanced HD Line* images are of high clinical value in diagnosing vitreoretinal adhesions, vitreoretinal traction, retinal tears in peripheral degenerations (Fig. 1.8), rhegmatogenous retinal detachment (Figs. 1.9 and 1.10), posterior

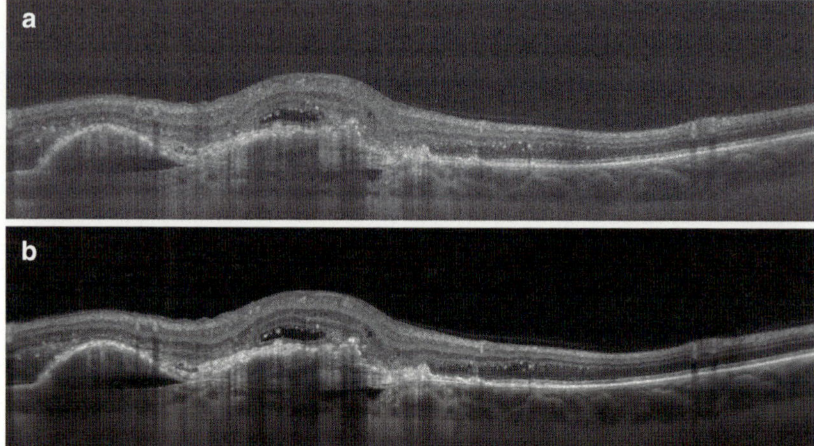

Fig. 1.6 The number of averaged scans and image quality; (**a**) 5 averaged scans; (**b**) 100 averaged scans (eye tracking enabled)

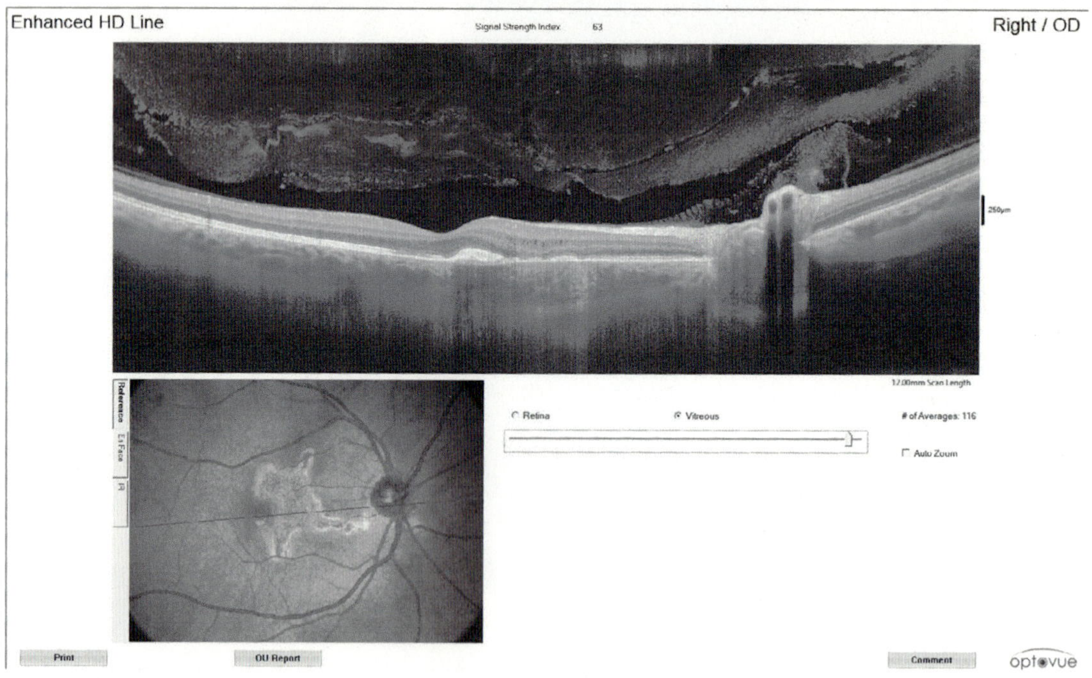

Fig. 1.7 OCT *Enhanced HD Line* scan of the vitreous in the central retina. Transverse scan length: 12 mm

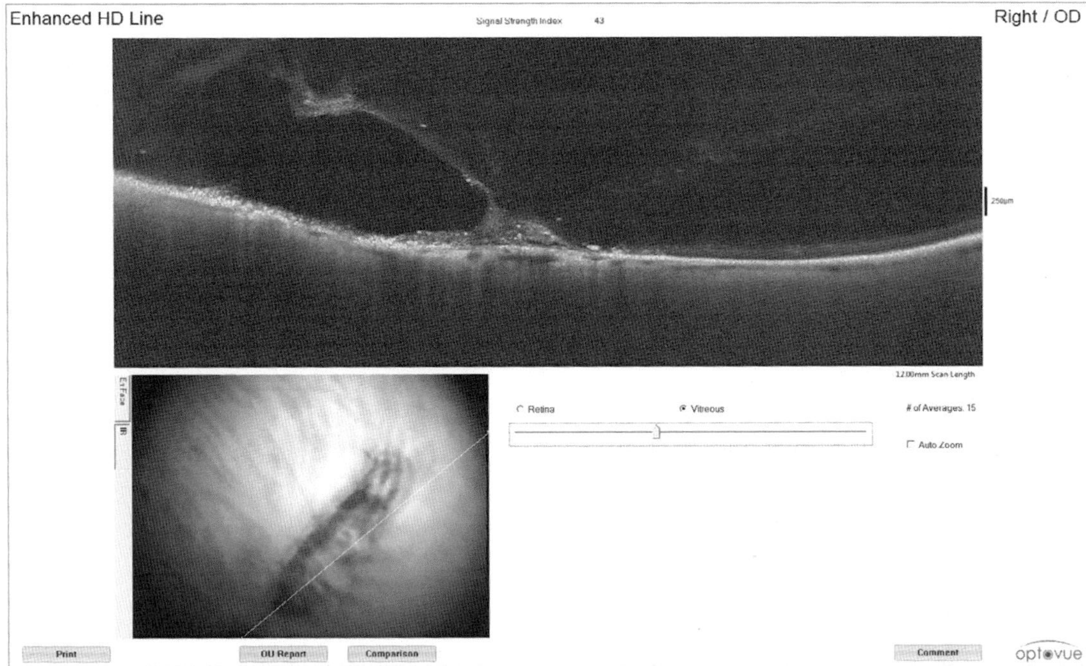

Fig. 1.8 OCT *Enhanced HD Line* scan of lattice degeneration. Transverse scan length: 12 mm. Marked site of vitreoretinal adhesion and tractions

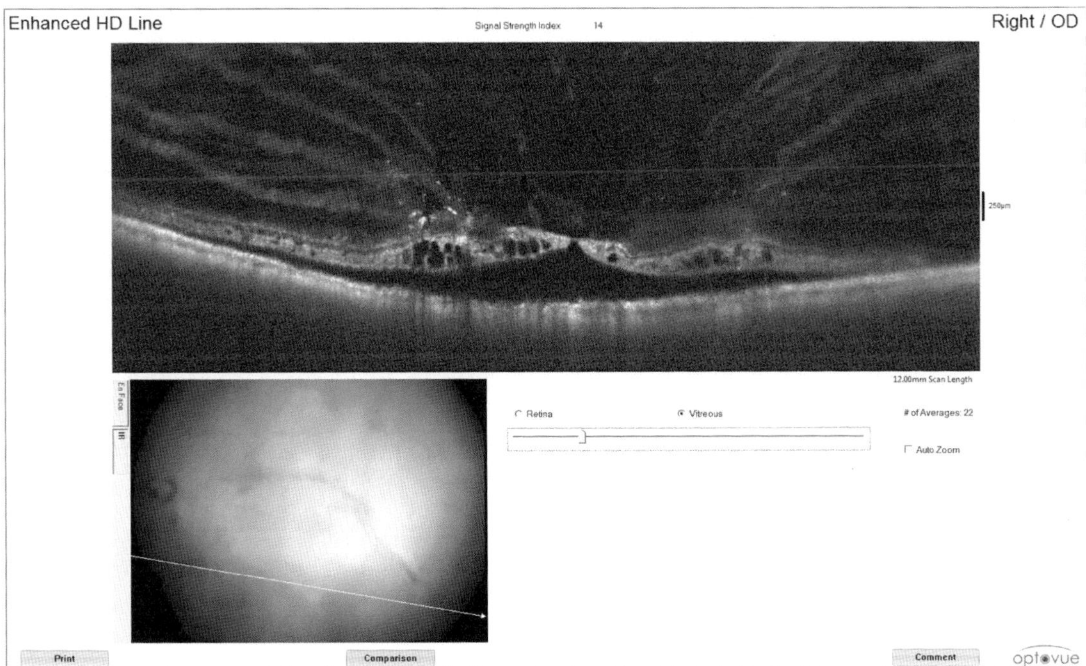

Fig. 1.9 OCT *Enhanced HD Line* scan of the inferior retinal periphery. Marked vitreoretinal adhesions and tractions over the demarcated shallow retinal detachment with a full-thickness tear

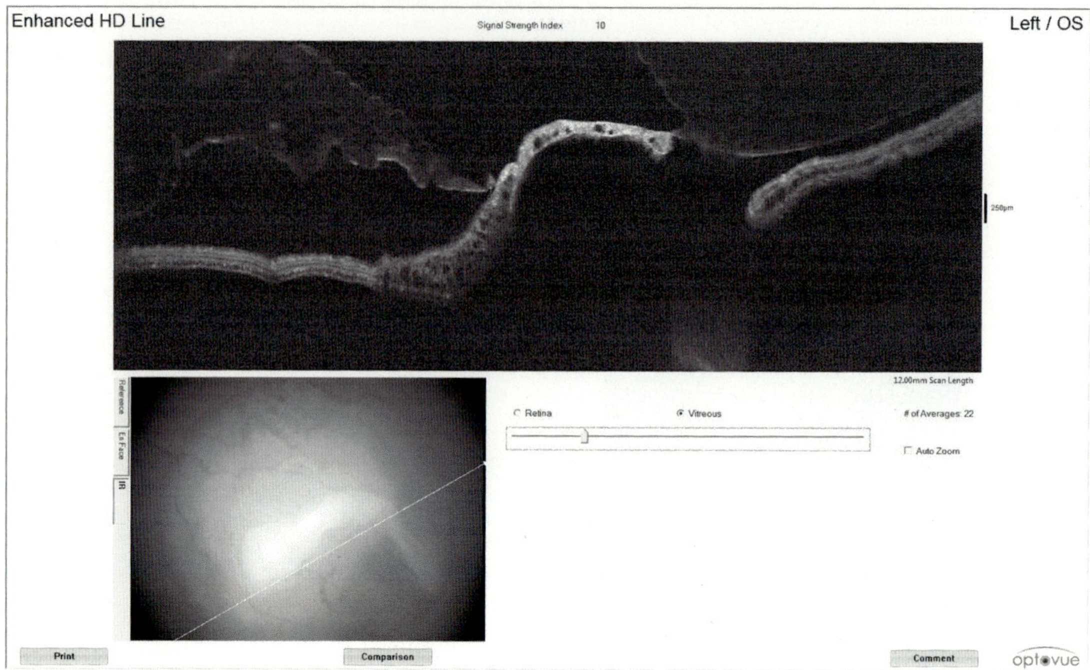

Fig. 1.10 OCT *Enhanced HD Line* scan of vitreoretinal adhesions with the edge of a flap tear in subtotal retinal detachment

vitreous detachment, and Weiss ring (Figs. 1.11 and 1.12). Similar to the *Line* protocol, the size of the scanning area in the axial direction is 3 mm, which allows to assess the vitreous cortex and its interrelations with the inner retinal layers. The figures demonstrate *Enhanced HD Line* images of retina and vitreous. Please note that the fundus camera (bottom left image) is an IR camera, and the image may differ from that seen during ophthalmoscopic examination.

Three-dimensional scans are obtained using two standard methods. The first method calculates a 3D scan from an array of 2D B-scans, with 141 parallel B-scans. The second one is a patent Motion Correction Technology (MCT) algorithm for correcting eye micro-movements. In the MCT-mode fundus is scanned four times: two horizontal and two vertical scans are performed to acquire a cubed dataset from four intermediate 3-D scans, with each scan compiled of 320 lines (B-scans), and each line compiled of 320 A-scans (a 320×320 3D cube). The MCT algorithm analyses and compares vascular maps for each of the four intermediate 3-D scans and reduces the effect of artifacts (image distortions, vascular "shifts" and "tears") associated with eye micro-movements. Quite importantly, the motional artifact correction is made in three dimensions - in plane and axial directions, thus increasing the quality of the *En Face* and ANGIO images. The 3D MCT image measures 12×9 mm. The vascular map obtained from the 3D MCT scan is used to match the associated retinal thickness maps and linear scans to the fundus (Fig. 1.13).

While performing peripheral retinal scanning, it is important to correlate the scan range with the degree of pupil dilation, distance from the scanning area to the fovea, and the location in the vertical and horizontal planes. Peripheral retinal scans are usually smaller than central retinal images.

The currently available tomographs provide both black and white (optical density coded in gray scale) and false color images (optical density coded in different colors). The eye-tracking system, which usually improves scanning quality, cannot always be used in peripheral retinal

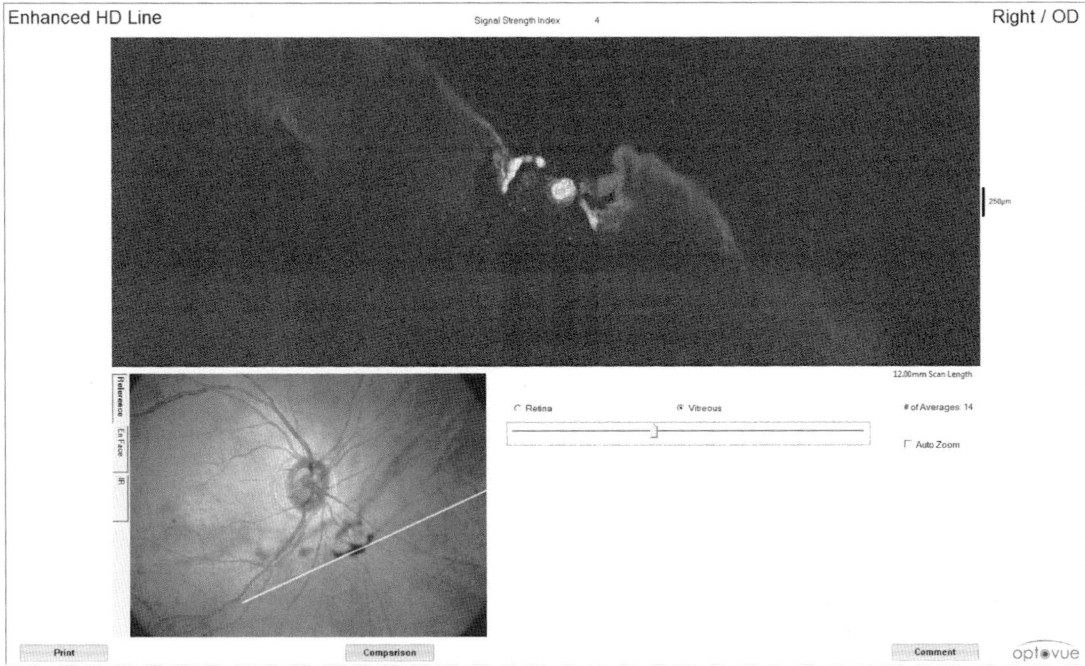

Fig. 1.11   OCT *Enhanced HD Line* scan of the Weiss ring structure in posterior vitreous detachment

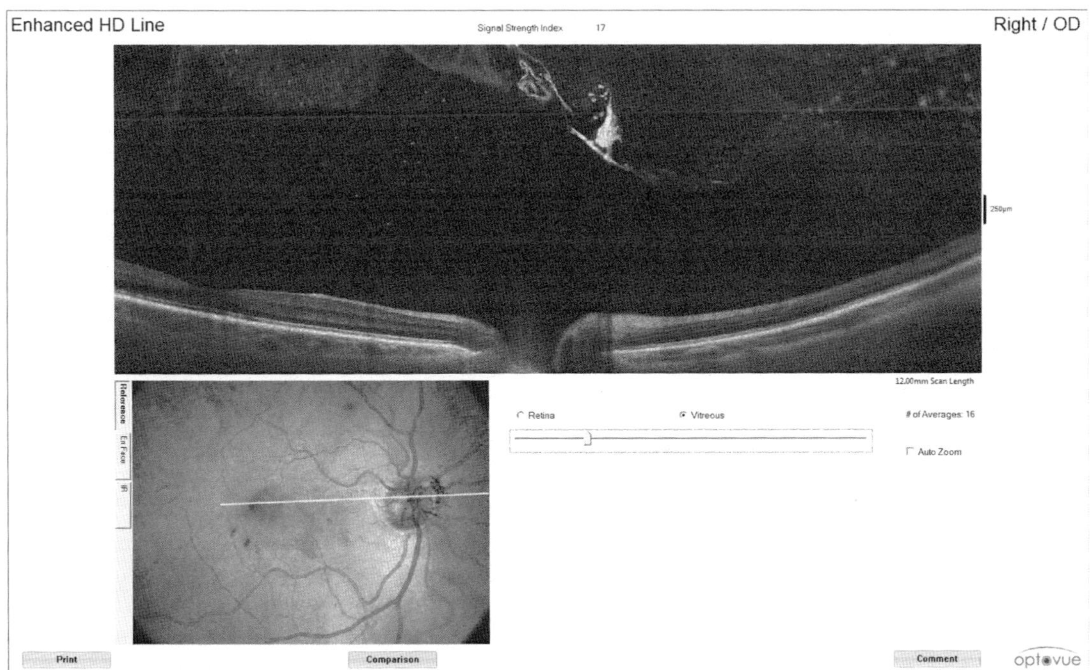

Fig. 1.12   OCT *Enhanced HD Line* scan of the complete PVD with Weiss ring

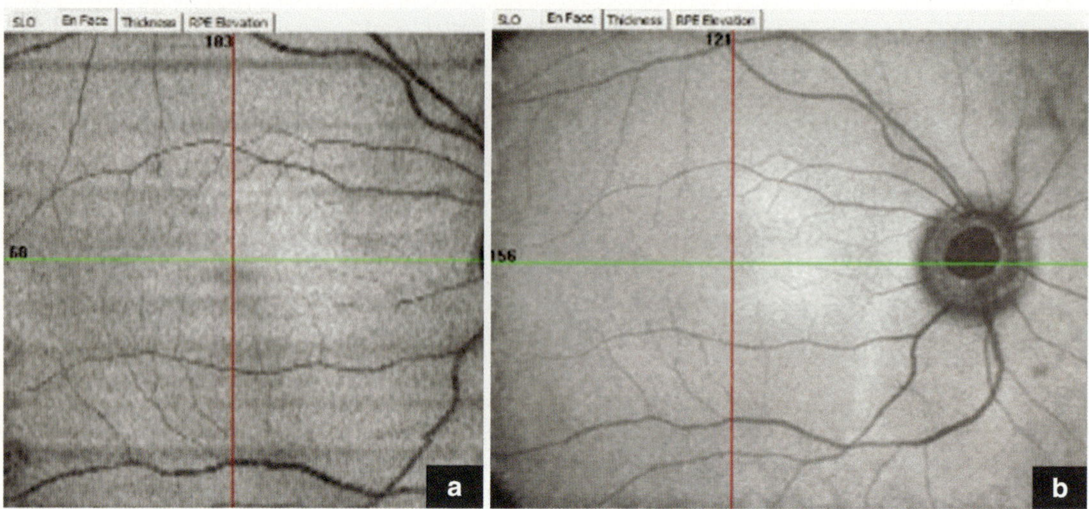

Fig. 1.13 An *En Face* image of the retinal vessels obtained with (**a**) An RTVue-100 scan in 3D Macular protocol and (**b**) An RTVue XR Avanti scan in 3D Widefield MCT protocol (true to scale)

scanning, as retinal periphery lacks high-contrast structures to track. Furthermore, peripheral scanning requires the patient's gaze point to be moved to the periphery, which often induces nystagmus and decreases the image quality even when the eye tracking is enabled. Both OCT models used in the present work have the autofocus function, which automatically adjusts the settings according to the patient's refraction and eye axis. In addition, the system optimizes the light polarization according to the predominant orientation of the collagen fibers in the cornea. The autofocus should be used not only during the primary procedure but also when changing the scanning region (from the center to the optical disc or from the center to the periphery).

B-scans allow to acquire cross-sectional images of eye structures in the axial direction. The *En Face* mode used in the Optovue tomographs enables to perform the cross-sectional follow-up of the tissue structure. *En Face* images are generated from 3D datasets through a special algorithm that identifies a tissue layer of a certain thickness (usually several dozen of microns) corresponding to a certain anatomical structure (e.g., pigment epithelium). The identified layer "outlines" the anatomical structure of interest, which gave the name to the term "*En Face*." The operator can manually examine the upper and lower layers of interest, thus evaluating over- and underlying structures. *En Face* images pro-

vide information on the irregularities of the assessed anatomical structures and the adjacent retina as well as on the location of pathological changes and their relation to the retina and vitreous, among other parameters. The quality (layer resolution) of *En Face* images depends on the number of B-scans in the 3D dataset. Each B-scan corresponds to a line in the *En Face* image, and the resolution increases with the increasing number of B-scans in the 3D scan. In some cases, only *En Face* images allow better understanding of the retinal structures.

En Face OCT images provide layer-by-layer information on the structural changes in the peripheral retinal degenerations (e.g., snail track degeneration). A *Line* scan of this degeneration is shown in Fig. 1.14a; the *En Face* image of this patient is shown in Fig. 1.14b–d.

The peripheral laser photocoagulation was performed using a diode-pumped frequency-doubled Nd:YAG laser GLX (IRIDEX, USA). The laser adapter (with a 50–500-μm retinal spot diameter), with parfocal revolving optics, was installed on the slit lamp SL 990 5x (CSO, Italy) with an overhead lightsource. The pulse power was set between 30 mW and 1.5 W (ranging mostly from 50 to 140 mW); the pulse duration was ≥30 ms depending on the desired laser spot diameter (100–150 ms in most cases). For the peripheral laser photocoagulation, the Goldmann and panfundus lenses were used.

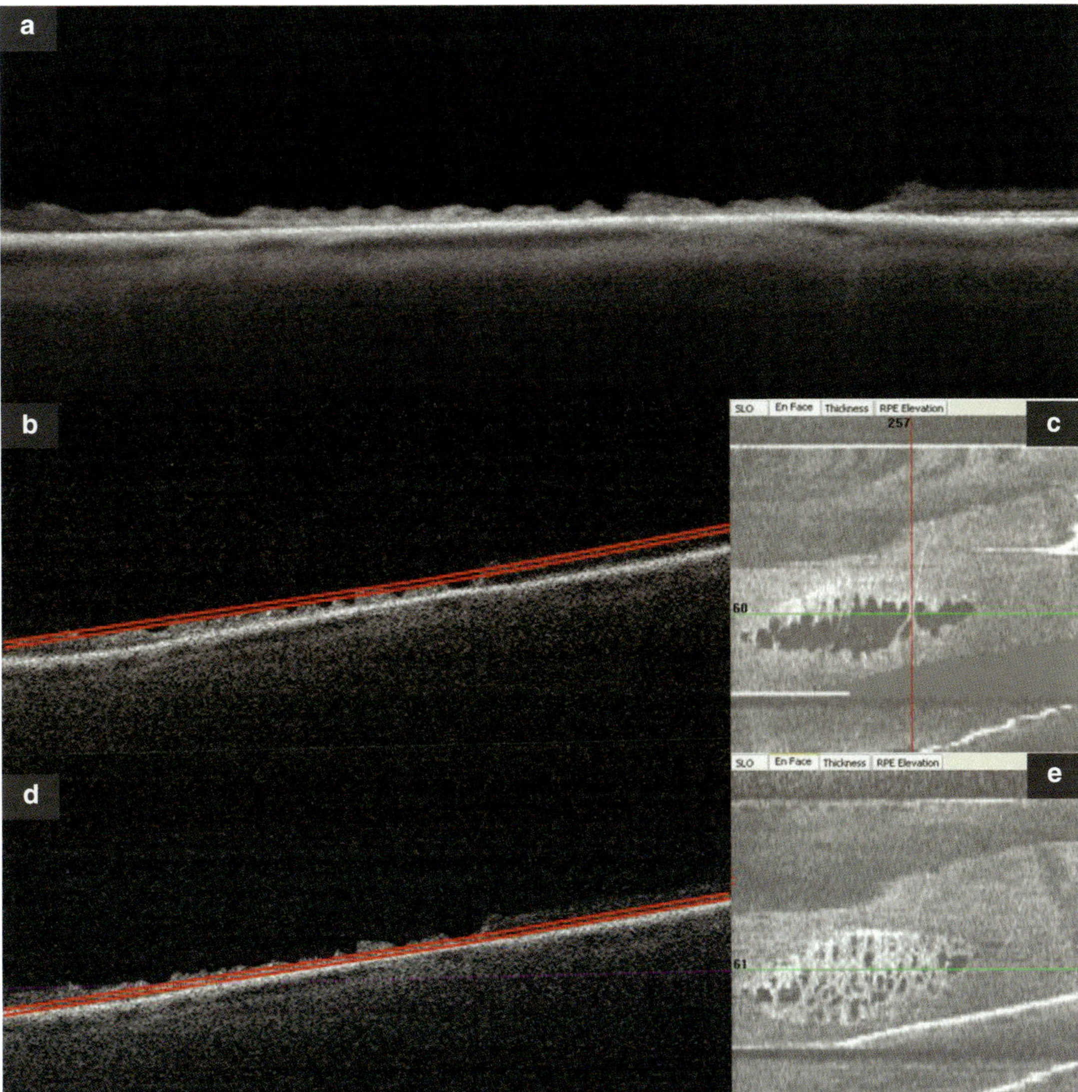

Fig. 1.14 (**a**) OCT *Line* image of a peripheral snail-track degeneration. The retinal surface within degeneration is irregular and jagged because of multiple atrophic holes in the neurosensory retina; (**b**) The double red line in the B-scan corresponds to the scanning *En Face* layer (the inner layers of the neurosensory retina); (**c**) OCT *En Face* image of the snail track degeneration. The multiple dark areas merge and correspond to the neurosensory retina thinning within the lesion. The *green line* corresponds to B-scan No 60 in (b); (**d**) The *double red line* in B-scan shows the outer layers of the neurosensory retina and indicates the position of the *En Face* image; (**e**) *En Face* image of snail track degeneration with multiple dark irregular areas, corresponding to atrophic retinal holes. The *green line* corresponds to B-scan No 61 in (d)

Optical Coherence Tomography of Peripheral Retina and Vitreoretinal Interface

Timur B. Shaimov and Venera A. Shaimova

Historical Overview of Optical Coherence Tomography in Diagnosing Peripheral Retinal Degenerations and Vitreoretinal Interface

Optical coherence tomography (OCT) is a high-speed visualization method that allows to acquire high-resolution cross-sectional images of ocular tissue microstructure in the anterior and posterior segments of the eye by detecting the reflections of infrared light [1]. Huang et al. were the first to obtain in vitro OCT-images of the peripapillary retina in 1991 [2]. The first in vivo OCT-scans of the optic disk and macular area were published in 1993 [3, 4]. Since then, macular and optic nerve pathology became the focus area of the OCT [5, 6, 7]. However, recent studies showed that OCT-imaging

T.B. Shaimov
Ophthalmology Department of Postgraduate Education Faculty, South Ural State Medical University, Chelyabinsk, Russian Federation

Center Zreniya Medical Clinic, LLC, Chelyabinsk, Russian Federation

V.A. Shaimova (✉)
Chelyabinsk State Laser Surgery Insitute, Chelyabinsk, Russian Federation

Center Zreniya Medical Clinic, LLC, Chelyabinsk, Russian Federation
e-mail: shaimova.v@mail.ru

may also be an accurate diagnostic tool for peripheral retinal degenerations [8].

Kamppeter and Jonas were the first to use OCT in vivo (OCT 3, Zeiss Humphrey Ophthalmic Systems, USA) to visualize peripheral retinal degenerations in 2004. The authors reported a case of peripheral retinoschisis with an outer retinal layer tear that was visualized with OCT, and showed the effectiveness of OCT in distinguishing choroidal nevus from choroidal melanoma, and retinoschisis from rhegmatogenous retinal detachment [9].

In 2006, Ghazi et al. studied histological sections from 11 enucleated eyes and presented OCT (Model number 3000, Carl Zeiss Ophthalmic Systems, USA) images of peripheral retinal lesions (cystoid degeneration, paving-stone degeneration and localized retinal detachment) that correlated with the histopathologic findings [10].

In 2010, Cheng et al. measured the central retinal thickness up to 40° from the fovea in both myopic and non-myopic eyes using OCT Stratus (Carl Zeiss Meditec, USA) [11]. The retinal thickness at 40° from the fovea was 7 % lower in myopic eyes than that in non-myopic eyes and did not depend on the presence of peripheral retinal degeneration (in both groups). The authors, however, did not make OCT scans of any peripheral retinal degenerations.

Muni et al. (2010) conducted a retrospective study of three patients (five eyes) with retinopathy of prematurity using a handheld (HHSD-OCT)

V.A. Shaimova (ed.), *Peripheral Retinal Degenerations*, DOI 10.1007/978-3-319-48995-7_2

spectral OCT (Envisu C2300, BIOPTIGEN). The authors found the device to be capable of assessing the structural properties of the vitreoretinal interface and the interactions of retina and vitreous in tractional retinoschisis and retinal detachment. The handheld SD-OCT proved to be of value in early detection of tractional retinoschisis, retinal tears, and retinal detachments as well as in defining the indications for laser photocoagulation in children [12].

Landa et al. (2010) in his rare clinical case reported OCT findings (OPKO/OTI spectral OCT, USA) in a patient with an inferonasal bullous retinoschisis in a 70-year old male that was seen as characteristic splitting of the outer plexiform layer and cystoid degeneration of the inner retinal layers [13].

Manjunath et al. (2011) examined patients with lattice degeneration in vivo using spectral domain (SD) Cirrus HD-OCT (Carl Zeiss Meditec, USA) and defined the main OCT signs of this type of retinal degeneration. They were also the first to perform morphometric analysis and to measure the length of subclinical retinal detachment [14]. SD-OCT was shown to be a useful tool for visualizing the vitreoretinal interface in lattice degeneration.

Stehouwer et al. (2011) explored the possibility of using an OCT device that was integrated into a slit-lamp (SL SCAN-1, Topcon Europe Medical BV, Netherlands) to visualize the retinal periphery through a three-mirror contact lens (HAAG-STREIT AG, Koeniz, Switzerland) and a handheld lens (Volk SuperField NC Lens) [15]. These lenses allowed to obtain good quality images of peripheral retinal tears, retinoschisis, retinal detachment after retinal laser photocoagulation. The authors showed high diagnostic performance of the OCT images similar to histological findings.

Oster et al. (2011) conducted a retrospective study on 11 patients (12 eyes) who underwent SLO/SD-OCT after scleral buckling surgery due to retinal detachment. The SD-OCT proved effective in evaluating surgery results, including residual retinal detachment, vitreoretinal traction, retinal tears, and subretinal fluid [16].

Kothari et al. (2012) published time-domain OCT (Stratus 3, Carl Zeiss Meditec, USA) and SD-OCT (Cirrus, Carl Zeiss Meditec, USA) in vivo scans of 36 eyes (28 patients) with various peripheral retinal degenerations (lattice, snail track, and paving-stone), retinal tears, senile retinoschisis, and choroidal nevus [17].

Shaimova et al. (2013) demonstrated OCT scanning results of peripheral retinal breaks (RTVue-100 (OPTOVUE, USA)) in a study involving 176 eyes [18] and peripheral retinal degenerations (lattice degeneration, snail track degeneration, cystoid degeneration, pathologic hyperpigmentation, retinoschisis, paving-stone degeneration) in a study involving 239 eyes [19].

The authors showed high diagnostic performance of OCT in detecting structural characteristics and shape of peripheral retinal degenerations and tears, vitreoretinal adhesions and tractions, and measuring morphometric parameters.

Fawzi et al. (2014) in their study showed that white-without-pressure degeneration is characterized by hyperreflectivity of the ellipsoid zone (EZ), and dark-without-pressure phenomenon causes hyporeflectivity of the EZ. One year follow-up examination showed no signs of progression [20].

Choudhry et al. (2016) have recently published a detailed analysis of high-resolution SD-OCT images of peripheral retinal degenerations and vitreoretinal interface combined with ultra-widefield color fundus photographs obtained with Optos Tx-200 (Optos, USA) [21].

All these international studies demonstrate the effectiveness of OCT in assessing peripheral retina in vivo with high quality scans similar to histologic images, which makes OCT a valuable tool in estimating the vitreoretinal interface, in the decision-making process, in treatment and follow-up.

OCT of Peripheral Retina in Emmetropic, Hyperopic, and Myopic Eyes

OCT enables detailed quantitative and qualitative analysis of the central retina. To assess the structural properties of the peripheral retina and the thickness of retinal layers, we performed OCT-scanning in various retinal regions (such as macula, equator, mid-periphery, and far periphery) in patients with emmetropia, moderate hyperopia, and moderate myopia. The procedure was performed on otherwise healthy volunteers.

Emmetropia

A 35-year-old male presenting with no complaints.

OD: VA, sc 20/20; axial length (AL), 23.5 mm. Clear media.

OCT Scan Description (Fig. 2.1)

Scan 1 Macular area The foveal pit retains a normal profile. All retinal layers are clearly distinguished. Retinal pigment epithelium (pigment epithelium) is smooth. Retinal vessels are observed as shadows parafoveally and perifoveally. The average foveal and parafoveal retinal thickness is 222 µm and 355 µm, respectively.

Scan 2 Equatorial area The retinal surface is smooth. Hyperreflective layers of the pigment epithelium, photoreceptors, and neuroepithelium are observed. Retinal vessels are observed as shadows. The posterior hyaloid membrane is adherent. Large choroidal vessels are identified. The average retinal thickness is 171 µm.

Scan 3 Mid-peripheral area The retinal surface is smooth. The inner and outer layers of the neuroepithelium are poorly distinguished. Retinal vessels are observed as shadows. The posterior hyaloid membrane is intact. Medium-sized choroidal vessels are identified. The average retinal thickness is 155 µm.

Scan 4 Far peripheral area The retinal surface is smooth. The inner and outer layers of the neuroepithelium are poorly distinguished. Retinal vessels and small choroidal vessels are identified. The average retinal thickness is 132 µm.

Conclusion

The retinal layers are more clearly distinguished in the central retina and equatorial area. The retinal thickness gradually decreases from the center to the periphery. The equatorial area is 2 times thinner, the mid-peripheral area is 2.3 times thinner, and the far-peripheral area is 2.7 times thinner than the parafoveal area.

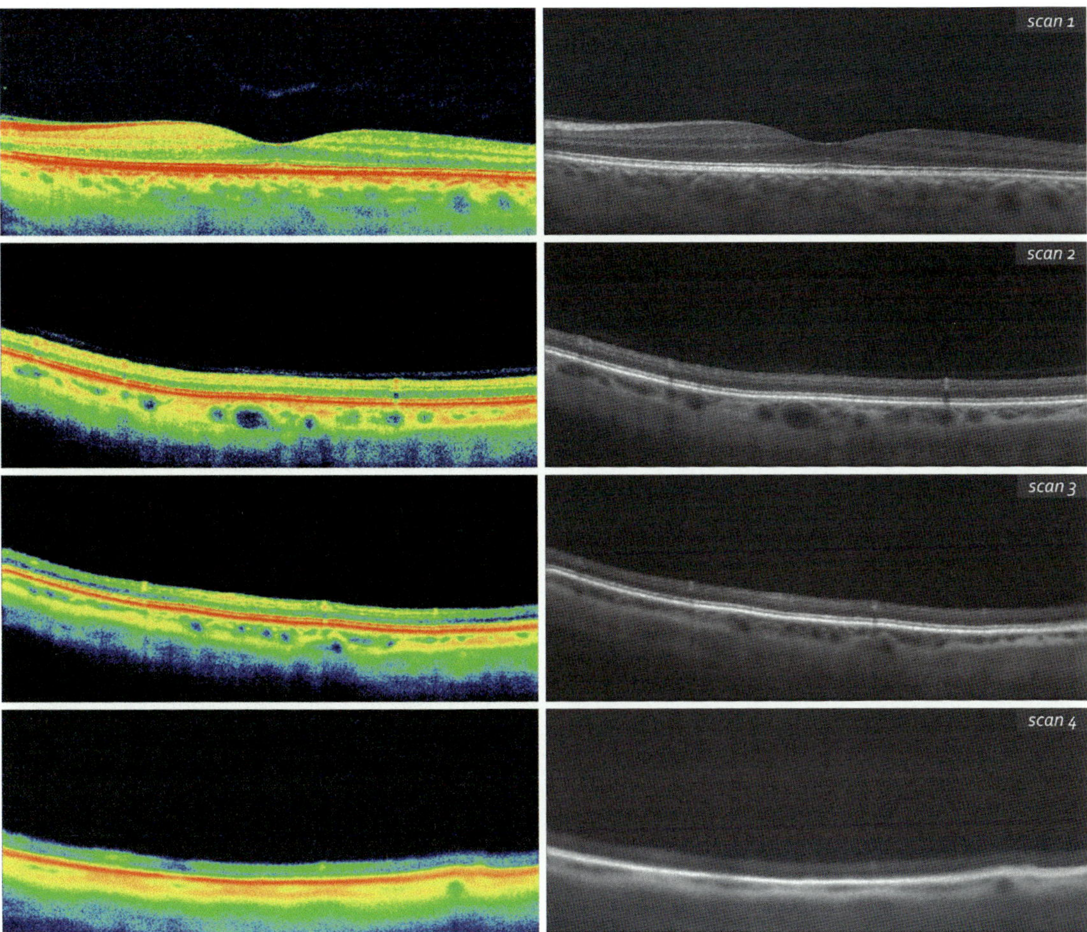

Fig. 2.1 OCT of the retina in emmetropic patient. **Scan 1** Macular area. The average foveal and parafoveal retinal thickness is 222 μm and 355 μm, respectively. **Scan 2** Equatorial area. The average retinal thickness is 171 μm. **Scan 3** Mid-peripheral area. The average retinal thickness is 155 μm. **Scan 4** Far peripheral area. The average retinal thickness is 132 μm

Moderate Hyperopia

A 37-year-old male complaining of deterioration of distance and near vision.

OD: VA, sc 20/200, cc 20/20 with +4.5 sph; AL, 21.9 mm.

OCT Scan Description (Fig. 2.2)

Scan 1 Macular area The foveal pit retains a normal profile. All retinal layers are clearly distinguished. The pigment epithelium is smooth. Retinal vessels are observed as shadows parafoveally and perifoveally. The average foveal and parafoveal retinal thickness is 245 μm and 375 μm, respectively.

Scan 2 Equatorial area The retinal surface is smooth. Hyperreflective layers of the pigment epithelium, photoreceptors, and neuroepithelium are observed. Retinal vessels are observed as shadows. Large and medium-sized choroidal vessels are identified. The average retinal thickness is 193 μm.

Scan 3 Mid-peripheral area The retinal surface is smooth. The inner and outer layers of the neuroepithelium are distinguishable. Retinal vessels are observed as shadows. Medium-sized choroidal vessels are identified. The average retinal thickness is 174 μm.

Scan 4 Far peripheral area The retinal surface is smooth. The inner and outer layers of the neuroepithelium are distinguishable. Retinal vessels and small choroidal vessels are identified. The average retinal thickness is 151 μm.

Conclusion

Retinal OCT in moderate hyperopia demonstrates decreasing retinal thickness from the center to the periphery. The equatorial area is 1.9 times thinner, the mid-peripheral area is 2.2 times thinner, and the far peripheral area is 2.5 times thinner than the central retina. Retinal thickness in patients with moderate hyperopia is 9 % higher in the foveal area, 5.4 % higher in the parafoveal area, 11.4 % higher in the equatorial area, 10.9 % higher in the mid-peripheral area, and 12.6 % higher in the far peripheral area than that in patients with emmetropia.

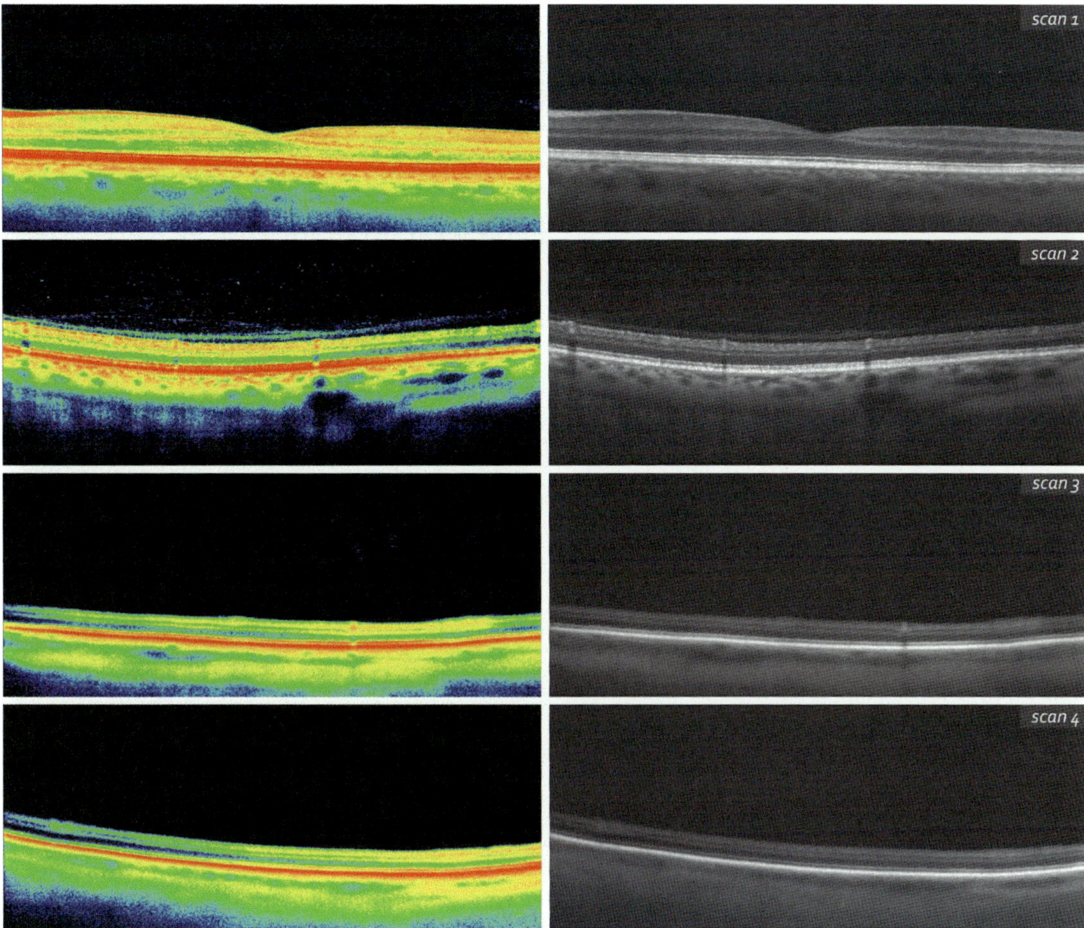

Fig. 2.2 OCT of the retina in hyperopic patient. **Scan 1** Macular area. The average foveal and parafoveal retinal thickness is 245 μm and 375 μm, respectively. **Scan 2** Equatorial area. The average retinal thickness is 193 μm. **Scan 3** Mid-peripheral area. The average retinal thickness is 174 μm. **Scan 4** Far peripheral area. The average retinal thickness is 151 μm

Moderate Myopia

An asymptomatic 36-year-old female complaining of low distance vision.

OD: VA, sc 20/200, cc 20/20 with −5.5 sph; AL, 25.8 mm.

OCT Scan Description (Fig. 2.3)

Scan 1 Macular area The foveal pit retains a normal profile. All retinal layers are clearly distinguished. Pigment epithelium is smooth. Retinal vessels are observed as shadows parafoveally and perifoveally. The average foveal and parafoveal retinal thickness is 208 μm and 302 μm, respectively.

Scan 2 Equatorial area The retinal surface is smooth. Hyperreflective layers of the pigment epithelium, photoreceptors, and neuroepithelium are observed. Retinal vessels are observed as shadows. The posterior hyaloid membrane is intact. Large choroidal vessels are identified. The average retinal thickness is 161 μm.

Scan 3 Mid-peripheral area The retinal surface is smooth. The inner and outer layers of the neuroepithelium are distinguishable. Retinal vessels are observed as shadows. The posterior hyaloid membrane is intact. Medium-sized choroidal vessels are identified. The average retinal thickness is 145 μm.

Scan 4 Far peripheral area The retinal surface is smooth. The inner and outer layers of the neuroepithelium are not distinguishable. Retinal vessels and small choroidal vessels are identified. The average retinal thickness is 126 μm.

Conclusion

Retinal OCT in moderate myopia demonstrates decreasing retinal thickness from the parafoveal area to the periphery. The equatorial area is 1.9 times thinner, the mid-peripheral area is 2.1 times thinner, and the far peripheral area is 2.4 times thinner than the central retina. The average retinal thickness in patients with moderate myopia is 6.3 % lower in the fovea, 14.9 % lower in the parafovea, 5.9 % lower in the equatorial area, 6.5 % lower in the mid-peripheral area, and 4.5 % lower in the far peripheral retina than that in patients with emmetropia.

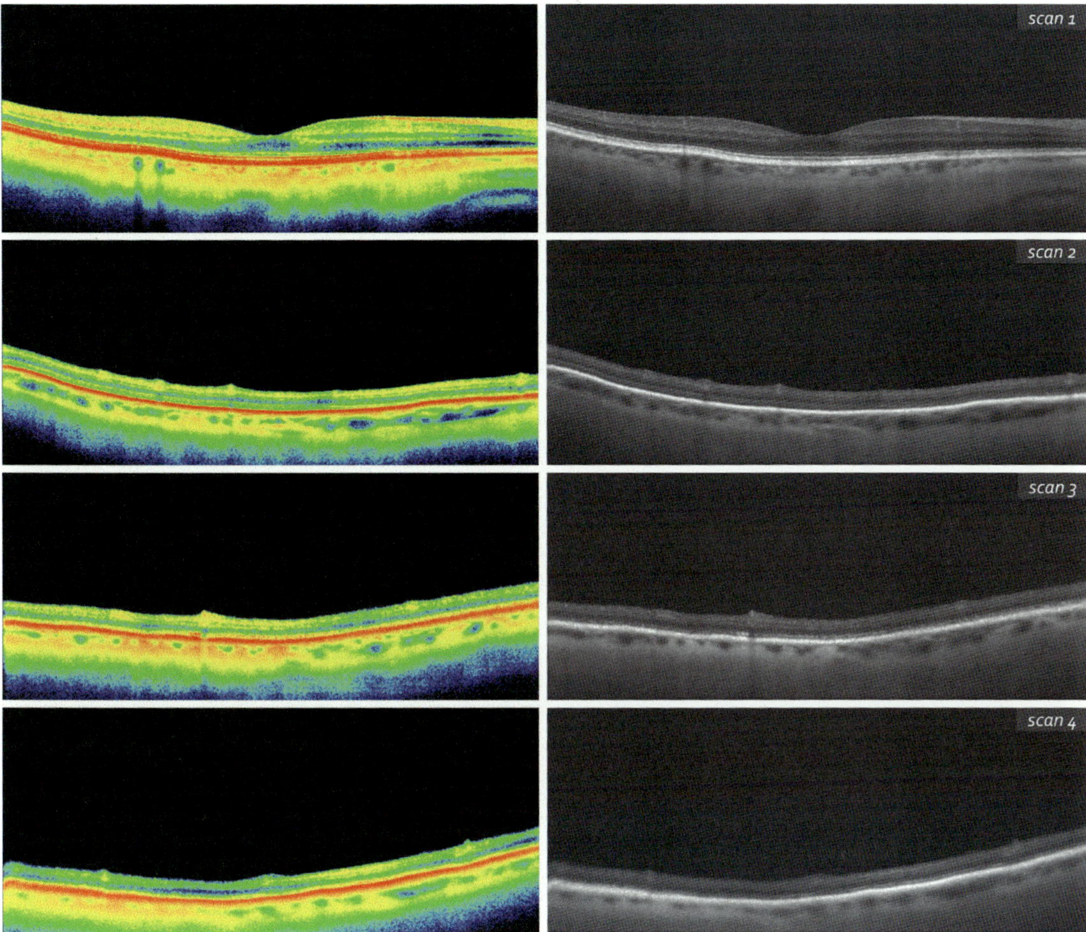

Fig. 2.3 OCT of the retina in myopic patient. **Scan 1** Macular area. The average foveal and parafoveal retinal thickness in is 208 μm and 302 μm, respectively. **Scan 2** Equatorial area. The average retinal thickness is 161 μm. **Scan 3** Mid-peripheral area. The average retinal thickness is 145 μm. **Scan 4** Far peripheral area. The average retinal thickness is 126 μm

OCT of Vitreoretinal Interface in Peripheral Retinal Degenerations

Pathologic changes of the vitreoretinal interface play an important role in the development of rhegmatogenous retinal detachment in patients with peripheral retinal degenerations [10, 21].

Normally, the vitreoretinal interface consists of the retinal internal limiting membrane and the tightly adjacent posterior hyaloid membrane. The results of morphohistological studies confirmed that the collagen fibrils of the posterior hyaloid membrane reach the sub-membrane space and penetrate in the internal limiting membrane, which is the basement membrane of the endfeet of the retinal Muller cells [22].

The use of OCT scanning provided invaluable data on normal and pathological conditions of the vitreoretinal interface in the central retina [5, 21]. In the recent years only few researches were made on the OCT-scanning of the peripheral retina and vitreoretinal interface [9, 18, 20, 21].

After a detailed analysis of OCT scans of the peripheral retina, the following vitreoretinal interface types were identified:

- Type 1 – transparent vitreous with no tractions (Fig. 2.4);
- Type 2 – partial posterior vitreous detachment (PVD) without vitreoretinal traction (Fig. 2.5);
- Type 3 – complete PVD without vitreoretinal traction (Fig. 2.6);
- Type 4 – vitreoretinal traction and locally liquefied vitreous (lacuna) above the degenerative lesion (Fig. 2.7);
- Type 5 – vitreoretinal adhesions, fibrotic folds, and pseudocysts (Fig. 2.8);
- Type 6 – pseudocysts with marked vitreoretinal traction (Fig. 2.9);
- Type 7 – atrophic retinal hole, marked traction, and vitreoretinal adhesions (Fig. 2.10);
- Type 8 – full-thickness operculated retinal tear (Fig. 2.11);
- Type 9 – flap tear with vitreoretinal traction (Fig. 2.12).

According to these types, three risk groups are distinguished depending on the risk of rhegmatogenous retinal detachment: group I with no risk of rhegmatogenous retinal detachment (types 1 and 3), group II with moderate (borderline) risk requiring follow-up (types 2, 4, and 8), and group III (types 5, 6, 7, and 9) with high risk requiring retinal laser photocoagulation.

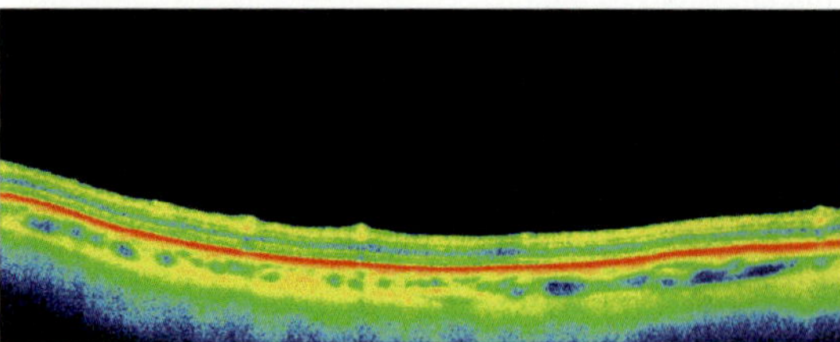
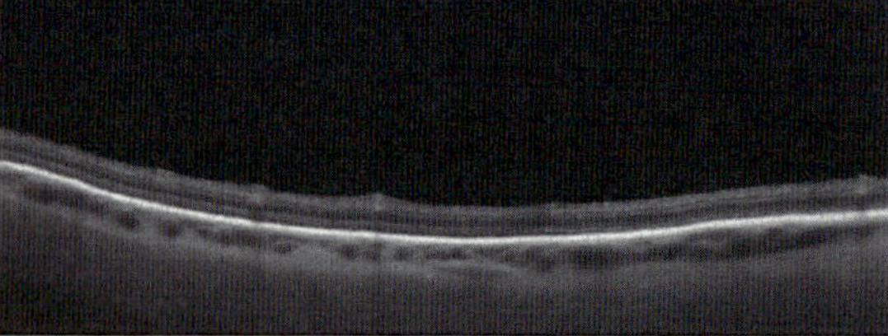

Fig. 2.4 Transparent vitreous with no vitreoretinal traction

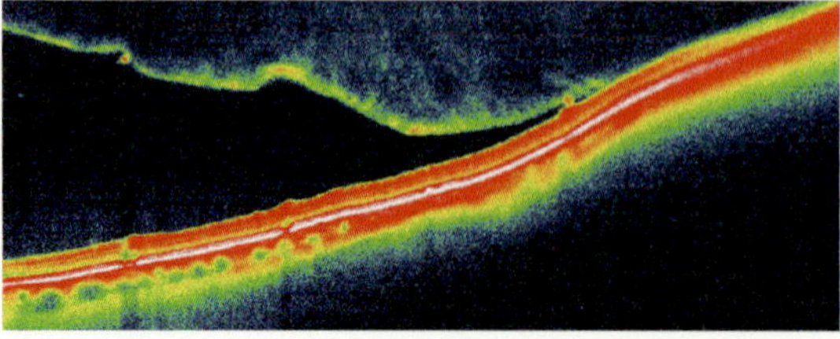
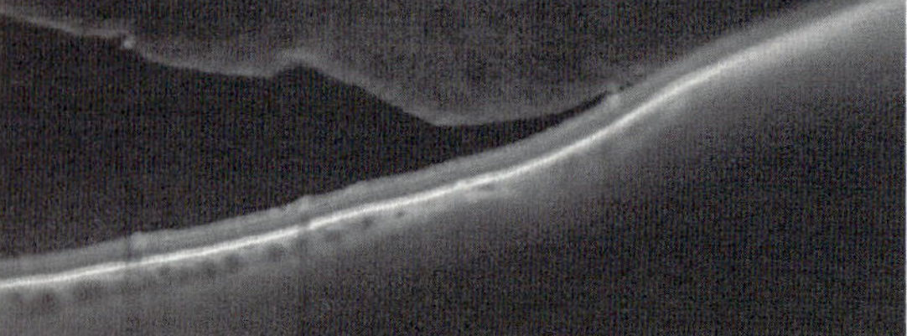

Fig. 2.5 Partial posterior vitreous detachment

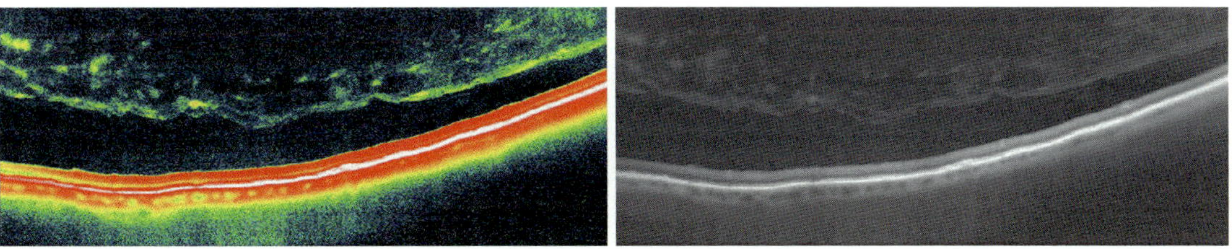

Fig. 2.6   Complete posterior vitreous detachment

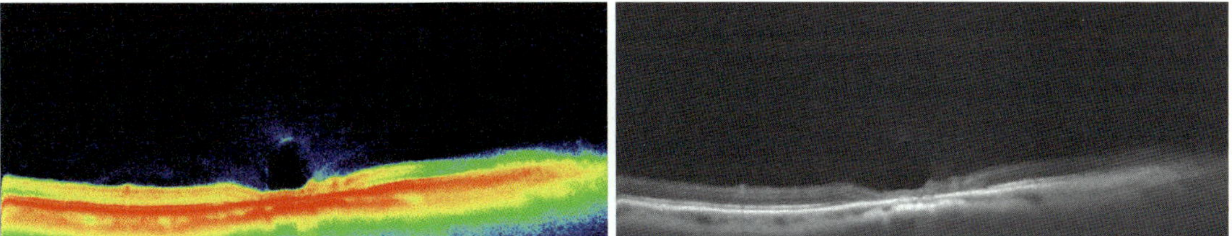

Fig. 2.7   Vitreoretinal tractions at the edge of the degenerative lesion

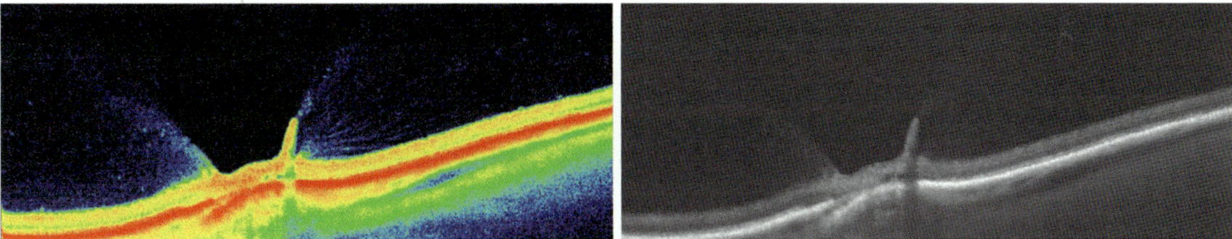

Fig. 2.8   Vitreoretinal adhesions and fibrotic folds

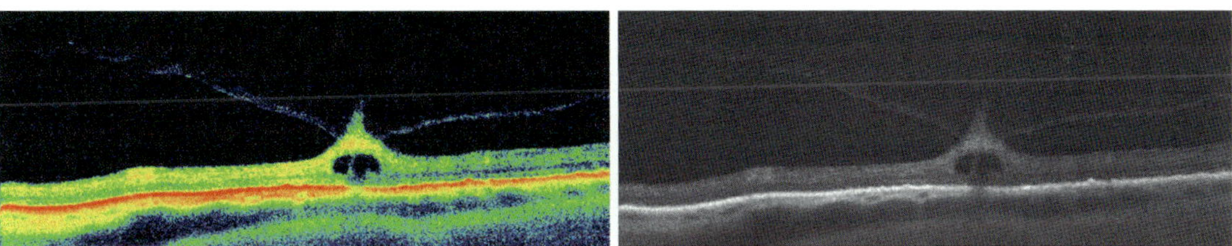

Fig. 2.9   Pseudocysts with severe vitreoretinal traction

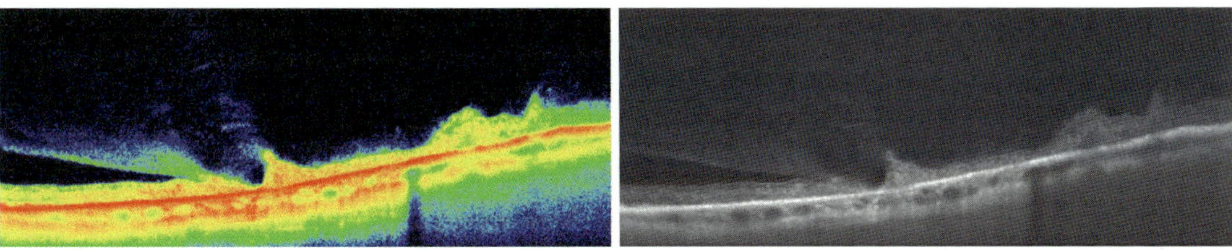

Fig. 2.10   Atrophic retinal hole, marked traction, and vitreoretinal adhesions

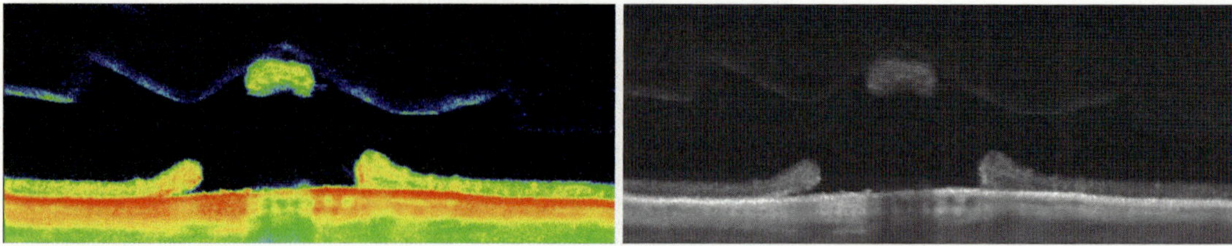

Fig. 2.11 Full-thickness operculated tear with an operculum attached to the posterior hyaloid membrane and floating in the vitreous; no traction near the tear

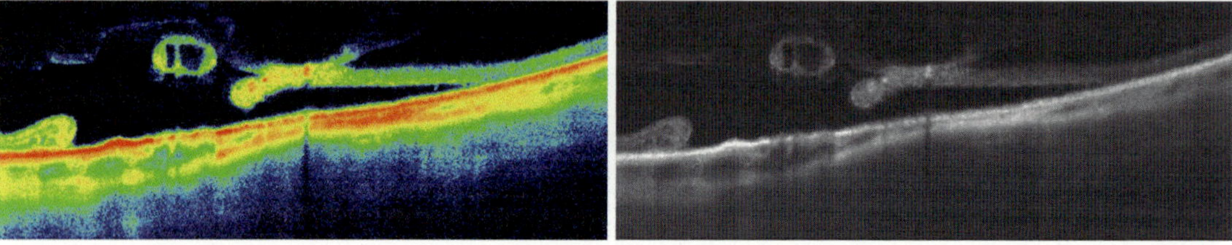

Fig. 2.12 Flap tear with a separated operculum, vitreoretinal traction and shallow retinal detachment

References

1. Fujimoto JG et al. Principles of optical coherence tomography. In: Schuman JS, editor. Optical coherence tomography of ocular diseases. 2nd ed. Thorofare: SLACK; 2004. p. 3–19.
2. Huang D, Swanson EA, Lin CP, et al. Optical coherence tomography. Science. 1991;254(5035):1178–81.
3. Fercher AF, Hitzenberger CK, Drexler W, et al. In vivo optical coherence tomography. Am J Ophthalmol. 1993;116:113–4.
4. Swanson EA, Izatt JA, Hee MR, et al. In vivo retinal imaging by optical coherence tomography. Opt Lett. 1993;18:1864–6.
5. Lumbroso B, Rispoli M. Practical handbook of OCT (retina, choroid, glaucoma). New Delhi: Jaypee Brothers Medical Publishers; 2012.
6. Lombardo M, Scarinci F, Giannini D, et al. High-resolution multimodal imaging after idiopathic epiretinal membrane surgery. Retina. 2016;36(1):171–80. doi:10.1097/IAE.0000000000000679.
7. Coscas G, Zhou Q, Coscas F, et al. Choroid thickness measurement with RTVue optical coherence tomography in emmetropic eyes, mildly myopic eyes, and highly myopic eyes. Eur J Ophthalmol. 2012;22(6):992–1000. doi:10.5301/ejo.5000189.
8. Kernt M, Kampik A. Imaging of the peripheral retina. Oman J Ophthalmol. 2013;6(Suppl 1):S32–5. doi:10.4103/0974-620X.122292.
9. Kamppeter BA, Jonas JB. Optical coherence tomography of a peripheral retinal schisis with an outer retinal layer break. Acta Ophthalmol Scand. 2004;82(5):574–5.
10. Ghazi NG, Dibernardo C. Optical coherence tomography of peripheral retinal lesions in enucleated human eye specimens with histologic correlation. Am J Ophthalmol. 2006;141(4):740–2.
11. Cheng SC, Lam CS, Yap MK. Retinal thickness in myopic and non-myopic eyes. Ophthalmol Physiol Opt. 2010;30:776–84.
12. Muni RH, Kohly RP, Charonis A, et al. Retinoschisis detected with handheld spectral-domain optical coherence tomography in neonates with advanced retinopathy of prematurity. Arch Ophthalmol. 2010;128(1):57–62.
13. Landa G, Shirkey L, Garcia PM. Acquired senile retinoschisis of the peripheral retina imaged by spectral domain optical coherence tomography: a case report. Eur J Ophthalmol. 2010;20(6):1079–81.
14. Manjunath V, Taha M, Fujimoto JG, et al. Posterior lattice degeneration characterized by spectral domain optical coherence tomography. Retina. 2011;31(3):492–6.
15. Stehouwer M, Verbraak FD, de Vries HR, et al. Scanning beyond the limits of standard OCT with a Fourier domain optical coherence tomography integrated into a slit lamp: the SL SCAN-1. Eye. 2011;25(1):97–104.
16. Oster SF, Mojana F, Freeman WR. Spectral-domain optical coherence tomography imaging of postoperative scleral buckles. Retina. 2011;31(8):1493–9.
17. Kothari A, Narendran V, Saravanan VR. In vivo sectional imaging of the retinal periphery using conventional optical coherence tomography systems. Indian J Ophthalmol. 2012;60:235–9.

18. Shaimova VA, Pozdeeva OG, Shaimov TB, et al. Optical coherence tomography in peripheral retinal tears diagnostics. Vestn Ophthalmol. 2013;6:51–66. (In Russian)
19. Shaimova VA, Pozdeeva OG, Shaimov TB, et al. Optical coherence tomography in peripheral vitreoretinal degenerations diagnostics. Ophthalmology. 2013;10(4):32–9. (In Russian)
20. Fawzi AA, Nielsen JS, Mateo-Montoya A, et al. Multimodal imaging of white and dark without pressure fundus lesions. Retina. 2014;34(12): 2376–87.
21. Choudhry N, Golding J, Manry MW, et al. Ultra-widefield steering-based spectral-domain optical coherence tomography imaging of the retinal periphery. Ophthalmology. (2016). doi: 10.1016/j.ophtha.2016.01.045. pii: S0161-6420(16)001512.
22. Worst JG, Los LI. Comparative anatomy of the vitreous body in rhesus monkeys and man. Doc Ophthalmol. 1992;82(1–2):169–78.

Peripheral Retinal Degenerations as a Risk Factor for Rhegmatogenous Retinal Detachment

3

Venera A. Shaimova

Peripheral retinal degenerations are considered a risk factor for rhegmatogenous retinal detachment [1, 2]. Rhegmatogenous retinal detachment (RRD) is the separation of the neurosensory retina from the retinal pigment epithelium by a thin layer of subretinal fluid. The annual incidence of RRD varies between 6.3 and 18.2 cases per 100,000, with an age-specific peak of 52.5 cases per 100,000 in the age group of 55–59 years [3–5].

According to the literature, retinal detachment can be caused not only by retinal tears, but also by the condition of vitreoretinal interface, and the presence of proliferative vitreoretinopathy [6–8]. Vitreoretinal interrelations include two antagonistic forces: vitreous changes on the one side, and choroidal pump (factors that keep the retina in its place) and interphotoreceptor matrix (that ensures close contact between cone and rod photoreceptor cells and pigment epithelium interface) on the other side. Choroidal pump consists of three factors: choroidal osmotic pressure, hydrostatic pressure of retinal vessels and active transport of substances through the pigment epithelium. Vitreous changes include vitreous syneresis, posterior vitreous detachment, and vitreous traction [9–11].

It is the interaction between vitreoretinal traction and a fragile area in the peripheral retina – a predisposing lesion – that causes retinal tears. The tear occurs at the sites of vitreoretinal adhesion in the peripheral retinal degeneration, when during anomalous posterior vitreous detachment, the liquefied synchytic fluid penetrates into the retrohyaloid space forcing down the solid vitreous gel. [5, 12].

At the same time, the shifted vitreous layers pull the site of vitreoretinal adhesion of the peripheral retinal degeneration, leading to a flap tear or an operculated tear [10]. Flap tears are associated with persistent retinal traction (Figs. 3.1a and 3.2a), in contrast to operculated tears, that are characterized by the absence of traction, which is eliminated when the site of vitreoretinal adhesion is torn away form the peripheral retinal degeneration (Figs. 3.1b and 3.2b). The retinal tear alone without at least partial vitreous liquefaction and tractions is not sufficient enough to cause retinal detachment [5].

The RRD develops when liquefied vitreous humor accelerated by rotary eye movements passes through the retinal tear or retinal holes (Fig. 3.3a) into the subretinal space and detaches (Fig. 3.3b) the neurosensory retina from the underlying pigment epithelium (Figs. 3.4, 3.5, and 3.6) [6, 10].

V.A. Shaimova
Chelyabinsk State Laser Surgery Institute, Chelyabinsk, Russian Federation

Center Zreniya Medical Clinic, LLC, Chelyabinsk, Russian Federation
e-mail: shaimova.v@mail.ru

© Springer International Publishing AG 2017
V.A. Shaimova (ed.), *Peripheral Retinal Degenerations*, DOI 10.1007/978-3-319-48995-7_3

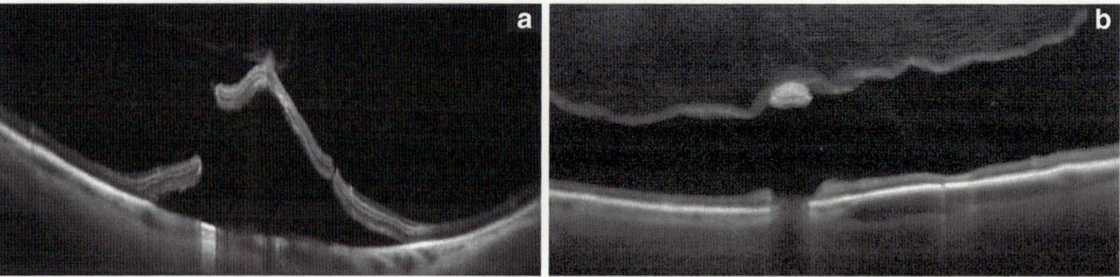

Fig. 3.1 OCT of peripheral retinal tears: (**a**) Flap tear; (**b**) Operculated tear

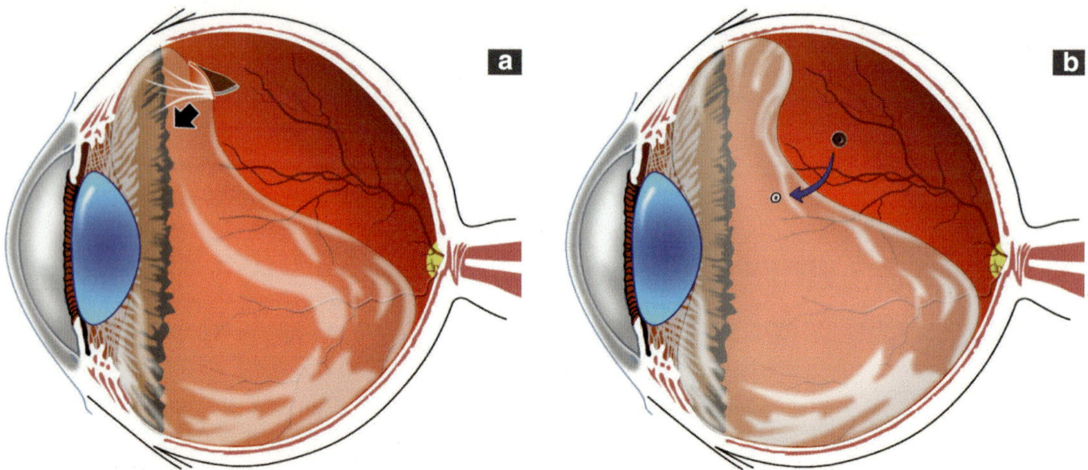

Fig. 3.2 Schematic image of peripheral retinal tears in PVD: (**a**) Flap tear; (**b**) Operculated tear

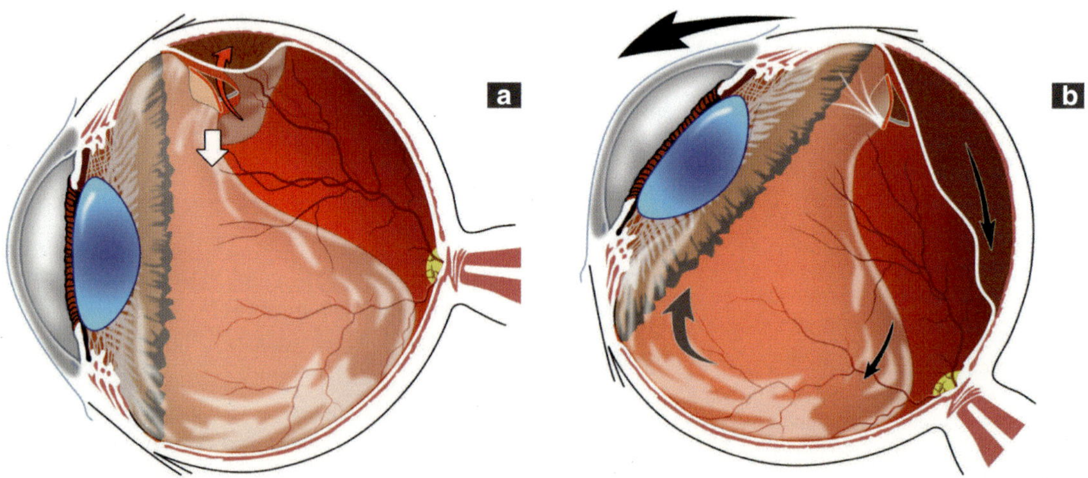

Fig. 3.3 Schematic image of RRD: (**a**) Local detachment; (**b**) Detachment progresses to the central retina

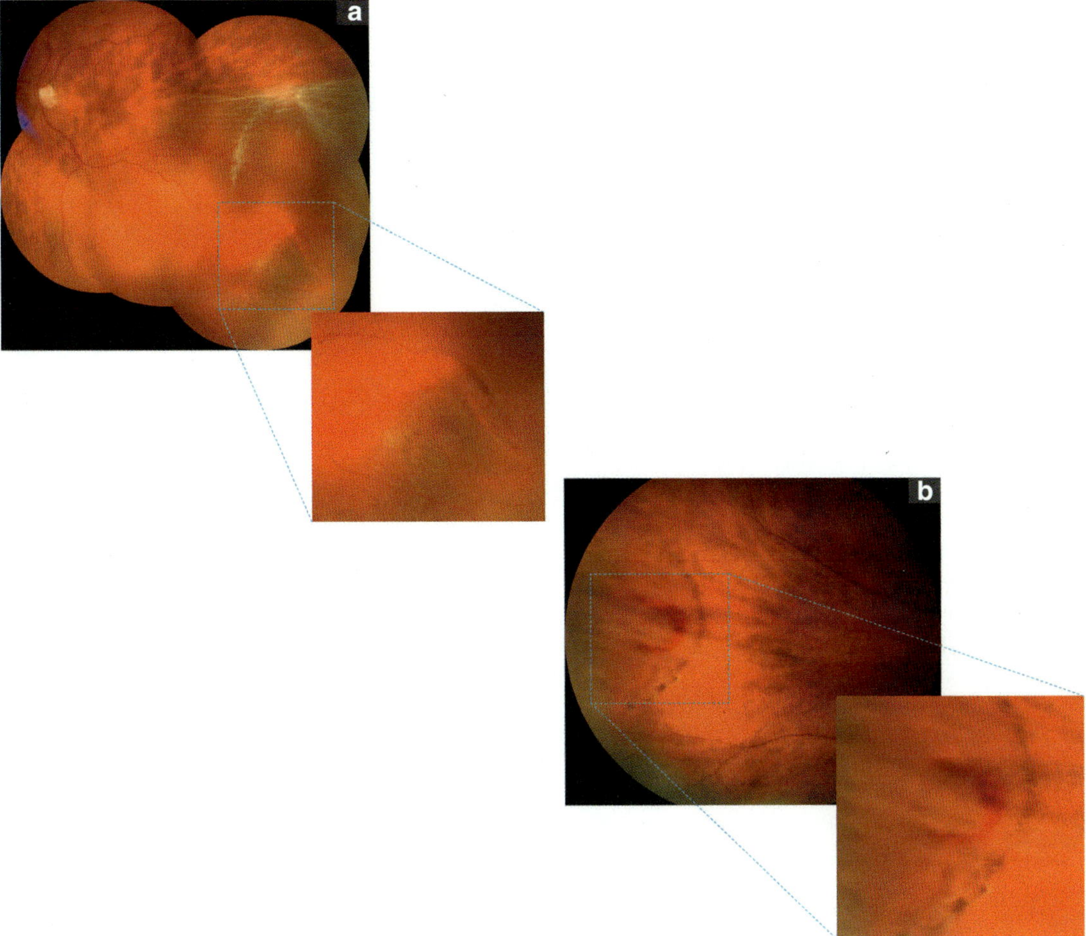

Fig. 3.4 Color fundus images: (**a**) Subtotal retinal detachment with a giant flap tear; (**b**) Local retinal detachment with a flap tear and a demarcation line

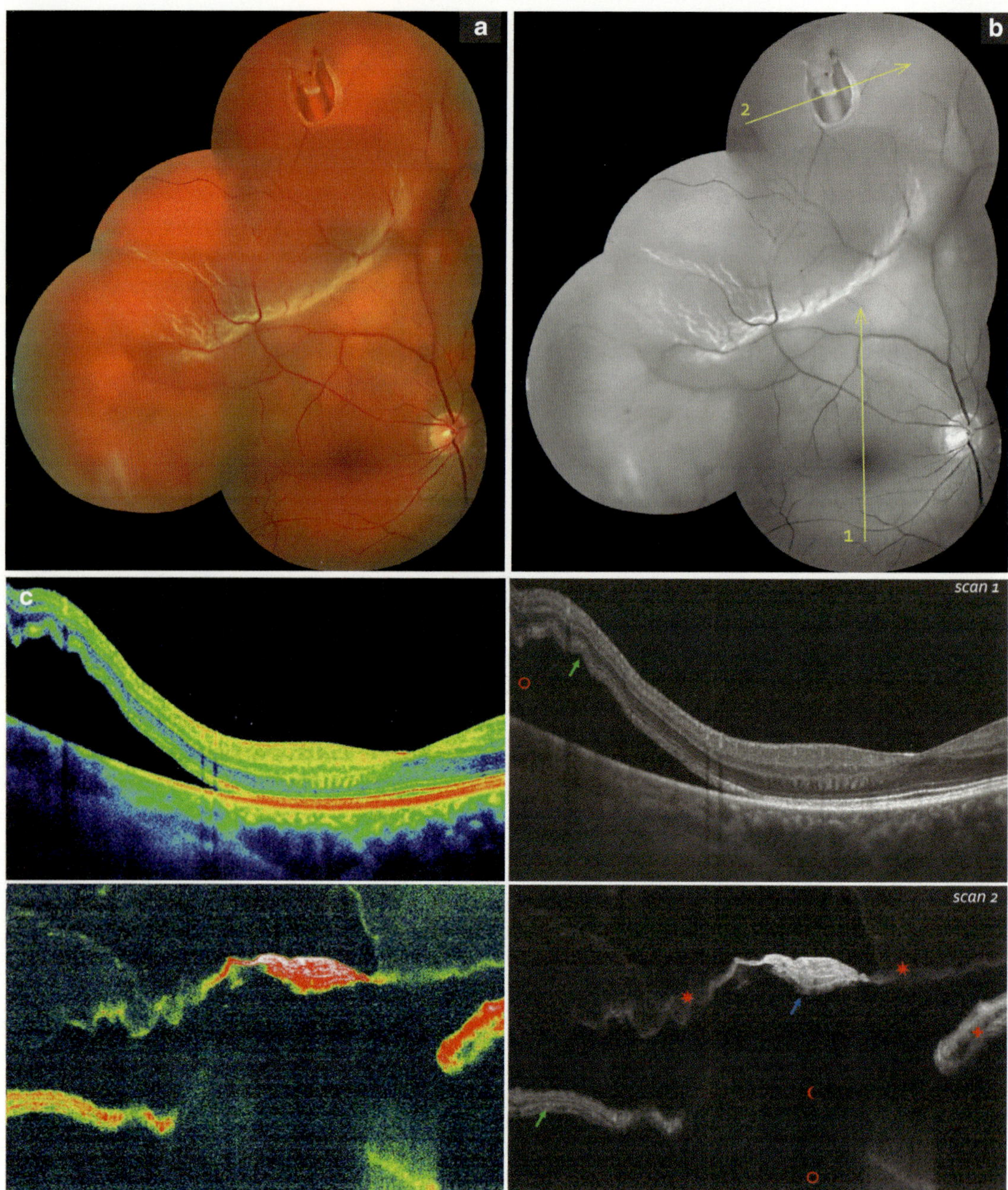

Fig. 3.5 (a) Color fundus image of the superior retinal detachment with a flap tear; (b) Scanning direction; (c) OCT images **Scan 1** Central retina. The detachment of para- and perifoveal neurosensory retina (*red circle*); multiple folds observed on the external retinal surface (*green arrow*); **Scan 2** Detached retina with an overhanging flap tear (*blue arrow*). Tear margins represented by the neurosensory retina (*green arrow*) with intraretinal cavities (*red cross*); retinal detachment cavity (*red circle*) and marked vitreoretinal adhesion with traction at the tear margins (*red asterisks*)

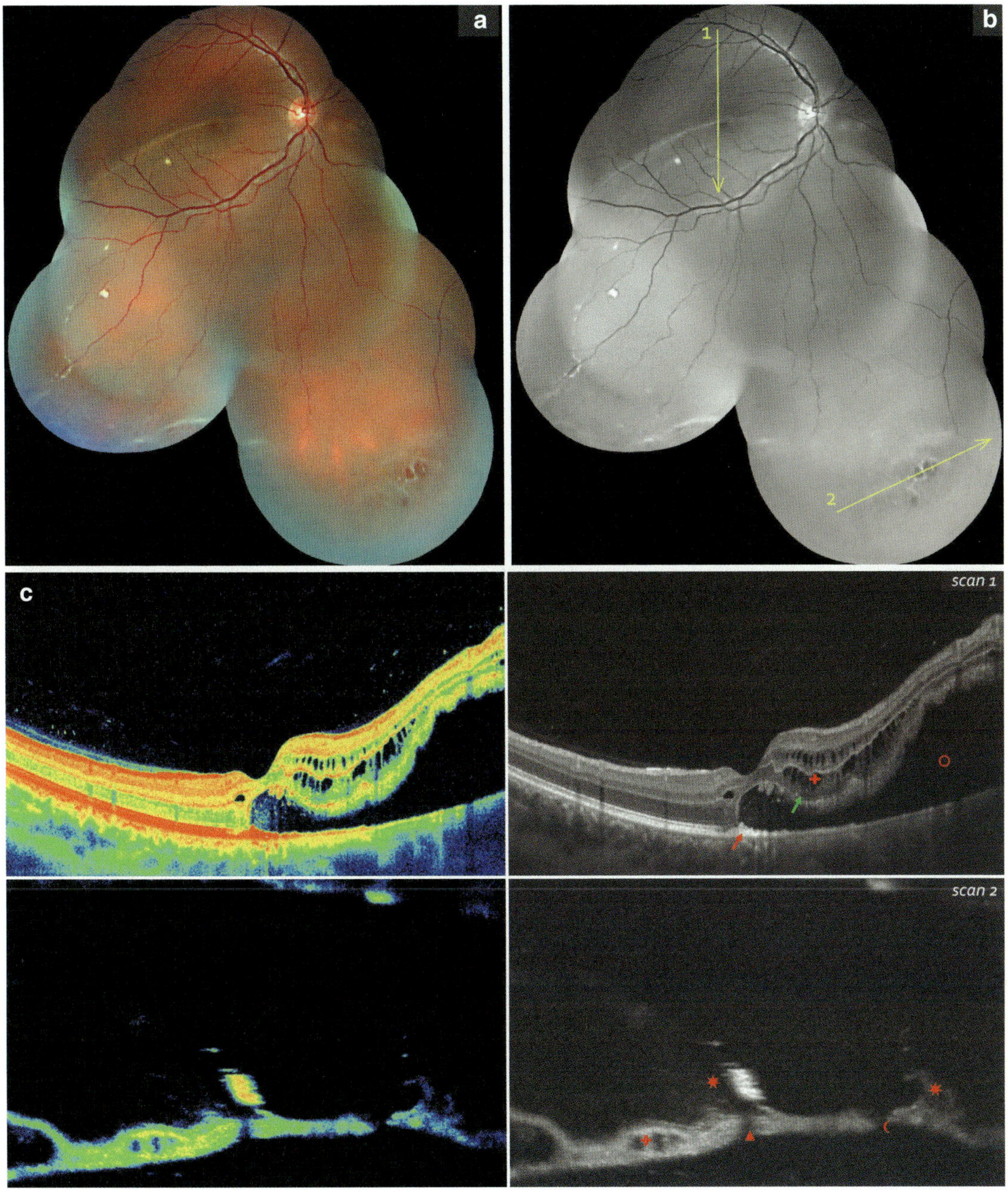

Fig. 3.6 (**a**) Color fundus image of retinal detachment with macula involved; lattice degeneration with multiple tears seen in the inferonasal retina; (**b**) Scanning direction; (**c**) OCT images **Scan 1** Neurosensory retina detached (*green arrow*) from the retinal pigment epithelium up to the macula, with a large cavity (*red circle*) between the layers. Multiple hyporeflective irregular cavities in the neuroepithelium (*red cross*). Dense retinal pigment epithelium at the fovea (*red arrow*). **Scan 2** Detached neuroepithelium corresponding to the lattice degeneration with tears (*red crescent*), intraretinal cavities in neurosensory retina (*red cross*), and marked vitreoretinal traction (*red asterisk*)

The most common risk factors for RRD include vitreous liquefaction, posterior vitreous detachment, retinal tears (flap tears, dialysis), lattice degeneration, cystic retinal tufts, degenerative retinoschisis, myopia, aphakia, pseudophakia, Nd:YAG laser posterior capsulotomy, RRD of the fellow eye, family history of RRD, systemic diseases, and peripheral vitreochorioretinal degenerations [1, 10].

The main causes for vitreous liquefaction (synchysis) are advanced age, myopia, eye injuries, and chronic inflammation [12]. Several studies claim that synchysis is associated with the depolymerization of hyaluronic acid leading to structural changes of the vitreous [13, 14]. Posterior vitreous detachment usually manifests with photopsias (flashing lights), floaters or blurry vision. Photopsias arise from the mechanical stimulation of vitreoretinal traction on the retina, and floaters are shadows on the retina cast by vitreous opacities: blood, glial cells, aggregated collagen fibers.

Peripheral retinal degenerations with vitreoretinal adhesions and tractions are associated with the highest risk of rhegmatogenous retinal detachment [8, 9, 15]. We can recognize these high-risk forms of degenerations if we perform a careful OCT study of their morphology and progression, thus preventing retinal detachment [16–20].

In this atlas we explore the interrelations between vitreous and retina in most common peripheral retinal degenerations by means of OCT imaging and reveal the most severe degenerations with increased risk of RRD.

Classifications of Peripheral Retinal Degenerations

The first classifications of peripheral retinal degenerations were proposed by Halpern [21] and Duke-Elder et al. [22]. These classifications were based on the histological studies of peripheral degenerations in asymptomatic patients published by Okun (1960, 1961) and Rutnin (1967) [23–26].

There is currently no universally accepted classification system of peripheral retinal degenerations.

Upon careful consideration of various published classifications, we have chosen several major features they all have in common. These features include:

1. Location: equatorial, peripheral, and combined degenerations [1].
2. Pathomorphology: trophic, tractional, trophic-tractional degenerations [27]; atrophic, tractional, and combined degenerations [28].
3. Depth of retinal changes: intraretinal, vitreoretinal, chorioretinal [2, 29]; retinal, vitreoretinal, chorioretinal [30]
4. Risk of retinal detachment: lesions predisposing to retinal detachment, lesions not predisposing to retinal detachment [11, 31, 32]; conditions that affect the outer retina (low risk of detachment) and conditions that affect the inner retina (high risk of detachment) [15].
5. Prognosis: progressive and stationary (non-progressive) [1].
6. Combined classification:
   (a) Pathomorphology: peripheral chorioretinal degenerations and peripheral vitreochorioretinal degenerations;
   (b) Degenerations with low (A), moderate (B), and high risk (C) of detachment and tears;
   (c) Degree of intensity of changes: grades I–V degenerations [33].

After many years of analyzing OCT images of peripheral retinal degenerations, we have come to the conclusion that classification based on the depth of retinal changes has proved to be the most useful and accurate in interpreting results of OCT scanning [2, 29, 30]. We use this layer-by-layer scanning principle to describe OCT-images and we offer the following types of peripheral retinal degenerations:

1. Intraretinal degenerations
  1.1. Senile retinoschisis
  1.2. White-without-pressure
  1.3. Dark-without-pressure
  1.4. Peripheral cystoid degeneration
  1.5. Snowflake degeneration
  1.6. Pearl degeneration

2. Vitreoretinal degenerations
  2.1. Snail-track degeneration
  2.2. Lattice degeneration
  2.3. Retinal tufts
  2.4. Peripheral retinal breaks

3. Chorioretinal degenerations
  3.1. Paving-stone degeneration
  3.2. Hypertrophy of the retinal pigment epithelium
  3.3. Honeycomb degeneration
  3.4. Peripheral retinal drusen

References

1. Saksonova EO, Zakharova GI, Platova LA, et al. Prevention of retinal detachment in patients with peripheral vitreochorioretinal dystrophies. Oftalmol Zh. 1983;38(3):151–5. (In Russian)
2. Conart JB, Baron D, Berrod JP. Degenerative lesions of the peripheral retina. J Fr Ophtalmol. 2014;37(1):73–80. doi:10.1016/j.jfo.2013.09.001.
3. Mitry D, Charteris D, Flec B. The epidemiology of rhegmatogenous retinal detachment geographical variation and clinical associations. Br J Ophthalmol. 2010;94(6):678–84.
4. Van de Put MA, Hooymans JM, Los LI. The incidence of rhegmatogenous retinal detachment in the Netherlands. Ophthalmology. 2013;120(3):616–22.
5. Kanski J, Bowling B. Clinical ophthalmology: a systematic approach. 7th ed. London: Butterworth Heinemann; 2011.
6. Feltgen N, Walter P. Rhegmatogenous retinal detachment – an ophthalmologic emergency. Dtsch Arztebl Int. 2014;111(1–2):12–21.
7. Snead MP, Snead DR, James S, et al. Clinicopathological changes at the vitreoretinal junction: posterior vitreous detachment. Eye. 2008;22(10):1257–62.
8. Sebag J. Anomalous posterior vitreous detachment: a unifying concept in vitreo-retinal disease. Graefes Arch Clin Exp Ophthalmol. 2004;242(8):690–8.
9. Jones WL et al. Care of the patient with retinal detachment and related peripheral vitreoretinal disease. St. Louis: American Optometric Association; 2004.
10. Brinton DA, Wilkinson CP. Retinal detachment: principles and practice. 3rd ed. Oxford: University Press in cooperation with American Academy of Ophthalmology; 2009.
11. Graue-Wiechers FA, Verduzco NS. Laser treatment for retinal holes, tears and peripheral. In: Boyd S, CP W, editors. Retinal detachment surgery and laser treatment. Panama: Jaypee Highlights Med Publ; 2009. p. 47–57.
12. Denniston A, Murray PI. Oxford handbook of ophthalmology. Oxford: Oxford Academ; 2014.
13. Foos RY, Wheeler NC. Vitreoretinal juncture: synchisis senilis and posterior vitrous detachment. Ophthalmology. 1982;89:1502–12.
14. Milston R, Madigan MC, Sebag J. Vitreous floaters: etiology, diagnostics, and management. Surv Ophthalmol. 2016;61(2):211–27.
15. Macaliester G, Sullivan P. Peripheral retinal degenerations. In: OT CET. 2011. http://goo.gl/PzTidM.
16. Choudhry N, Golding J, Manry MW, et al. Ultra-widefield steering-based spectral-domain optical coherence tomography imaging of the retinal periphery. Ophthalmology. 2016;23(6):1368–74. doi:10.1016/j.ophtha.2016.01.045.
17. Stehouwer M, Verbraak FD, de Vries HR, et al. Scanning beyond the limits of standard OCT with a Fourier domain optical coherence tomography integrated into a slit lamp: the SL SCAN-1. Eye. 2011;25(1):97–104.
18. Oster SF, Mojana F, Freeman WR. Spectral-domain optical coherence tomography imaging of postoperative scleral buckles. Retina. 2011;31(8):1493–9.
19. Fawzi AA, Nielsen JS, Mateo-Montoya A, et al. Multimodal imaging of white and dark without pressure fundus lesions. Retina. 2014;34(12):2376–87.
20. Shaimova VA, Pozdeeva OG, Shaimov TB, et al. Optical coherence tomography in peripheral retinal tears diagnostics. Vestn Ophthalmol. 2013;129(6):51–66. (In Russian)
21. Halpern JI. Routine screening of the retinal periphery. Am J Ophthalmol. 1966;62(1):99–102.
22. Duke-Elder S, Dobree JH. Diseases of the retina. In: Duke-Elder S, editor. System of ophthalmology, vol. 10. London: Henry Kimpton; 1967, p. 126–7.
23. Okun E. Gross and microscopic pathology in autopsy eyes. Part II. Peripheral chorioretinal atrophy. Am J Ophthalmol. 1960;50:574–83.
24. Okun E. Gross and microscopic pathology in autopsy eyes. III. Retinal breaks without detachment. Am J Ophthalmol. 1961;51:369–91.

25. Okun E. Gross and microscopic pathology in autopsy eyes. IV. Pars plana cysts. Am J Ophthalmol. 1961;51:1221–8.
26. Rutnin U, Schepens CL. Fundus appearance in normal eyes: III. Peripheral degenerations. Am J Ophthalmol. 1967;64(6):1063–9.
27. Zinn K, Tilden D. Clinical atlas of peripheral retinal disorders. New York: Springer; 1988.
28. Antelava DI, et al. Primary retinal detachment. Tbilisi (In Russian): Sabchota Sakartvelo; 1986. Boyd S, Cortez R, Sabates N. Retinal and vitreoretinal diseases and surgery. Clayton: Jaypee Highlights Medical Publishers; 2010.
29. Chhablani J, Bagdi AB. Peripheral retinal degenerations. In: Eye Wiki. 2015. http://eyewiki.aao.org/Peripheral_Retinal_Degenerations. Accessed 17 Oct 2015.
30. Franchuk AA. The clinical characteristics of different types of peripheral retinal degeneration and their relationship to retinal breaks and detachment. Oftalmol Zh. 1989. 8:451–4.
31. Engstrom RS Jr, Glasgow BR, Foos RY, et al. Degenerative diseases of the peripheral retina. In: Duane's ophthalmology on CD-ROM. 2006. http://www.oculist.net/downaton502/prof/ebook/duanes/pages/v3/v3c026.html.
32. Skuta GL, Cantor LB, Weiss JS. Basic and clinical science course, retina and vitreous. American Academy of Ophthalmology: San Francisco; 2011.
33. Ivanishko YA, Miroshnikov VV, Nesterov EA. Primary peripheral retinal degenerations. Working classification. Indications for laser retinopexy. Okulist. 2003;44(4):6. (In Russian)

Intraretinal Degenerations

First Group of Peripheral Retinal Degenerations

Timur B. Shaimov and Venera A. Shaimova

T.B. Shaimov
Ophthalmology Department of Postgraduate
Education Faculty, South Ural State Medical
University, Chelyabinsk, Russian Federation

Center Zreniya Medical Clinic, LLC,
Chelyabinsk, Russian Federation

V.A. Shaimova (⬚)
Center Zreniya Medical Clinic, LLC,
Chelyabinsk, Russian Federation

Chelyabinsk State Laser Surgery Institute,
Chelyabinsk, Russian Federation
e-mail: shaimova.v@mail.ru

© Springer International Publishing AG 2017
V.A. Shaimova (ed.), *Peripheral Retinal Degenerations*, DOI 10.1007/978-3-319-48995-7_4

Senile Retinoschisis

Senile retinoschisis (SR, degenerative, or acquired retinoschisis) is splitting of the neurosensory retina into layers separated by thick fluid [1–3]. Retinoschisis develops as a progression of peripheral cystoid degeneration in the outer plexiform or inner nuclear layer when the glial supporting elements stretch, Müller cells break and there appear shallow cavities splitting the retina [4–9].

SR (Table 4.1) is estimated to affect 1.6–7 % of general population and is more commonly found in patients aged 40 and older [10–12]. This condition mostly affects hyperopic eyes (70 %), is usually bilateral, asymptomatic and found in the inferotemporal, or less commonly in the superotemporal quadrants [3, 12, 13].

There is currently no universally accepted classification of retinoschisis. Astakhov et al. (2004) proposed the classification of the SR based on the following features [4]:

1. Presence of retinal tears: in the inner, outer, or both layers, and without tears
2. Disease progression: non-progressive with retinal scarring, progressive without demarcation, complicated (vitreous haemorrhage, intracystic hemorrhage, and retinal detachment)

3. Development: primary or secondary
4. Location: central, peripheral, or combined
5. Type: flat or bullous
6. Affected side: unilateral or bilateral

SR may be associated with retinal detachment. According to various authors, SR is found in rhegmatogenous retinal detachment in 2.5–10.5 % of cases [4, 6], but may be considered the primary cause in only 0.05–2.5 % of cases [11, 14].

At the present moment there is no consensus on the best treatment of senile retinoschisis [15]. The majority of authors consider that retinoschisis should be treated in case of symptomatic, progressive retinal detachment threatening the macula [11, 14]. The lateral and central barring or treatment of the margins of an outer retinal break should be avoided [16]. Some experts strongly advocate individual approach in treating retinoschisis [17].

There are several studies claiming that high resolution OCT may be successfully used for the timely diagnosis of retinoschisis, differentiating it from retinal detachment and identifying breaks in its layers [18–20].

Table 4.1   Diagram of peripheral retinal degenerations

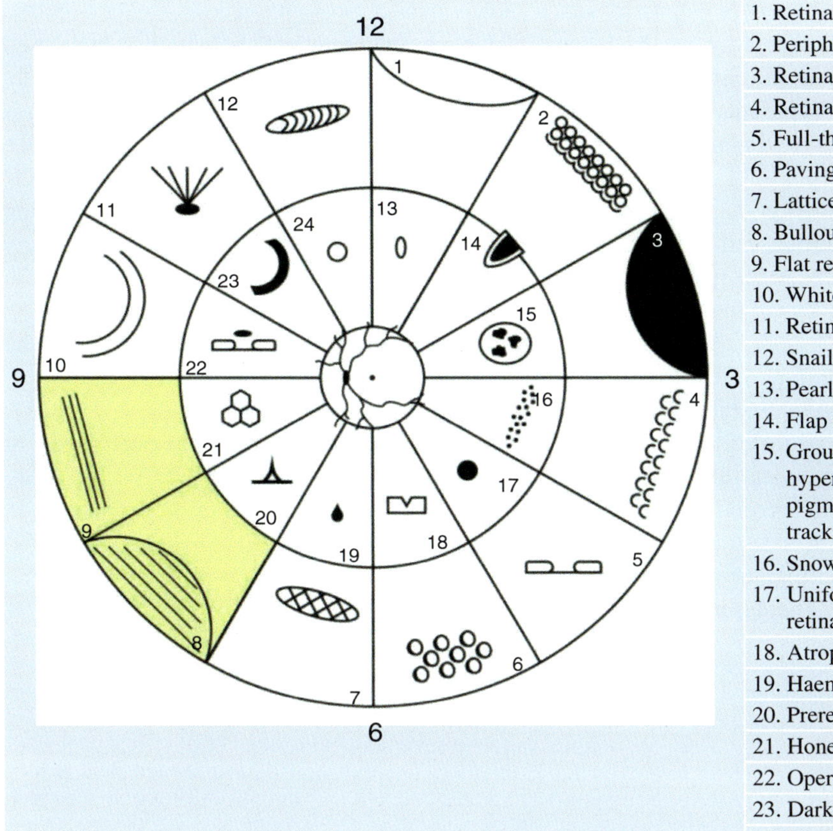

1. Retinal dialysis
2. Peripheral cystoid degeneration
3. Retinal detachment
4. Retinal drusen
5. Full-thickness tear
6. Paving-stone degeneration
7. Lattice degeneration
8. Bullous retinoschisis
9. Flat retinoschisis
10. White-without-pressure
11. Retinal tuft
12. Snail-track degeneration
13. Pearl degeneration
14. Flap tear
15. Grouped congenital hypertrophy of the retinal pigment epithelium ("bear tracks")
16. Snowflake degeneration
17. Unifocal hypertrophy of the retinal pigment epithelium
18. Atrophic retinal hole
19. Haemorrhage
20. Preretinal fibrosis
21. Honeycomb degeneration
22. Operculated retinal tear
23. Dark-without-pressure
24. Unifocal atrophy of the retinal pigment epithelium

Degenerative retinoschisis is highlighted in yellow: sector 8 – bullous retinoschisis; sector 9 – flat retinoschisis

Case 1. Flat Two-Layer Retinoschisis

A 54-year-old male patient was referred for decreased visual acuity in his left eye. During examination, moderate hyperopia and flat retinoschisis in his left eye were diagnosed.

Ophthalmoscopic Findings (Fig. 4.1a, b)

A slightly elevated whitish retinal area with blurred borders is observed in the peripheral temporal quadrant (2–4 o'clock) of the left eye.

OCT Scan Description (Fig. 4.1c, d)

The retinal profile is irregular. Intraretinal hyporeflective cavities split the neurosensory retina into two layers: the inner layer and the outer layer. Presumably, elongated Müller cells are seen in the cavity. Pigment epithelium is destroyed and thickened. The vitreous has irregular density and is detached from the retina. There is no vitreoretinal traction.

OCT Scan Details (Fig. 4.1c, d)

★ Layers of moderate reflectivity (increased density) in the vitreous over the split retina

➤ Elevated inner layers of the neurosensory retina

+ Intraretinal hyporeflective cavities separating the inner and outer layers of the neurosensory retina

➤ Areas of thickening and redistribution of the pigment epithelium

◆ Irregular and jagged layer in the outer layers of the neurosensory retina

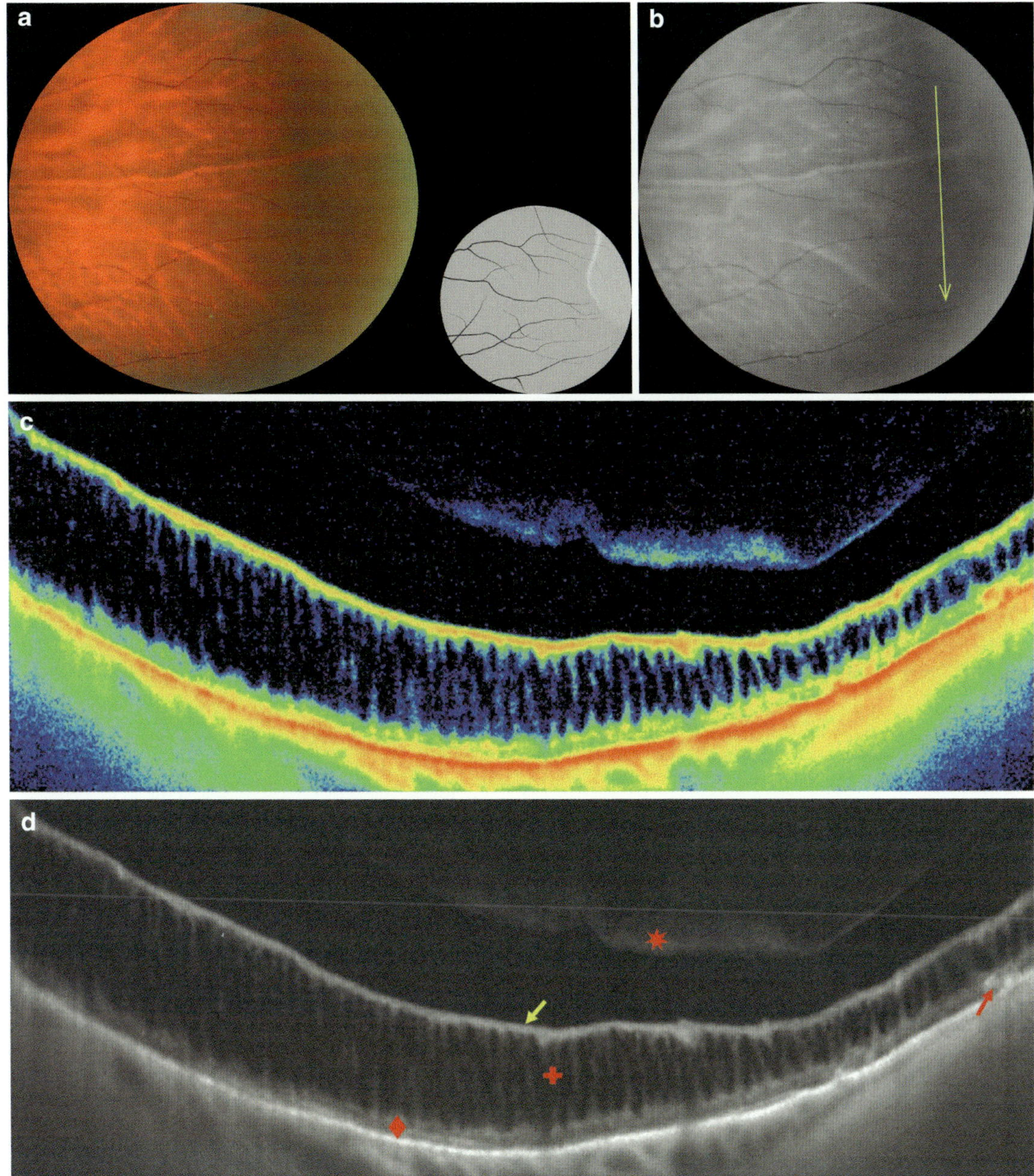

Fig. 4.1 (**a**) Flat retinoschisis. (**b**) Scanning (*yellow line*) of the elevated area in the temporal peripheral retina, left eye. (**c, d**) OCT-scanning line corresponding to the elevated area

Case 2. Flat Retinoschisis with Snowflake Degeneration

A 37-year-old female patient with bilateral moderate hyperopia and incomplete posterior vitreous detachment presented with the main complaint of floaters affecting her both eyes.

Ophthalmoscopic Findings (Fig. 4.2a, b)

An elevated grayish retinal area with blurred borders is observed in the inferior quadrant of the mid-peripheral retina of the right eye. Multiple white deposits are scattered over the degenerated surface and look like "snowflakes".

OCT Scan Description (Fig. 4.2c)

Scan 1 The retinal surface is smooth and thickened. Multiple hyporeflective cylindrical cavities splitting the retina into two layers are seen in the center of the scan.

Scan 2 The retinal surface is smooth, the elevated area enlarged. There are multiple intraretinal hyporeflective cylindrical cavities between the inner and outer layers of the neurosensory retina. Multiple hyperreflective deposits in the outer plexiform layer are present. Destructive changes are seen in the vitreous, and there is no vitreoretinal traction.

OCT Scan Details (Fig. 4.2c)

- Layers of increased density in the vitreous

- Elevated inner layers of the neurosensory retina

- Irregular and jagged surface of the outer layers of the neurosensory retina

- Intraretinal hyporeflective cavities separating the inner and outer layers of the neurosensory retina

- Dense outer plexiform layer with hyperreflective spot-like deposits

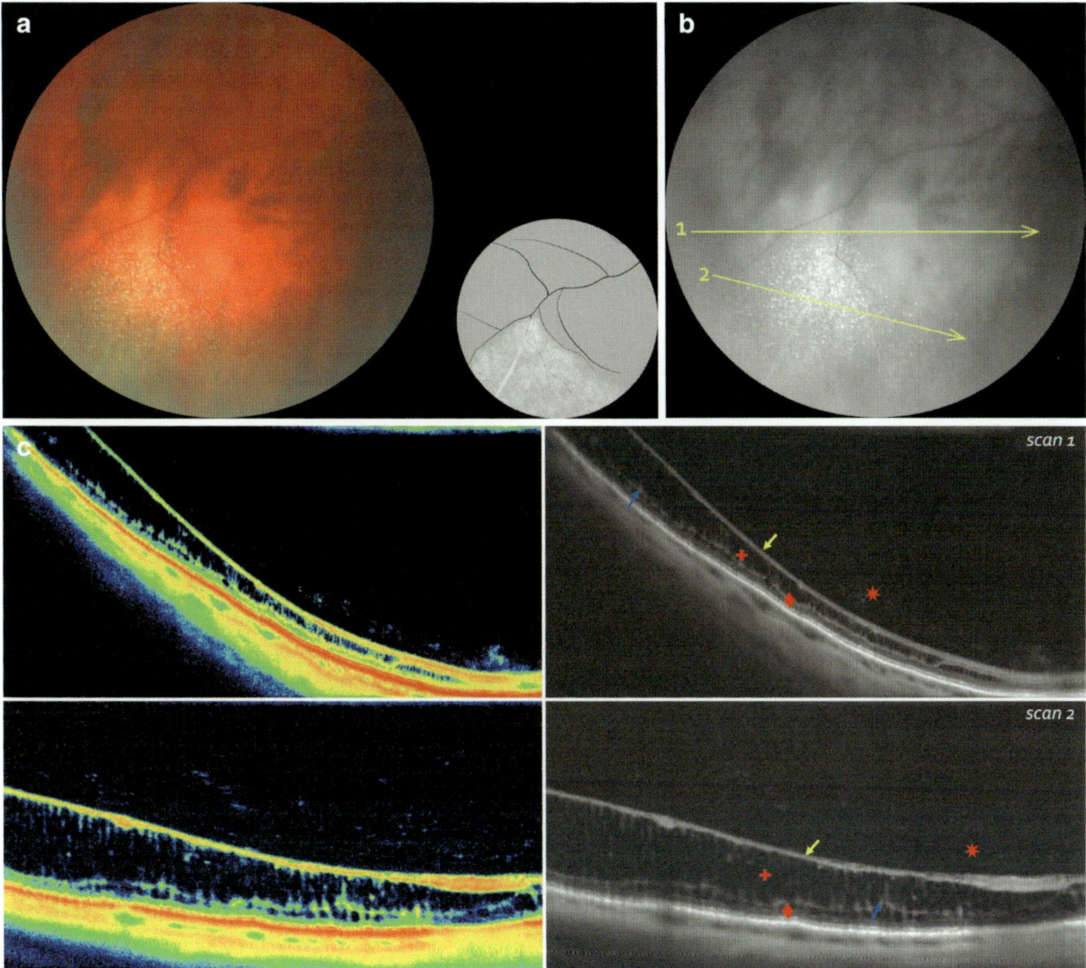

Fig. 4.2 (**a**) Flat retinoschisis with snowflake degeneration. (**b**) *Lines* indicate OCT-scanning direction. (**c**) OCT-scanning results according to the lines direction in (b)

Case 3. Flat Three-Layer Retinoschisis

A 56-year-old female patient was referred for low vision in her right eye. Ocular examination revealed mild hyperopia, early-stage cortical cataract, and bilateral retinoschisis.

Ophthalmoscopic Findings (Fig. 4.3a, b)

A grayish line of a slightly elevated retina is observed in the far peripheral temporal retina of the right eye.

OCT Scan Description (Fig. 4.3c)

Scan 1 The OCT scan shows retinoschisis secondary to cystoid degeneration. The retina is slightly elevated because of multiple hyporeflective cylindrical cavities in the inner plexiform layer of the neurosensory retina, that pass into splitting (schisis) of the retina into two layers: the inner and outer layers of the neurosensory retina. Vitreoretinal traction is not seen.

Scan 2 Three-layer retinoschisis. The retina is elevated because of three-layer splitting: multiple intraretinal cavities in the inner and outer nuclear layers separated by the dense outer plexiform layer.

OCT Scan Details (Fig. 4.3c)

Dense inner layers of the neurosensory retina

Intraretinal hyporeflective cavities separating the inner and outer layers of the neurosensory retina

Dense outer plexiform layer separated from other layers of the neurosensory retina by hyporeflective cavities

Photoreceptor layer destruction. As intraretinal cavities grow in size, this destruction becomes more distinct

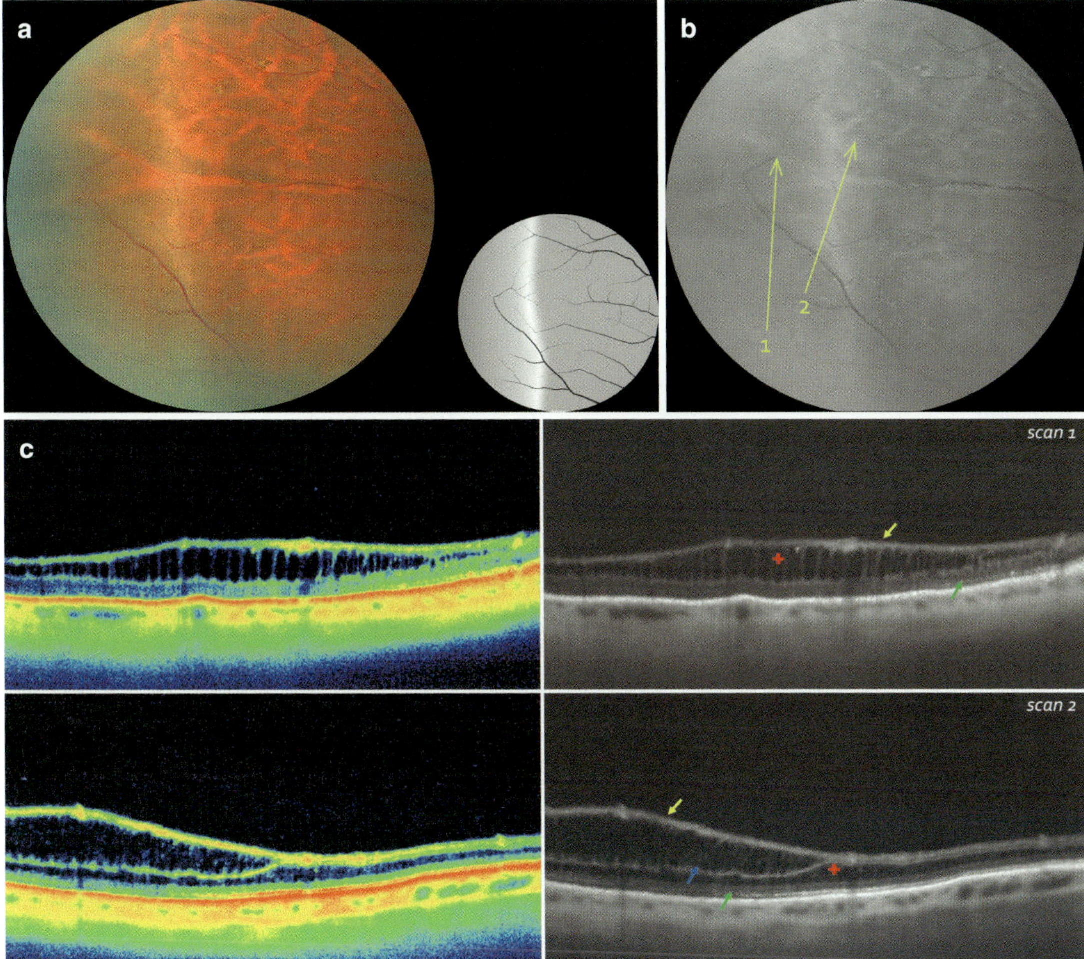

Fig. 4.3 (**a**) Flat retinoschisis. (**b**) *Lines* indicate OCT-scanning direction. (**c**) OCT-scanning results according to the lines direction in (b)

Case 4. Bullous Retinoschisis

A 35-year-old male patient with moderate hyperopia and incomplete posterior vitreous detachment presented with complaints about mild floaters affecting his both eyes.

Ophthalmoscopic Findings (Fig. 4.4a, b)

A clearly outlined, elevated cystoid area darker than the adjacent retina is seen in the temporal quadrant of the left eye. The retinal vessels are seen over the surface of the bullous formation.

OCT Scan Description (Fig. 4.4c, d)

The retinal surface is slightly elevated by multiple cylindrical cavities with hyporeflective content in the neurosensory retina. There is a clearly seen flat splitting into inner and outer layers of the neurosensory retina. This splitting progresses into a large cavity with hyperreflective content separated from the underlying tissues by what supposedly is the dense outer plexiform layer.

Multiple dense and slightly elevated pigment epithelium areas are seen at the borders of degeneration. The ellipsoid zone is destructed. No vitreoretinal traction is seen.

OCT Scan Details (Fig. 4.4c, d)

Elevated inner layers of the neurosensory retina

Large hyporeflective cavity between the inner and outer layers of the neurosensory retina

Photoreceptor layer destruction in the area of the hyporeflective cavity

Intraretinal hyporeflective cavities splitting the inner and outer layers of the neurosensory retina

Dense outer plexiform layer separated from other neurosensory retinal layers by hyporeflective cavities

Areas of increased density and slight elevation of the pigment epithelium

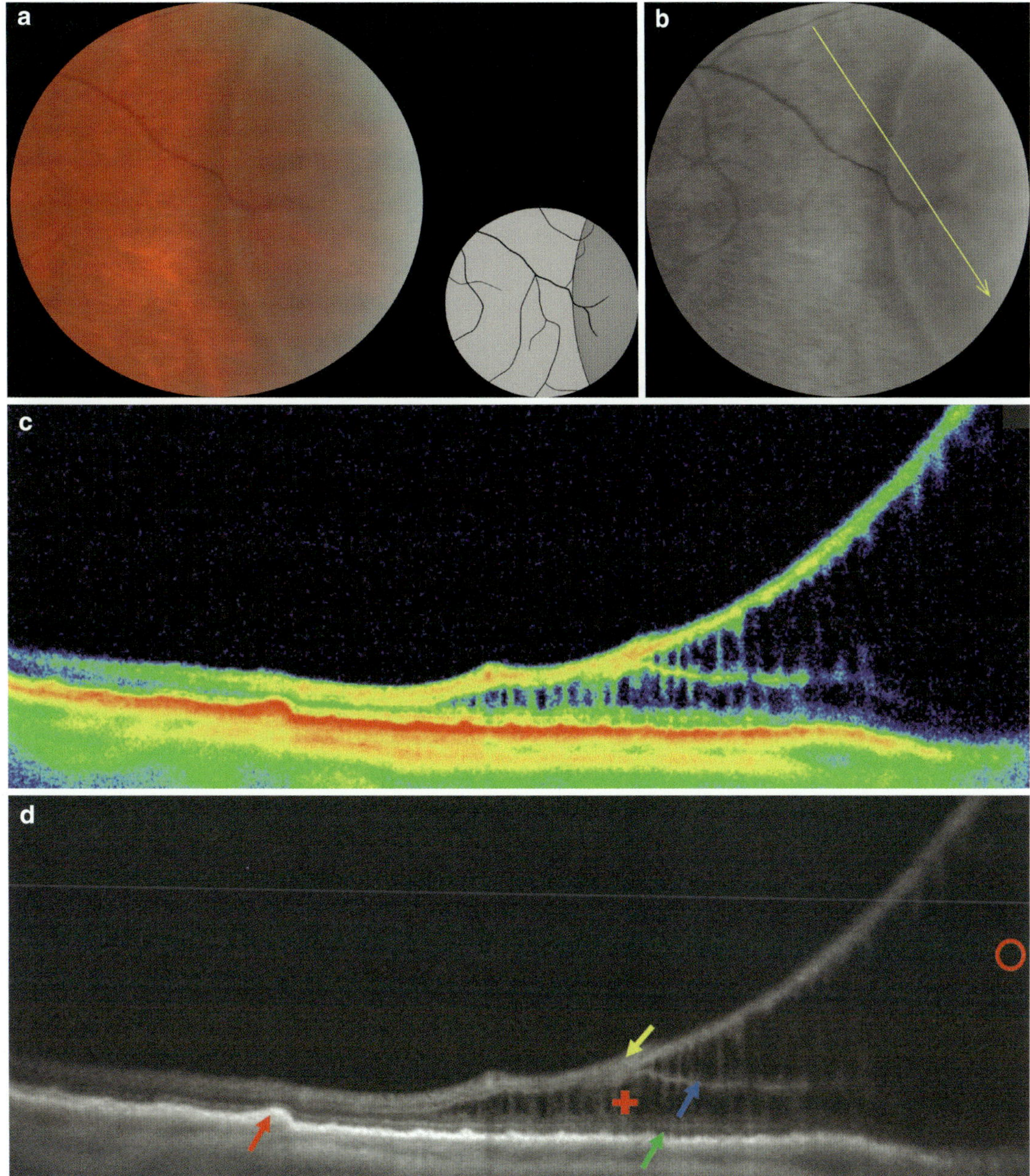

Fig. 4.4 (**a**) Bullous retinoschisis. (**b**) *Line* indicates OCT-scanning direction. (**c**, **d**) OCT-scanning results according to the line direction in (b)

Case 5. Flat Retinoschisis with Subclinical Retinal Detachment

A 49-year-old male patient complained of central vision loss in his right eye. During examination, moderate myopia, early-stage cortical cataract, and far peripheral retinoschisis with subclinical retinal detachment were diagnosed.

Ophthalmoscopic Findings (Fig. 4.5a, b)

A slightly elevated grayish area with blurred borders is observed in the far peripheral retina of the inferotemporal quadrant of the right eye. Laterally, there is a clearly outlined red area imitating a giant retinal tear.

OCT Scan Description (Fig. 4.5c)

Scan 1 The outer retinal layers are irregular. Two cavities separated by a thin layer of neurosensory retina are observed. The cavity on the right developed from the splitting of the neurosensory retina, whereas the one on the left resulted from the complete detachment of the neurosensory epithelium layer from the pigment epithelium.

Scan 2 The transition of retinoschisis to retinal detachment (left part of the scan) is shown, the detached retina is dense. There are no signs of vitreoretinal tractions and adhesions. Local area of destructive changes in the pigment epithelium and hyperreflective choroid in the area of retinoschisis are observed.

OCT Scan Details (Fig. 4.5c)

◯ Large hyporeflective cavity between the inner and outer layers of the neurosensory retina

◆ The outer layers of the neurosensory retina with irregular, jagged surface

↗ Destroyed photoreceptor layer next to retinoschisis border

▲ Hyporeflective outer retinal layers, pigment epithelium, and choroid, at the level of presumably retinal vessels and dense parts in the inner retinal layers

✚ Intraretinal hyporeflective cavities splitting the inner and outer layers of the neurosensory retina

↗ Detached and dense neurosensory retina

↗ Areas of dense and slightly elevated pigment epithelium

↖ Elevated and dense inner layers of the neurosensory retina separated from the outer layers by a hyporeflective cavity

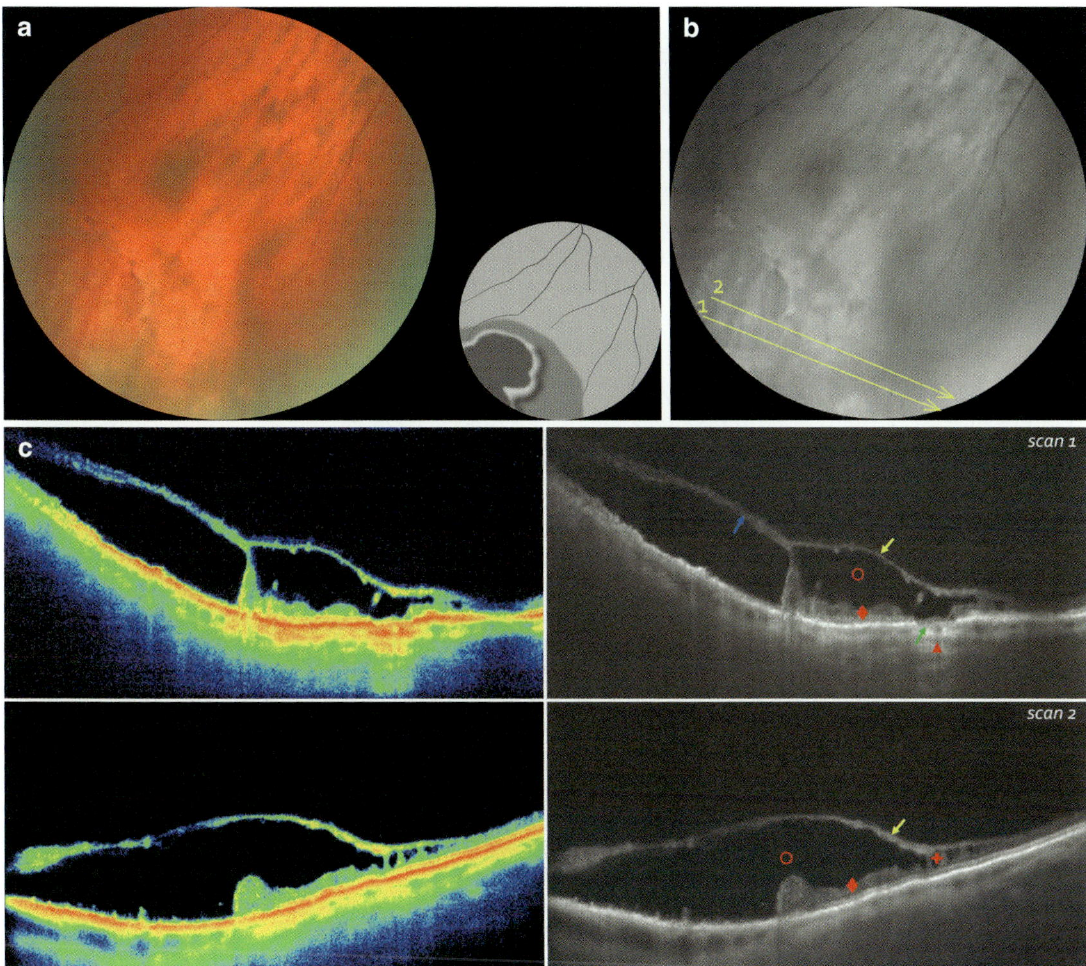

Fig. 4.5 (**a**) Flat retinoschisis with subclinical detachment of the neurosensory epithelium. (**b**) *Lines* indicate OCT-scanning direction. (**c**) OCT-scanning results according to the line direction in (b)

Case 6. Bullous Retinoschisis Progressing into a Retinal Detachment with Fibrosis

A 67-year-old female patient presented with complaints about floaters and occasional flashes of light affecting her right eye for 2 days. During examination, pseudophakia was diagnosed, OD: VA, sc 20/20.

Ophthalmoscopic Findings (Fig. 4.6a, b)

An elevated area of the split retina extending to the mid- and far peripheral retina is observed at the equator and inferotemporal quadrant of the right eye. The medial border of the retinal split is white-gray and clearly outlined with the area of grayish and loose retina seen at its periphery.

OCT Scan Description (Fig. 4.6c)

Scan 1 The retinal surface is raised up. Medially, there are multiple cylindrical elongated cavities at the neurosensory retina level and a schisis of the outer and inner layers progressing into a large hyporeflective cavity.

Scan 2 There is a tear of the outer layer of the neuroepithelium in the area of retinoschisis. The retina is detached.

OCT Scan Details (Fig. 4.6c)

Elevated inner layers of the neurosensory retina

Large hyporeflective cavity between the inner and outer layers of the neurosensory retina

Inner layers of the neurosensory retina with irregular, jagged surface

Pigment epithelium destruction at the retinoschisis border

Intraretinal hyporeflective cavities splitting the inner and outer layers of the neurosensory retina

Detached and dense neurosensory retina

The tear of the outer layers of the neurosensory retina

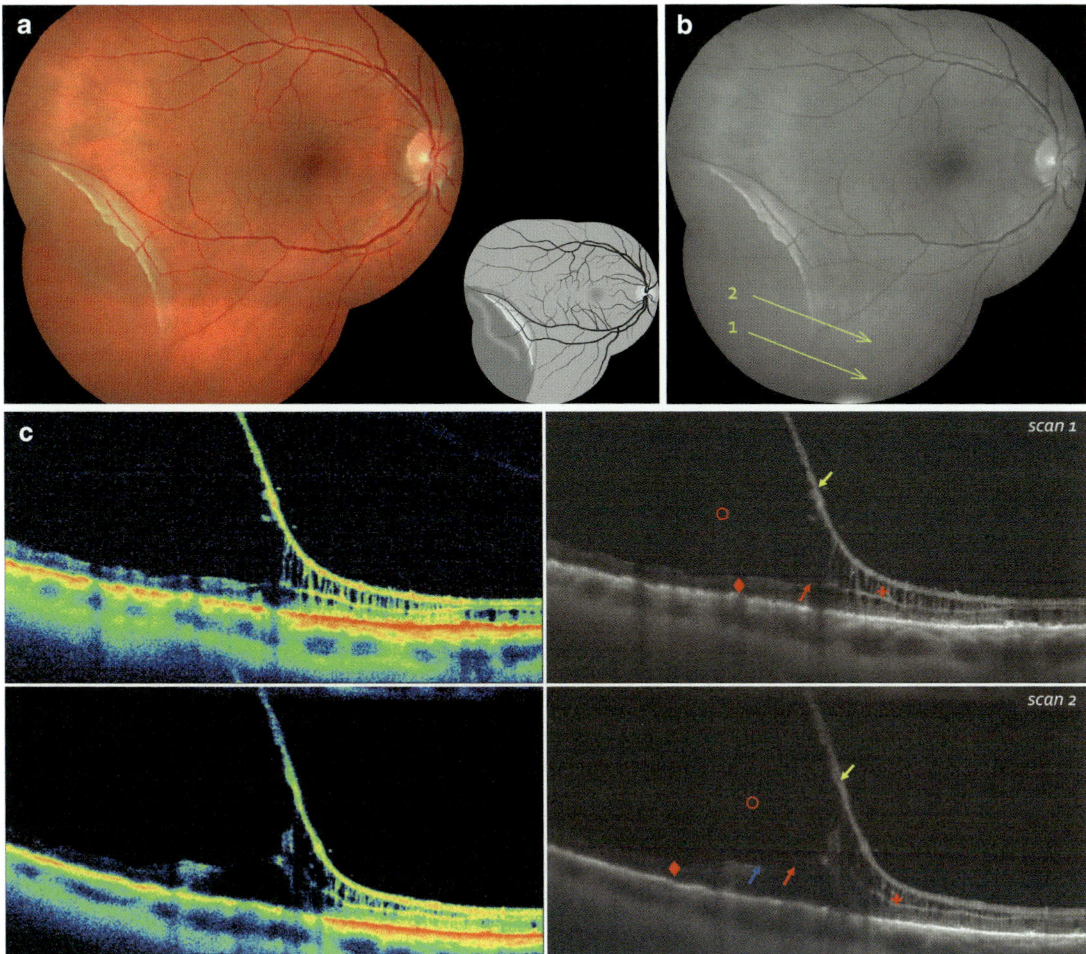

Fig. 4.6 (**a**) Bullous retinoschisis progressing into a retinal detachment. (**b**) *Lines* indicate OCT-scanning direction. (**c**) OCT-scanning results according to the lines direction in (b)

White-Without-Pressure Degeneration

White-without-pressure degeneration (Table 4.2) is an optical phenomenon in retinal periphery characterized by the fundus color change from orange-red to translucent white without a mechanical stimulus [21]. This degeneration is commonly found in the post equatorial area at the base of the vitreous and ora serrata, and may be focal or affect the entire segment of the peripheral retina [22].

Different sources give different data on the prevalence of white-without-pressure degeneration. Some authors report that this degeneration is found in up to 30 % of normal eyes and is usually bilateral [10]. Other authors claim that white-without-pressure is more frequently diagnosed in young individuals (less than 19 years of age – 36 %, 20–39 years of age – 35 %) and there is a definite correlation with the axial length: there were no cases of degeneration in eyes with the shortest axial length of 21 mm and a 54 % incidence in eyes with axial length of >33 mm [22].

This degeneration is widespread, its occurrence in the peripheral retina was first described by Rutnin and Schepens (1967) and Nagpal (1976), however, the clinicopathologic interrelations in this group still remain unclear [23–25]. According to some authors the changes of retina color from orange-red to translucent white or gray-white are due to vitreous traction, and

appear more often in African-Americans [1, 26], whereas other authors explain the retina whitening by increased density of collagen fibrils at the inner retinal surface [10].

There are reports of a circumferential dark-red band around the area of degeneration that may give a false impression of linear retinal tear [21].

Currently there is no universally accepted classification of white-without-pressure. This degeneration is considered by some authors to be benign [27], with no risk of rhegmatogenous retinal detachment [21]. Other experts consider it a trophic-tractional phenomenon [28], or vitreoretinal degeneration [29] with the risk of linear and giant retinal tears along the posterior margin of the lesion [3].

OCT imaging plays an important role in studying white-without-pressure degeneration. OCT-scanning results have shown that the whitish areas in equatorial and peripheral retina correspond to hyperreflective outer retinal layers and ellipsoid zone with no signs of vitreous traction [25, 30].

It is therefore ascertained that white-without-pressure is not associated with vitreoretinal traction and increased risk of retinal detachment, so this degeneration is not considered an indication for prophylactic laser photocoagulation [10, 21, 31]. The patient should be routinely examined every 1–2 years, informed about the symptoms of a retinal tear or detachment and asked to have his retina examined if these symptoms occur [21].

Table 4.2 Diagram of peripheral retinal degenerations

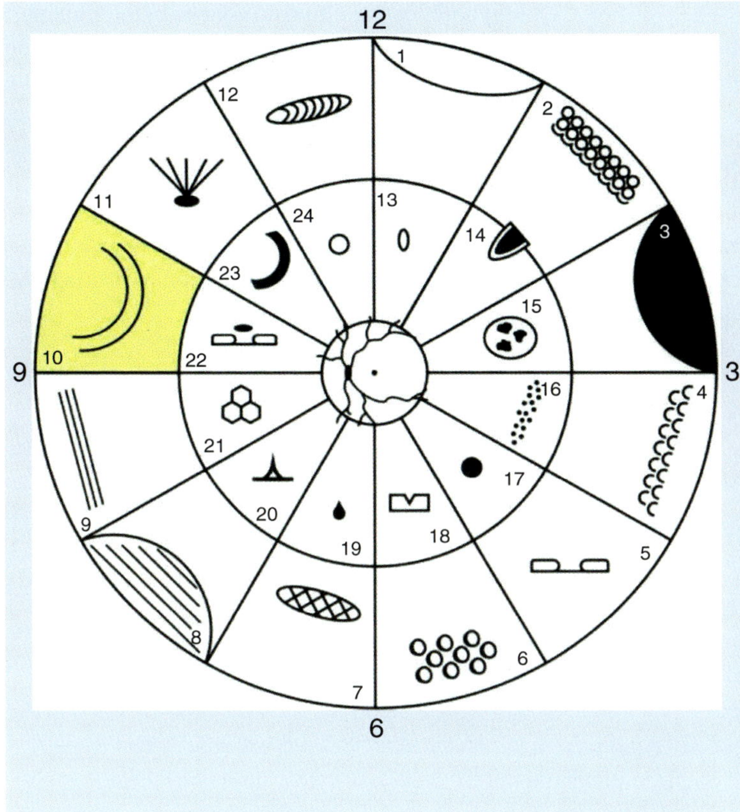

1. Retinal dialysis
2. Peripheral cystoid degeneration
3. Retinal detachment
4. Retinal drusen
5. Full-thickness tear
6. Paving-stone degeneration
7. Lattice degeneration
8. Bullous retinoschisis
9. Flat retinoschisis
10. White-without-pressure
11. Retinal tuft
12. Snail-track degeneration
13. Pearl degeneration
14. Flap tear
15. Grouped congenital hypertrophy of the retinal pigment epithelium ("bear tracks")
16. Snowflake degeneration
17. Unifocal hypertrophy of the retinal pigment epithelium
18. Atrophic retinal hole
19. Haemorrhage
20. Preretinal fibrosis
21. Honeycomb degeneration
22. Operculated retinal tear
23. Dark-without-pressure
24. Unifocal atrophy of the retinal pigment epithelium

White-without-pressure degeneration in sector 10 is highlighted in yellow

Case 7. White-Without-Pressure

An asymptomatic 25-year-old female patient with mild myopia. Degeneration was diagnosed during routine examination.

Ophthalmoscopic Findings (Fig. 4.7a, b)

A wide, white retinal band without a clear border is seen in the mid-peripheral retina of the superotemporal quadrant of the right eye. The retinal vessels are not changed in terms of direction, caliber, and color.

OCT Scan Description (Fig. 4.7c, d)

The retinal surface is smooth. A hyperreflective ellipsoid zone is in the left part of the scan corresponding to the white-without-pressure lesion. A hyporeflective ellipsoid zone is in the right part of the scan corresponding to the normal retina. In the center of the scan, there is a border where the hyperreflective layer changes into hyporeflective. No vitreoretinal tractions or adhesions are seen.

OCT Scan Details

Layer of moderate reflectivity indicating the ellipsoid zone

Marked hyperreflectivity of the ellipsoid zone

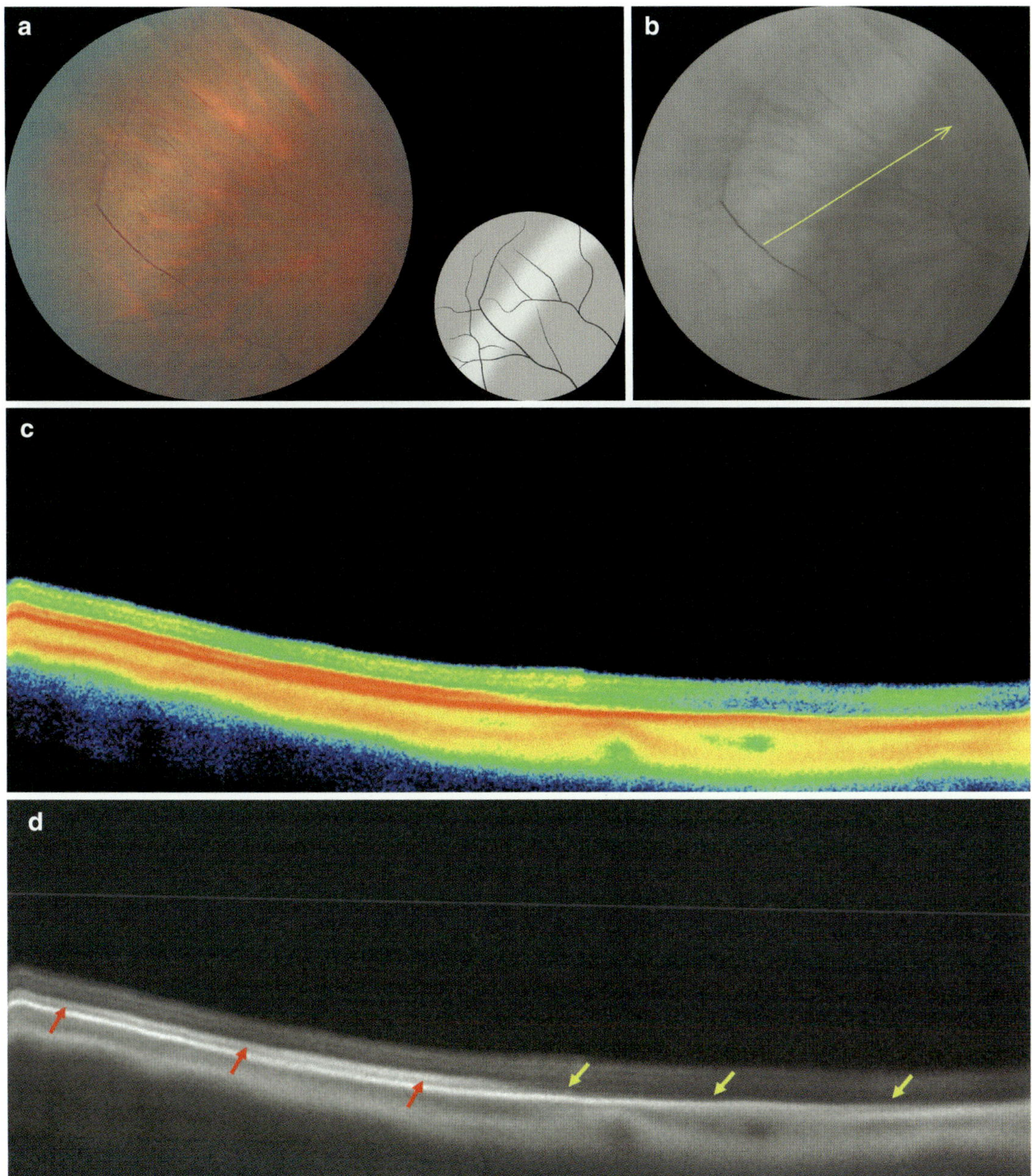

Fig. 4.7 (**a**) White-without-pressure. (**b**) *Line* indicates OCT-scanning direction. (**c**, **d**) OCT-scanning results according to the position of the line in (b)

Case 8. White-Without-Pressure with Pigmented Demarcation Line

An asymptomatic 20-year-old male patient with moderate myopia. Degeneration was diagnosed during routine examination.

Ophthalmoscopic Findings (Fig. 4.8a, b)

An area of degeneration is seen in the mid-peripheral retina of the inferotemporal quadrant of the right eye. The retina appears pale and elevated, with a clearly outlined dark demarcation line.

OCT Scan Description (Fig. 4.8c, d)

The retinal surface is smooth. The ellipsoid zone in the center of the scan is slightly elevated and hyperreflective. The ellipsoid zone interrupts at the level of the demarcation line (where the degenerated area changes into normal retina). The ellipsoid zone at the borders of the retinal degeneration is intact. The choroidal thickness is normal, and no vitreoretinal tractions or adhesions are seen.

OCT Scan Details (Fig. 4.8c, d)

Hyperreflectivity indicating the ellipsoid zone

Marked hyperreflectivity of the ellipsoid zone

No ellipsoid zone is seen

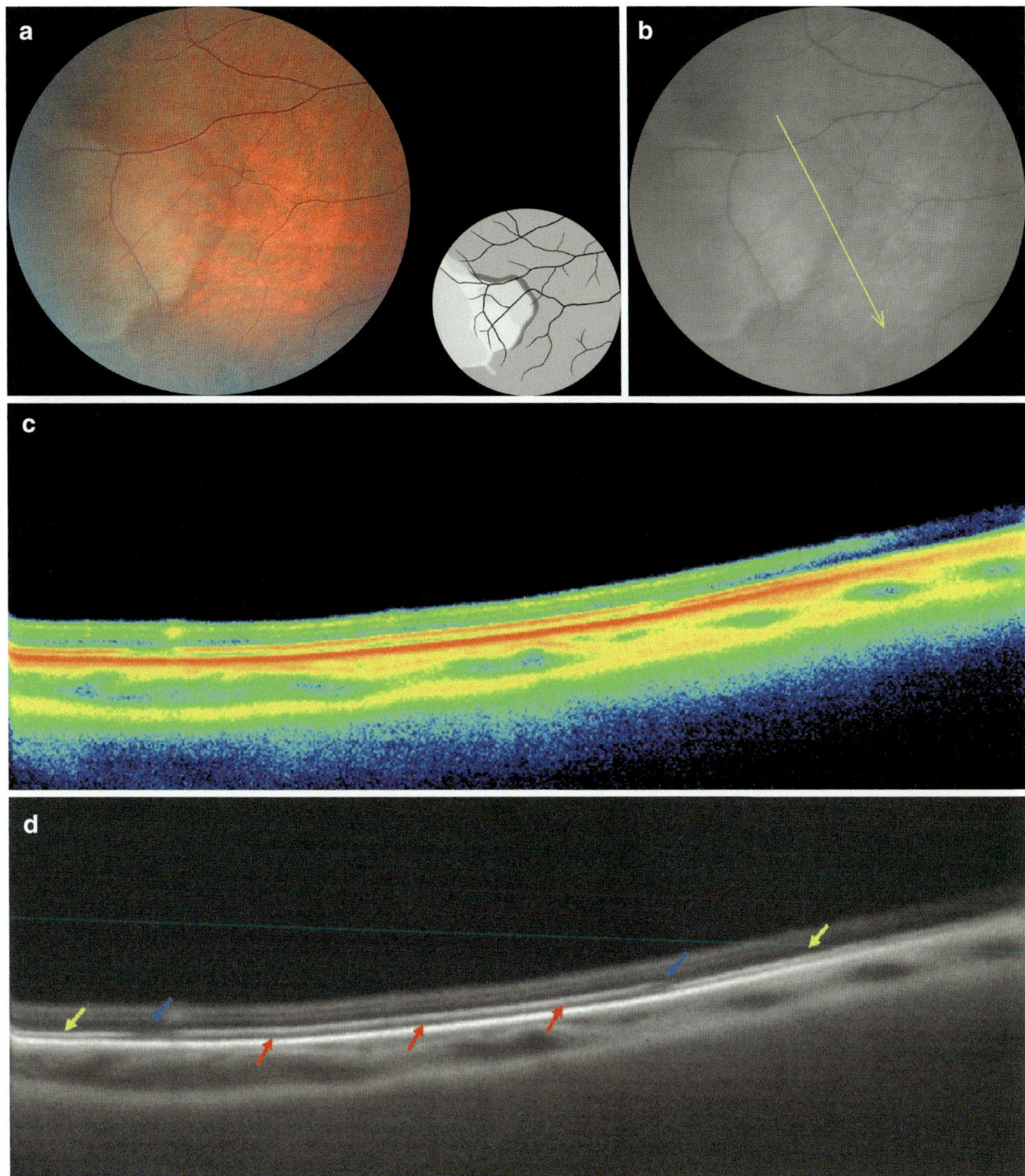

Fig. 4.8 (a) White-without-pressure with a demarcation line. (b) *Line* indicates OCT-scanning direction. (c, d) OCT-scanning results according to the position of the line in (b)

Dark-Without-Pressure Degeneration

Dark-without-pressure (Table 4.3) is a fundus lesion that looks like a flat brown area with well-defined margins of different forms, usually located in the equator of the peripheral retina. This degeneration was initially found in dark-skinned patients and in patients with sickle cell retinopathy [32].

According to the literature [21], dark-without-pressure can be found immediately posterior to an area of white-without-pressure, often as a small dark red zone or a circumferential band around white-without-pressure degeneration that may give a false impression of a retinal tear. Dark-without-pressure is generally found posteriorly to the ora serrata (no more than 3 disc diameters), although it may extend as far as the temporal arcades. This degeneration is presumed to have the same nature as the white-without-pressure lesion.

Some authors [32] consider dark-without-pressure as a reflectivity change of retinal pigment epithelium in the internal limiting membrane or in other fundus areas. However, it is still unknown what factors lead to these changes. No vascular changes in the area of degeneration were seen in fluorescent angiography, no vitreoretinal traction was identified, and no structural changes of the vitreous above the area of degeneration were observed.

There are usually no symptomatic complaints in patients with dark-without-pressure and there are no signs of pathological changes in peripheral and central vision.

OCT provides new possibilities for diagnosing dark-without-pressure. OCT imaging showed hyporeflectivity of the ellipsoid zone, whereas no changes in the vitreoretinal interface, neurosensory retina layers, and choroid were observed. One year follow-up showed no signs of progression [24, 33].

Table 4.3 Diagram of peripheral retinal degenerations

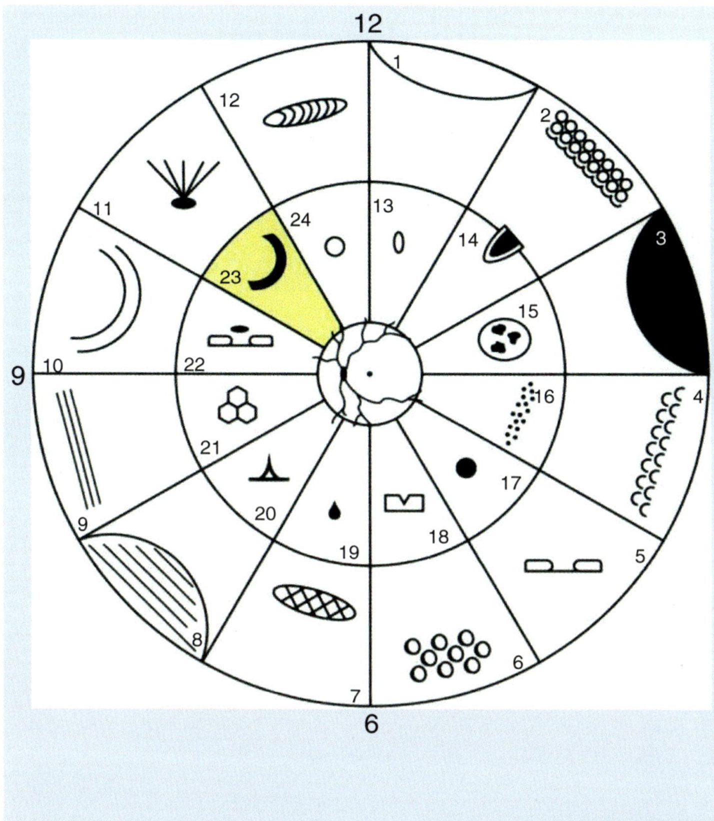

1. Retinal dialysis
2. Peripheral cystoid degeneration
3. Retinal detachment
4. Retinal drusen
5. Full-thickness tear
6. Paving-stone degeneration
7. Lattice degeneration
8. Bullous retinoschisis
9. Flat retinoschisis
10. White-without-pressure
11. Retinal tuft
12. Snail-track degeneration
13. Pearl degeneration
14. Flap tear
15. Grouped congenital hypertrophy of the retinal pigment epithelium ("bear tracks")
16. Snowflake degeneration
17. Unifocal hypertrophy of the retinal pigment epithelium
18. Atrophic retinal hole
19. Haemorrhage
20. Preretinal fibrosis
21. Honeycomb degeneration
22. Operculated retinal tear
23. Dark-without-pressure
24. Unifocal atrophy of the retinal pigment epithelium

Dark-without-pressure degeneration in sector 23 is highlighted in yellow

Case 9. Dark-Without-Pressure

A 23-year-old dark-skinned male patient with severe myopia complained about low vision in both eyes.

Ophthalmoscopic Findings (Fig. 4.9a, b)

A dark brown non-elevated area with well-defined borders is seen in the mid-peripheral retina of the inferior quadrant of the left eye. The retina outside the dark brown area is of characteristic white, silvery color.

OCT Scan Description (Fig. 4.9c, d)

The retinal surface is smooth with no vitreoretinal traction. Hyperreflective ellipsoid zone corresponds to the normal retina, and hyporeflective ellipsoid zone corresponds to the dark-without-pressure lesion.

OCT Scan Details (Fig. 4.9c, d)

Hyperreflective ellipsoid zone

Marked hyporeflectivity of the ellipsoid zone in the area of the dark-without-pressure lesion

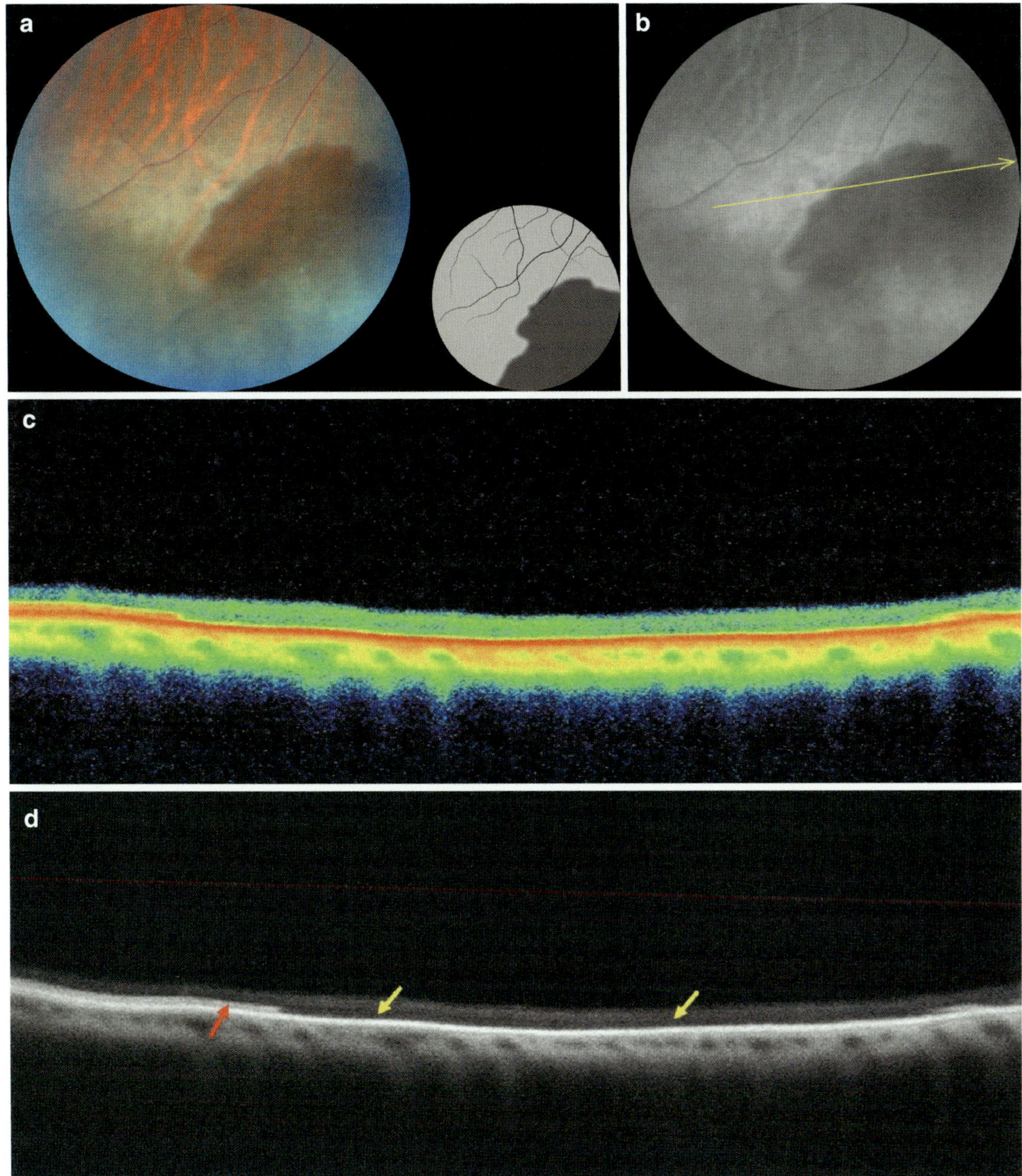

Fig. 4.9 (**a**) Dark-without-pressure. (**b**) *Line* indicates OCT-scanning direction. (**c**, **d**) OCT-scanning results according to the line direction in (b)

Case 10. Combined Lesion: Dark-Without-Pressure and White-Without-Pressure

An asymptomatic 26-year-old fair-skinned female patient with mild myopia came for a routine examination. White-without-pressure and dark-without-pressure degenerations were revealed on the mid-peripheral retina of her right eye.

Ophthalmoscopic Findings (Fig. 4.10a, b)

In the mid-peripheral retina of the temporal quadrant of the right eye, normal retinal tissue transforms into a wide white band and then into a well-demarcated dark brown area. The white zone appears elevated, while the dark area seems to be retracted, imitating a retinal tear.

OCT Scan Description (Fig. 4.10c)

Scan 1 The change of the intact retinal tissue into the white-without-pressure lesion – there is a distinct difference in the photoreceptor layer where the normal ellipsoid zone becomes hyperreflective, indicating the white-without-pressure lesion.

Scan 2 The scan through the white-without-pressure – there is an increased hyperreflectivity of the ellipsoid zone.

Scan 3 The border between the dark-without-pressure and white-without-pressure degenerations is seen as a change of photoreceptor layer reflectivity: the hyporeflective ellipsoid zone in the dark-without-pressure becomes hyperreflective in the white-without-pressure area.

OCT Scan Details (Fig. 4.10c)

Moderate reflectivity layer corresponding to the ellipsoid zone

Sharply increased reflectivity of the ellipsoid zone in the whitish area of retina

Decreased reflectivity of the ellipsoid zone in the dark-without-pressure area

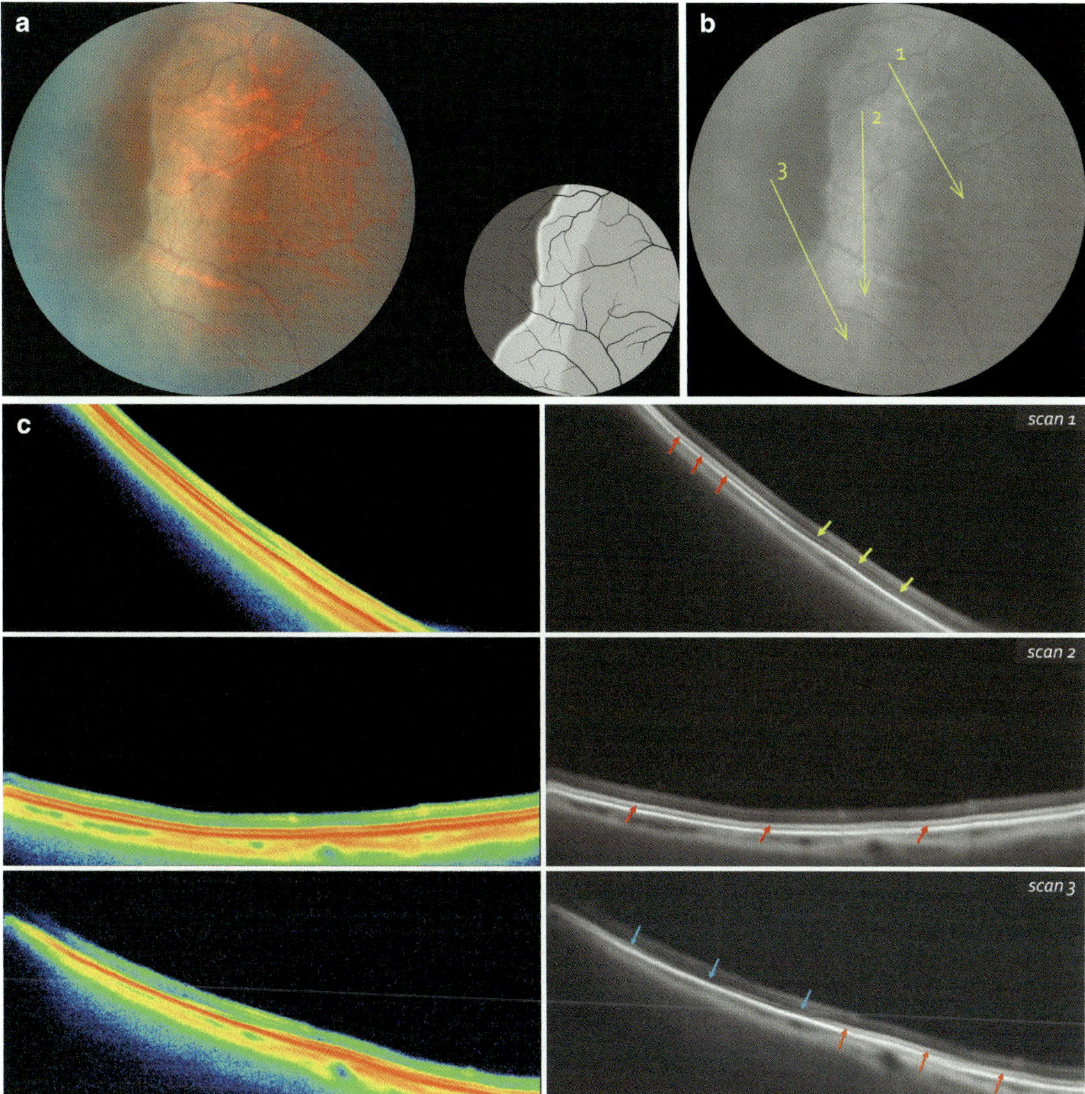

Fig. 4.10 (**a**) Dark-without-pressure and white-without-pressure. (**b**) OCT-scanning positions indicated by *lines*. (**c**) OCT-scanning results according to the lines direction in (b)

Peripheral Cystoid Degeneration

Peripheral cystoid degeneration (Blessing-Iwanoff microcystoid degeneration) is characterized by multiple tiny intraretinal microcystoid cavities that may be found in all retinal quadrants, but more frequently occur in the temporal half of the peripheral retina [21, 23, 28, 34].

Cystoid degeneration (Table 4.4) appears as minute yellowish vesicles with blurred borders on a greyish-white background that make the retina look thickened [3, 10]. In advanced cases these vesicles can merge, become pink, irregular in shape and have more clearly defined borders [27]. The newly formed cystoid degeneration is usually localized immediately posterior to the ora serrata and progresses posteriorly up to the equator in more advanced cases [5].

There are two types of peripheral cystoid degeneration: typical and reticular. Typical cystoid degeneration occurs in all adults [3, 28]. Reticular cystoid degeneration may be found in 18 % of individuals in general population; in 41 % it is bilateral [21, 28, 34]. A histological study showed the 17 % incidence of reticular cystoid degeneration, which was bilateral in 44 % of cases [35].

Typical cystoid degeneration may lead to the fusion of cysts and cavities, and to the flat senile retinoschisis in the outer plexiform layer. Reticular cystoid degeneration is often complicated by bullous retinoschisis [3, 4].

The majority of experts believe that cystoid degeneration seldom causes clinically significant retinal tears or detachment. Therefore, this degeneration does not require prophylactic laser photocoagulation [3, 5, 10, 27].

Table 4.4 Diagram of peripheral retinal degenerations

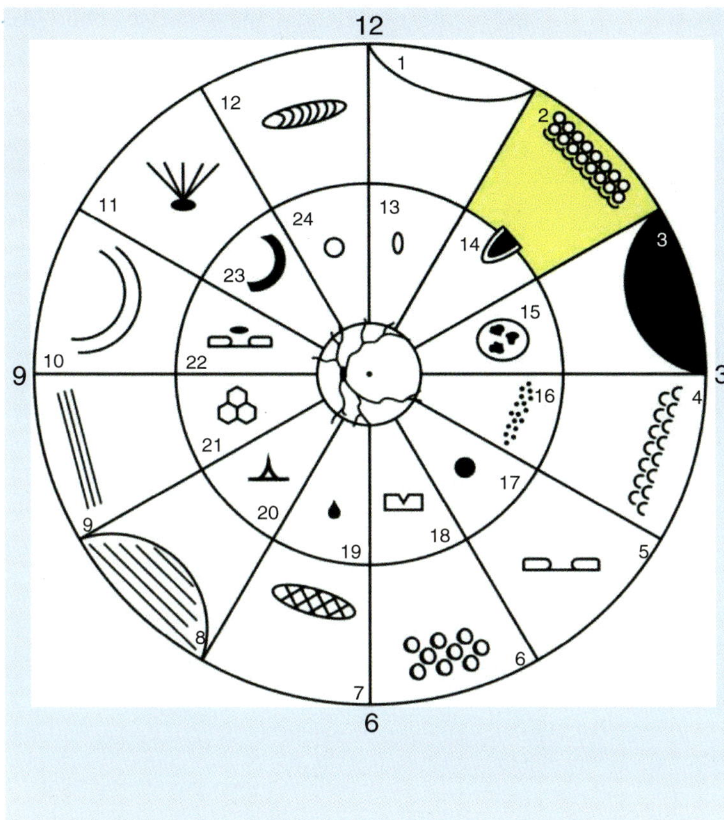

1. Retinal dialysis
2. Peripheral cystoid degeneration
3. Retinal detachment
4. Retinal drusen
5. Full-thickness tear
6. Paving-stone degeneration
7. Lattice degeneration
8. Bullous retinoschisis
9. Flat retinoschisis
10. White-without-pressure
11. Retinal tuft
12. Snail-track degeneration
13. Pearl degeneration
14. Flap tear
15. Grouped congenital hypertrophy of the retinal pigment epithelium ("bear tracks")
16. Snowflake degeneration
17. Unifocal hypertrophy of the retinal pigment epithelium
18. Atrophic retinal hole
19. Haemorrhage
20. Preretinal fibrosis
21. Honeycomb degeneration
22. Operculated retinal tear
23. Dark-without-pressure
24. Unifocal atrophy of the retinal pigment epithelium

Peripheral cystoid degeneration in sector 2 is highlighted in yellow

Case 11. Peripheral Cystoid Degeneration without Vitreous Traction

A 23-year-old male patient with moderate myopia and no symptomatic complaints.

Ophthalmoscopic Findings (Fig. 4.11a, b)

A wide, slightly elevated area of retina with multiple intraretinal tiny oval cystoid cavities is seen in the far periphery of the temporal quadrant of the right eye. The retina is pale gray and spongy.

OCT Scan Description (Fig. 4.11c, d)

The retinal surface is irregular, with multiple separated and confluent intraretinal cavities filled with hyporeflective fluid. Hyperplasia of the retinal pigment epithelium and decreased choroidal reflectivity are seen. There are no signs of vitreoretinal traction.

OCT Scan Details (Fig. 4.11c, d)

★ Layers of moderate and high reflectivity in the vitreous

✛ Multiple large hyporeflective intraretinal cavities

◤ Dense area of the pigment epithelium

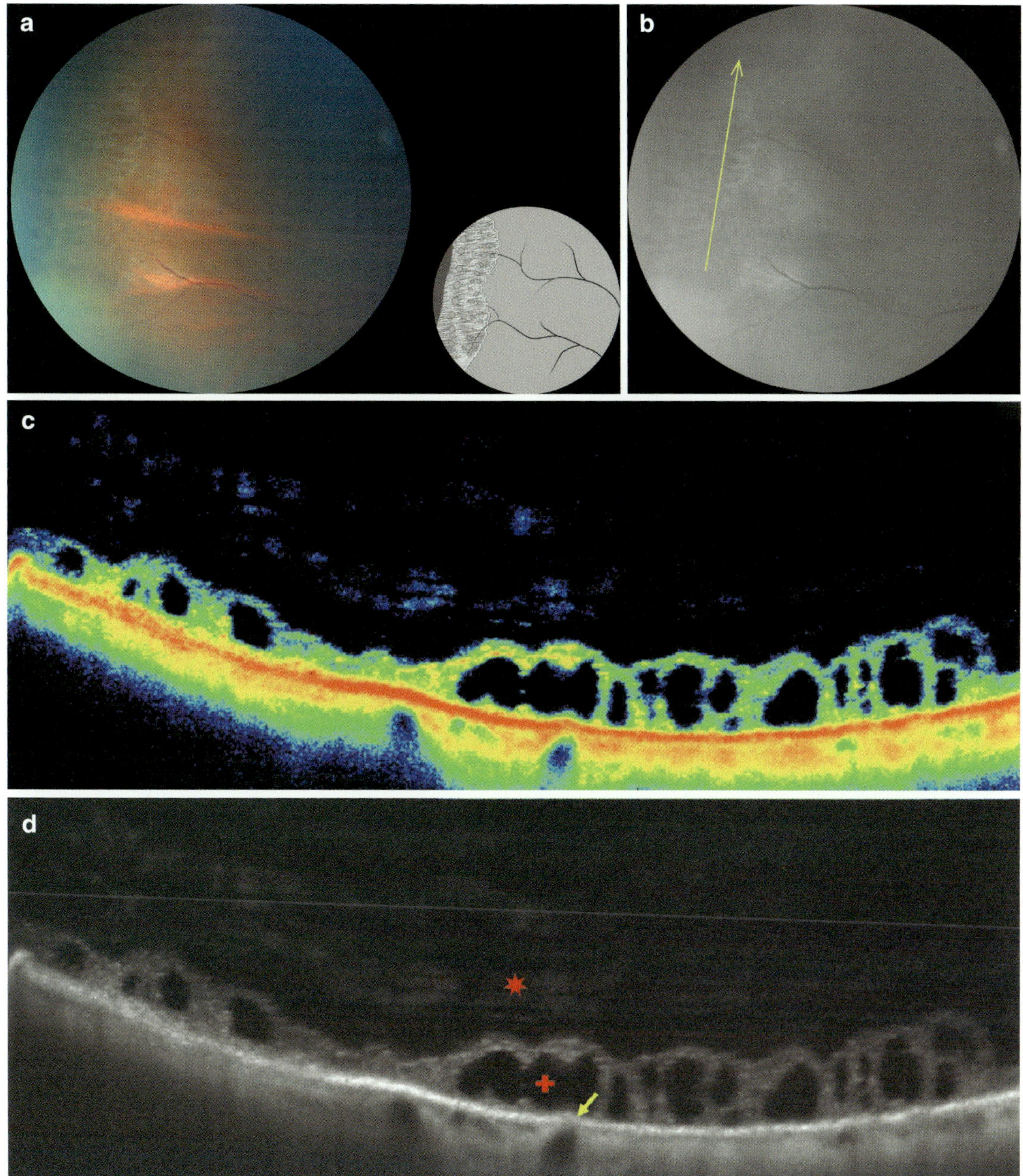

Fig. 4.11 (**a**) Peripheral cystoid degeneration without traction. (**b**) *Line* indicates OCT-scanning direction. (**c, d**) OCT-scanning results according to the line direction in (b)

Case 12. Peripheral Cystoid Degeneration with Vitreous Traction

A 34-year-old male patient with low hyperopia and no symptomatic complaints.

Ophthalmoscopic Findings
(Fig. 4.12a, b)

An elevated lesion with multiple intraretinal cavities is seen in the far periphery of the temporal quadrant of the right eye. The retina appears pale gray and spongy. Retina overhang, signs of vitreoretinal traction, and decreased media transparency are seen at the ora serrata.

OCT Scan Description (Fig. 4.12c, d)

The retinal surface is irregular and elevated. Multiple intraretinal hyporeflective cavities are seen in the neurosensory retina. The vitreous is dense, there are vitreoretinal adhesions and tractions. The pigment epithelium is irregular, with multiple dense areas.

OCT Scan Details (Fig. 4.12c, d)

✳ Large area of condensed vitreous and vitreoretinal adhesions with traction

✚ Multiple large hyporeflective intraretinal cavities

◤ Dense areas of the pigment epithelium

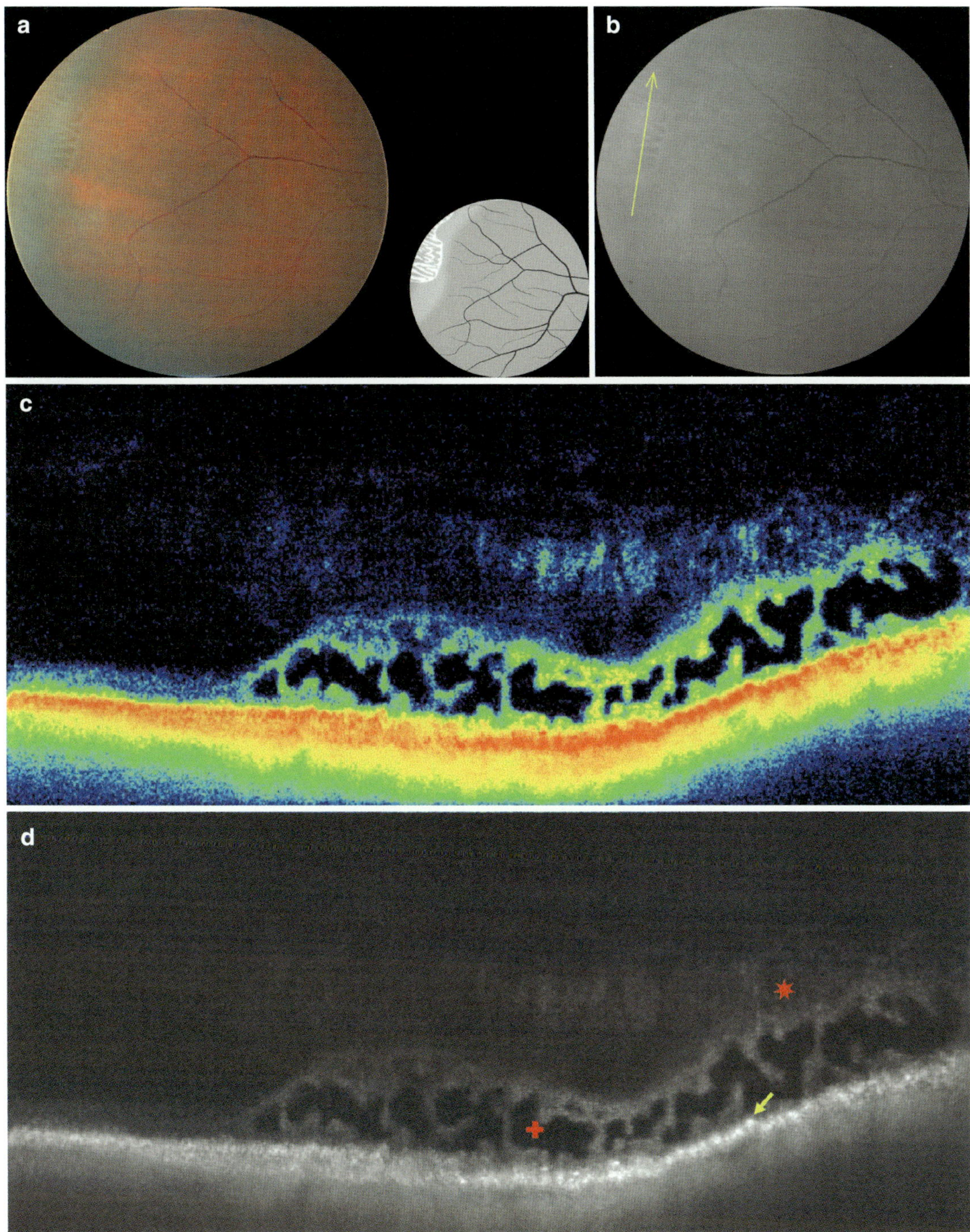

Fig. 4.12 (a) Peripheral cystoid degeneration with traction. (b) *Line* indicates OCT-scanning direction. (c, d) OCT-scanning results according to the line direction in (b)

Case 13. Peripheral Cystoid Degeneration Parallel to the Ora Serrata

A 27-year-old male patient with low hyperopia and no symptomatic complaints.

Ophthalmoscopic Findings (Fig. 4.13a, b)

A clearly outlined, cord-like cystoid lesion with pigmentation is seen across the far periphery of the left eye. Multiple red-colored cavities mimicking retinal tears are seen in the area of degeneration.

OCT Scan Description (Fig. 4.13c, d)

The retinal surface is irregular with multiple intraretinal hyporeflective cavities. Vitreoretinal adhesion is seen over the lesion as layers of consolidated vitreous with moderate to high reflectivity. Destructive changes are seen in the ellipsoid zone and the pigment epithelium.

OCT Scan Details (Fig. 4.13c, d)

★ Layers of moderate and high reflectivity in the vitreous; large areas of vitreoretinal adhesions

+ Multiple large hyporeflective intraretinal cavities separated by irregular septums

◤ Areas of increased density of the pigment epithelium

➤ Pigment epithelium and photoreceptor layer destruction

◆ Increased reflectivity of choroidal vessels in the area of pigment epithelium destruction

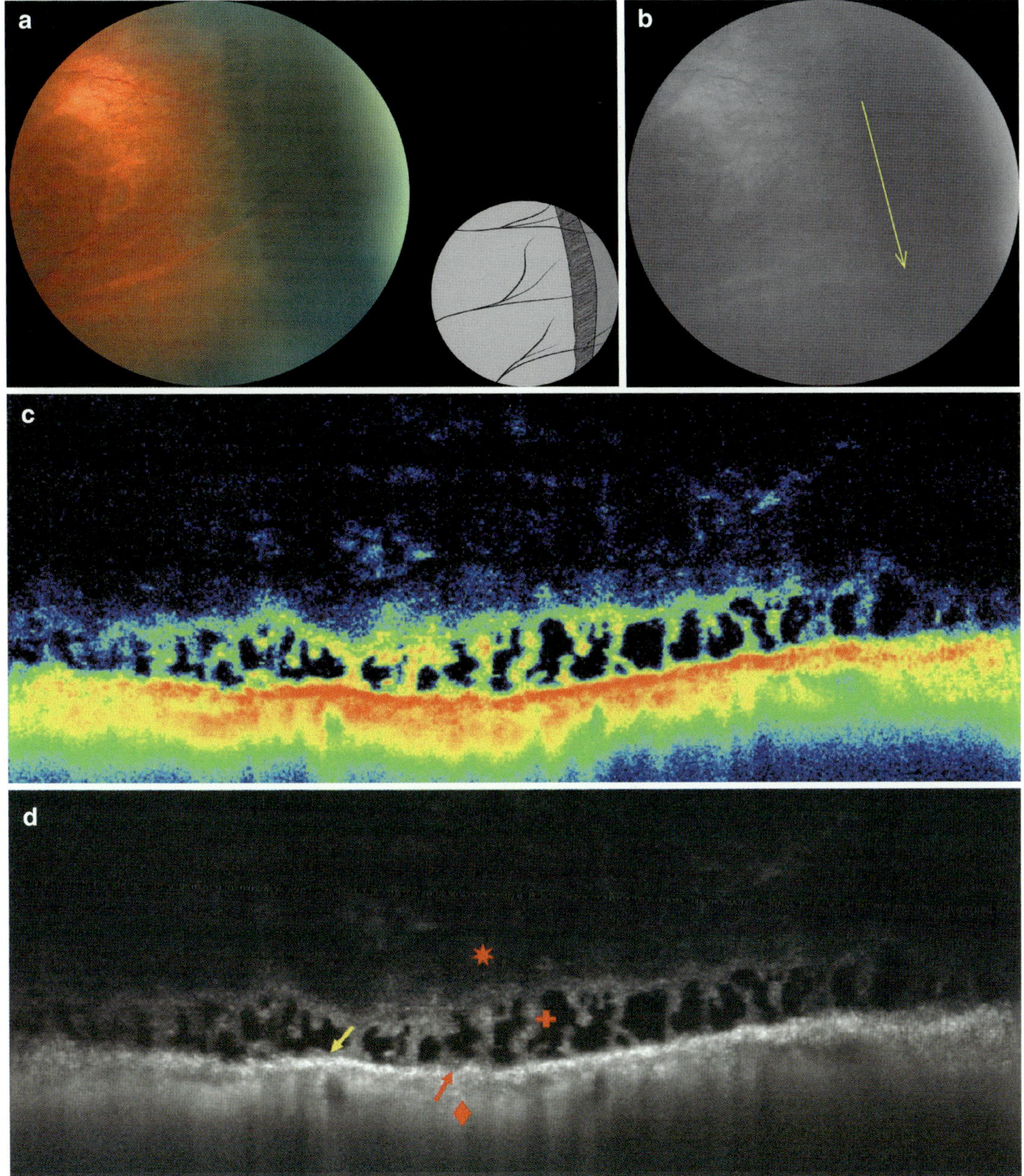

Fig. 4.13 (**a**) Peripheral cystoid degeneration parallel to the ora serrata. (**b**) *Line* indicates OCT-scanning direction. (**c, d**) OCT-scanning results according to the line direction in (b)

Snowflake Degeneration

Snowflake degeneration (Table 4.5) was first described by Hirose et al. in 1974 [36, 37]. This degeneration appears as little white-yellow dots or ovals in the peripheral retina. They often appear crystalline because of light reflection [21].

Snowflake degeneration may be found either as an isolated entity or as combined with other degenerations, like retinoschisis, lattice degeneration, and white-without-pressure [21, 36].

Snowflake degeneration may appear as a wide band (1–3 disc diameters), and may be located in one or more retinal quadrants. This lesion may also be distributed circumferentially around the retina. Snowflake degeneration is located mostly in the superotemporal quadrant (95 %) and less frequently in the inferior quadrant [37].

Snowflake degeneration is a rare condition in general population [38]. This degeneration has an autosomal dominant inheritance pattern [36, 38, 39], but it is considered to be a clinically and genetically independent condition [40].

Hirose et al. gave four stages of the disease progression [41]:

- Stage 1. Peripheral white-with-pressure degeneration with minimal vitreous changes;
- Stage 2. Snowflake-like inclusions appearing in the retinal periphery up to the ora serrata;
- Stage 3. Sheathing of retinal vessels and hyperpigmentation;
- Stage 4. Increased pigmentation and occlusion of the retinal vessels. The progression of chorioretinal atrophy. Destructive changes in the vitreous.

Snowflake degeneration can lead to retinal breaks (holes and flap tears), and subsequent retinal detachment [3, 21]. There have been reports of retinal detachment secondary to snowflake degeneration in 17–20 % eyes in one family [37, 40].

A wide range of evidence suggests prophylactic laser surgery of retinal tears associated with snowflake degeneration. In these cases, laser photocoagulation or cryopexy are indicated [21, 42].

Table 4.5 Diagram of peripheral retinal degenerations

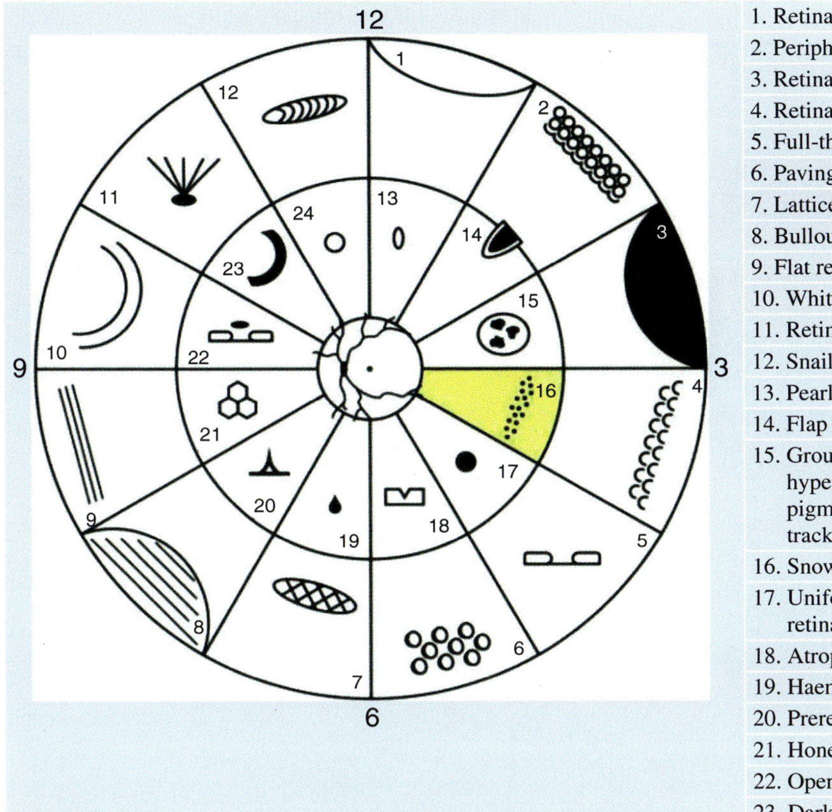

1. Retinal dialysis
2. Peripheral cystoid degeneration
3. Retinal detachment
4. Retinal drusen
5. Full-thickness tear
6. Paving-stone degeneration
7. Lattice degeneration
8. Bullous retinoschisis
9. Flat retinoschisis
10. White-without-pressure
11. Retinal tuft
12. Snail-track degeneration
13. Pearl degeneration
14. Flap tear
15. Grouped congenital hypertrophy of the retinal pigment epithelium ("bear tracks")
16. Snowflake degeneration
17. Unifocal hypertrophy of the retinal pigment epithelium
18. Atrophic retinal hole
19. Haemorrhage
20. Preretinal fibrosis
21. Honeycomb degeneration
22. Operculated retinal tear
23. Dark-without-pressure
24. Unifocal atrophy of the retinal pigment epithelium

Snowflake degeneration in sector 16 is highlighted in yellow

Case 14. Snowflake Degeneration with Multiple Tiny Deposits (without Traction)

A 35-year-old emmetropic female patient with no symptomatic complaints. Retinal changes were revealed during routine examination.

Ophthalmoscopic Findings (Fig. 4.14a, b)

A wide band of multiple white dots and tiny deposits in the superficial layers of the retina is observed in the far peripheral retina of the temporal quadrant of the right eye. Pigment is redistributed.

OCT Scan Description (Fig. 4.14c, d)

Retinal surface appears smooth with multiple hyperreflective deposits in the neuroepithelium. Layers of moderate reflectivity are seen in the vitreous. There are no signs of vitreoretinal traction. Posterior hyaloid membrane is fully detached.

OCT Scan Details (Fig. 4.14c, d)

- Multiple intraretinal hyperreflective deposits

- Increased density (hyperreflectivity) of all layers of the neurosensory retina

- Layers of moderate reflectivity in the vitreous; no signs of vitreoretinal adhesion

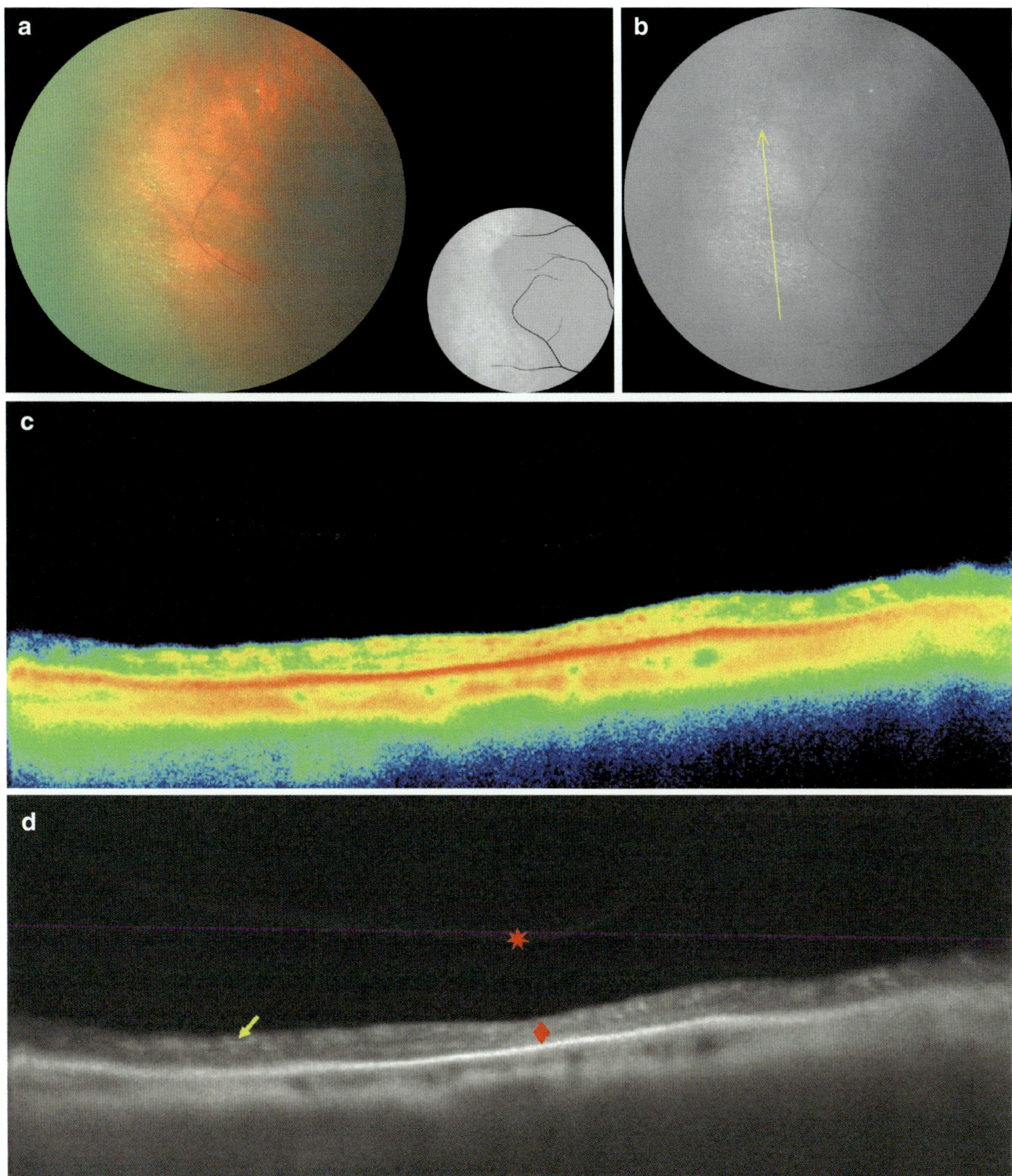

Fig. 4.14 (**a**) Snowflake degeneration without vitreous traction. (**b**) *Line* indicates OCT-scanning direction. (**c**, **d**) OCT-scanning results according to the line direction in (b)

Case 15. Snowflake Degeneration with Large Intraretinal Deposits (without Traction)

A 26-year-old emmetropic female patient with no symptomatic complaints. Snowflake degeneration was diagnosed during routine examination.

Ophthalmoscopic Findings (Fig. 4.15a, b)

Multiple white dots with metallic sheen are observed in the far peripheral retina of the inferior quadrant of the left eye. The lesions are round in shape and have clear borders.

OCT Scan Description (Fig. 4.15c, d)

The retinal surface is smooth; the neuroepithelium is of normal thickness. Three round hyperreflective deposits causing a shadow effect on the underlying tissues are seen in the neurosensory retina. The pigment epithelium is intact. Vitreous structure is uneven, with areas of increased reflectivity. No signs of vitreoretinal traction are present.

OCT Scan Details (Fig. 4.15c, d)

★ Layers of moderate reflectivity (increased density) in the vitreous

↙ Intraretinal hyperreflective round-shaped deposits

+ Area of increased density (hyperreflectivity) of all layers of the neurosensory retina

▲ Decreased reflectivity of the choroid at the level of the hyporeflective deposits in the neurosensory retina

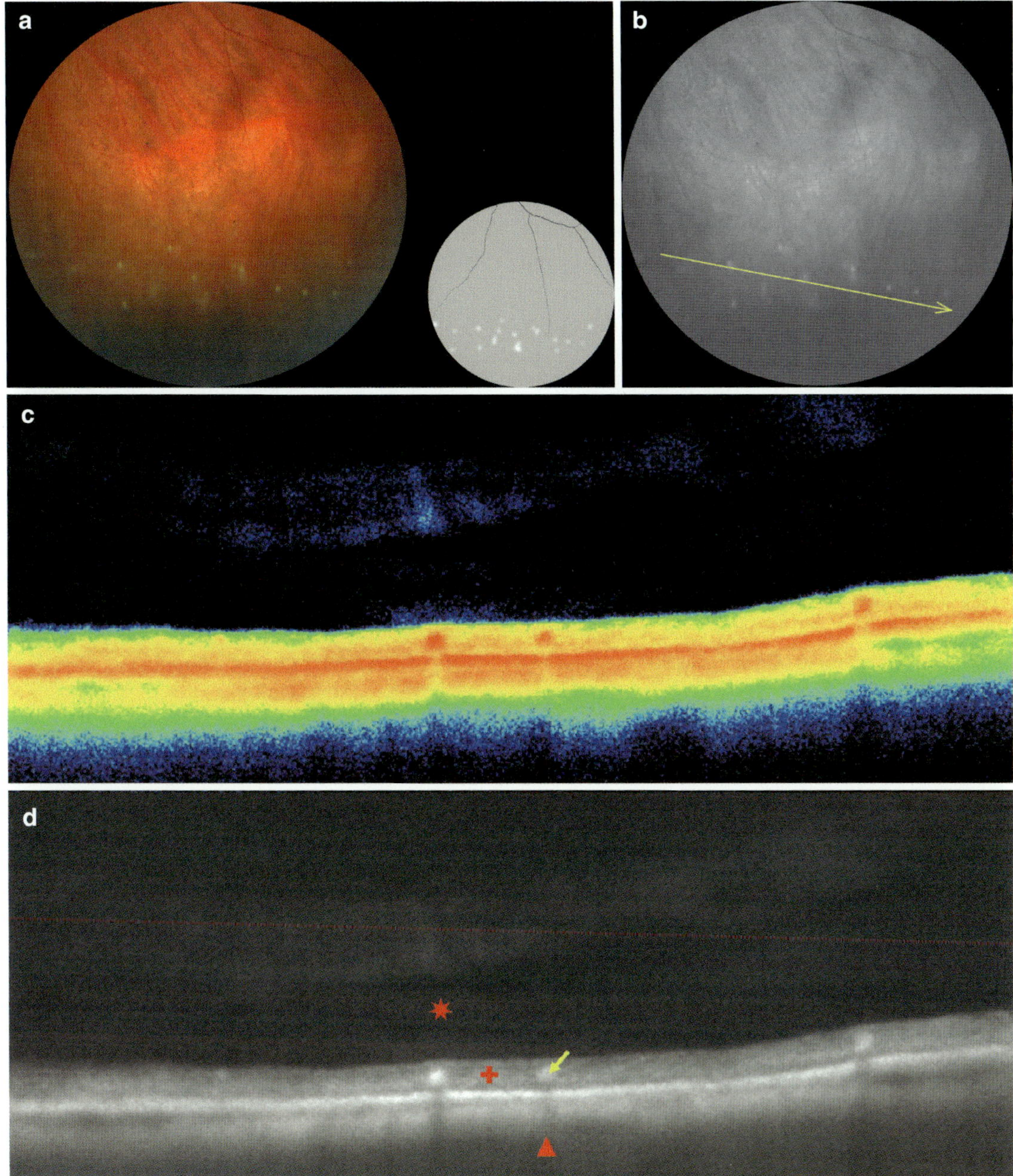

Fig. 4.15 (**a**) Snowflake degeneration with large intraretinal deposits. (**b**) *Line* indicates OCT-scanning direction. (**c**, **d**) OCT-scanning results according to the line direction in (**b**)

Case 16. Complicated Snowflake Degeneration (with Vitreoretinal Traction and Retinoschisis)

A 49-year-old moderately myopic female patient with an early stage cortical cataract and partial posterior vitreous detachment presented with complaints of flashes of light, floaters, and decreased visual acuity affecting her left eye for the last 2 months.

Ophthalmoscopic Findings (Fig. 4.16a, b)

Multiple crystalline white-colored thread-like deposits are seen in the far peripheral retina of the superotemporal quadrant of the left eye. The retinal surface is blurred, because the transparency of the media is reduced.

OCT Scan Description (Fig. 4.16c)

Scan 1 Retina profile is irregular because of vitreoretinal adhesions. Consolidated vitreous is partially attached to the retina. The neuroepithelium is thickened, there are multiple intraretinal cavities of various size.

Scan 2 The retinal profile is altered by vitreoretinal adhesions and vitreous traction. Intraretinal cavities enlarged. There are multiple hyperreflective deposits in the neurosensory retina.

OCT Scan Details (Fig. 4.16c)

* Vitreous layers of moderate and high reflectivity, and vitreoretinal adhesions

* Multiple intraretinal hyperreflective deposits

* Multiple intraretinal cavities filled with hyporeflective fluid

* Increased density (hyperreflectivity) of all layers of the neurosensory retina

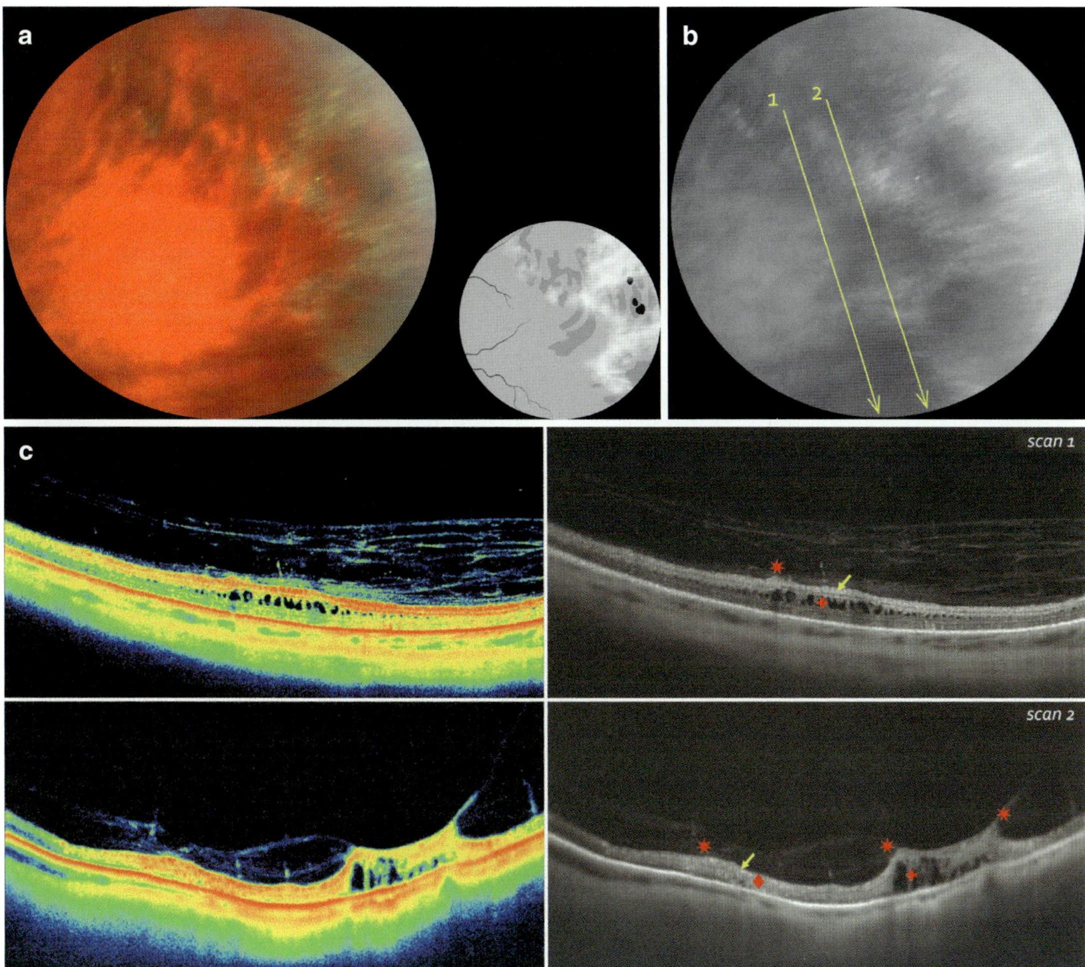

Fig. 4.16 (**a**) Complicated snowflake degeneration. (**b**) *Lines* indicate OCT-scanning direction. (**c**) OCT-scanning results according to the lines direction in (b)

Pearl Degeneration

Pearl degeneration (ora pearls, pearls of the ora serrata) is a rare congenital pathology of the peripheral retina [3] that may look like white beads resembling retinal drusen [27]. There is at present no universal term for this entity. Ora pearls (Table 4.6) appear as milk-white dense glistening spheroids located at the ora serrata or pars plana [31, 43]. There is usually a single isolated pearl, less frequently – multiple pearls that are bilateral and symmetrical.

According to some authors, ora pearls may be found in up to 20 % of patients of both sexes and all age groups; however, this degeneration is diagnosed more frequently with age [44]. Other authors claim that this degeneration is not associated with age and may have developmental origin [23].

Histological studies showed that ora pearls can be described as large retinal drusen located between the pigment epithelium and Bruch's membrane or "freely floating" over the pigment epithelium, depending on the stage of degeneration. In early stages, ora pearls are attached to the Bruch's membrane, and are dark brown, because of pigment epithelium covering. In advanced stages, they become white because of the pigment epithelium thinning [21, 44].

Many authors consider pearl degeneration to be benign and not requiring prophylactic laser treatment [3, 21, 45].

There have recently appeared first OCT scans of the ora pearl describing it as a hyporeflective cavity (cystoid content) in the neurosensory retina with the vitreous cortical layers attached to the top of the lesion [46]. The silvery outer "coating" is hyperreflective and shadows the choroid [33].

Table 4.6 Diagram of peripheral retinal degenerations

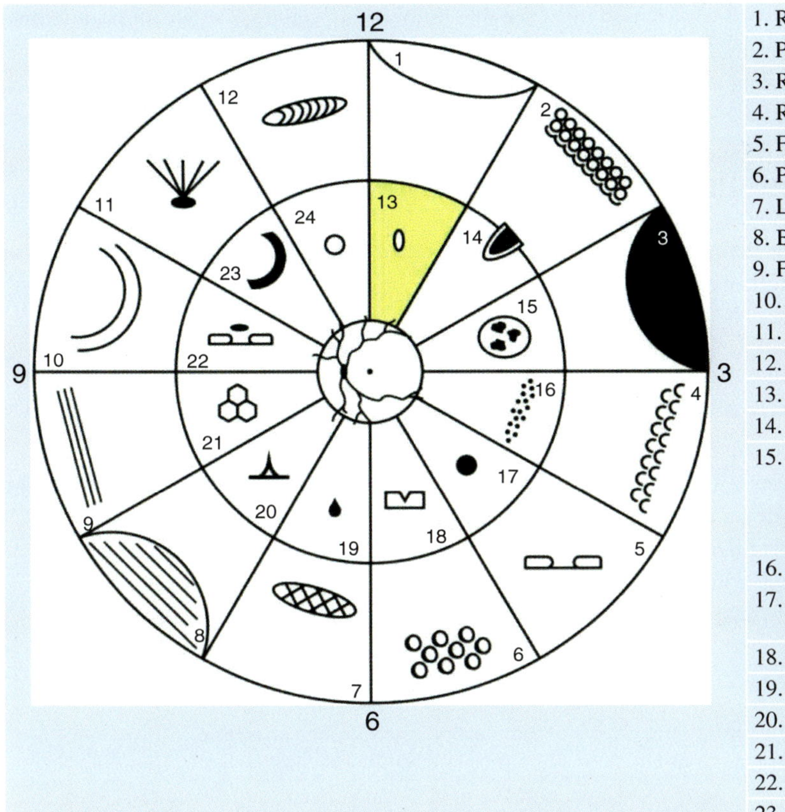

1. Retinal dialysis
2. Peripheral cystoid degeneration
3. Retinal detachment
4. Retinal drusen
5. Full-thickness tear
6. Paving-stone degeneration
7. Lattice degeneration
8. Bullous retinoschisis
9. Flat retinoschisis
10. White-without-pressure
11. Retinal tuft
12. Snail-track degeneration
13. Pearl degeneration
14. Flap tear
15. Grouped congenital hypertrophy of the retinal pigment epithelium ("bear tracks")
16. Snowflake degeneration
17. Unifocal hypertrophy of the retinal pigment epithelium
18. Atrophic retinal hole
19. Haemorrhage
20. Preretinal fibrosis
21. Honeycomb degeneration
22. Operculated retinal tear
23. Dark-without-pressure
24. Unifocal atrophy of the retinal pigment epithelium

Pearl degeneration in sector 13 is highlighted in yellow

Case 17. Pearl Degeneration

An asymptomatic 20-year-old male patient with mild myopia. Degeneration was diagnosed during routine examination.

Ophthalmoscopic Findings (Fig. 4.17a, b)

A metalescent, white, pearl-like spheroid is seen at 9 o'clock position in the far peripheral retina of the right eye. The pearl is slightly elongated. The surrounding retinal surface is grayish and irregular.

OCT Scan Description (Fig. 4.17c, d)

The retina is dome-shaped because of the clearly outlined local hyperreflective cystoid lesion in the neuroepithelium that shadows the underlying structures. The lesion cavity is filled with hyporeflective content. Vitreoretinal adhesion without traction is seen at the top of the lesion. There are small intraretinal cavities with hyporeflective content in the peripheral parts of the scan.

OCT Scan Details (Fig. 4.17c, d)

Intraretinal cavity with hyperreflective walls

Hyporeflective content of the intraretinal cavity

Vitreoretinal adhesions

Multiple small intraretinal cavities

Hyporeflective choroid at the level of the intraretinal cavity

Areas of thickened pigment epithelium

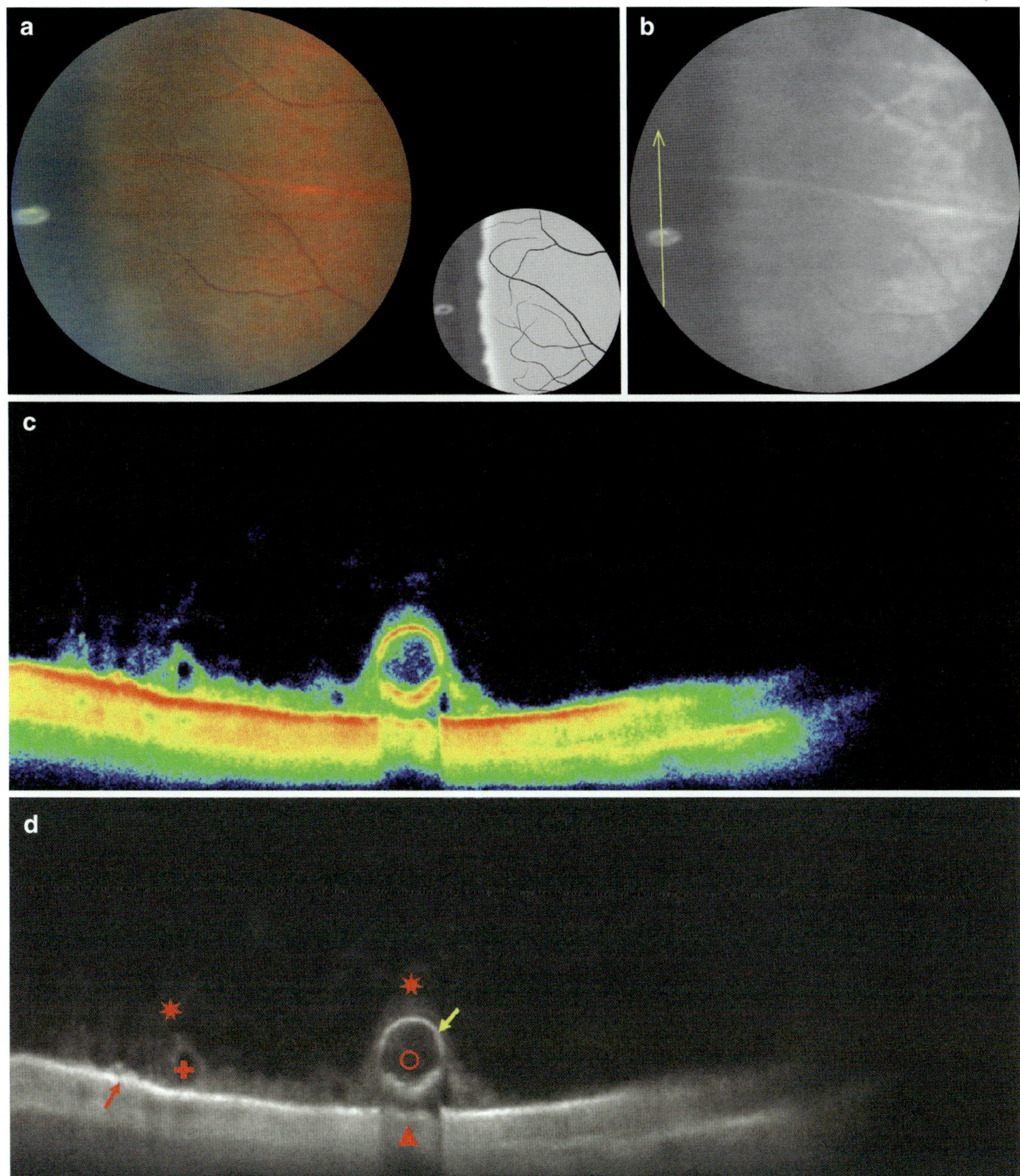

Fig. 4.17 (**a**) Pearl degeneration. (**b**) *Line* indicates OCT-scanning direction. (**c**, **d**) OCT-scanning results according to the line direction in (b)

References

1. Jones WL et al. Care of the patient with retinal detachment and related peripheral vitreoretinal disease. St. Louis: American Optometric Association; 2004.
2. Stehouwer M, Tan SH, van Leeuwen TG, et al. Senile retinoschisis versus retinal detachment, the additional value of peripheral retinal OCT scans (SL SCAN-1, Topcon). Acta Ophthalmol. 2014;92(3):221–7. doi:10.1111/aos.12121.
3. Kanski JJ, Bowling B. Clinical ophthalmology: a systematic approach. 7th ed. Edinburgh: Elsevier/Saunders; 2011.
4. Astakhov IS, Lukovskaya NG. Retinoschisis. Part I. Diagnosis, classification, investigation methods. Vestn ophthalmol. 2004;120(1):26–9. (In Russian)
5. Brinton DA, Wilkinson CP. Retinal detachment: principles and practice. 3rd ed. Oxford: Oxford University Press; 2009.
6. Graue-Wiechers FA, Verduzco NS. Laser treatment for retinal holes, tears and peripheral. In: Boyd S, Wilkinson CP, editors. Retinal detachment surgery and laser treatment. Panama: Jaypee Highlights Med Publ; 2009. p. 47–57.
7. Foos RY. Senile retinoschisis. Relationship to cystoid degeneration. Trans Am Acad Ophthalmol Otolaryngol. 1970;74:33–51.
8. Mitry D. Primary rhegmatogenous retinal detachment: clinical epidemiology and genetic aetiology. Dissertation, University of Edinburgh; 2012.
9. Onofrey BE et al. Ocular therapeutics handbook: a clinical manual. Philadelphia: Lippincott Williams & Wilkins; 2005.
10. Macaliester G, Sullivan P. Peripheral retinal degenerations. In: OT CET. 2011. http://www.optometry.co.uk/uploads/exams/articles/cet_30_09_2011_macalistersullivancorrect.pdf. Accessed 30 Sept 2011.
11. Byer NE. The long-term natural history of senile retinoschisis with implications for management. Ophthalmology. 1986;93(9):1127–37.
12. Buch H, Vinding T, Nielsen NV. Prevalence and long-term natural course of retinoschisis among elderly individuals: the Copenhagen city eye study. Ophthalmology. 2007;114(4):751–5.
13. Landa G, Shirkey L, Garcia PM. Acquired senile retinoschisis of the peripheral retina imaged by spectral domain optical coherence tomography: a case report. Eur J Ophthalmol. 2010;20(6):1079–81.
14. Lewis H. Peripheral retinal degenerations and the risk of retinal detachment. Am J Ophthalmol. 2003;136(1):155–60.
15. Suzuki AC, Zacharias LC, Tanaka T, et al. Case report: pneumatic retinopexy for the treatment of progressive retinal detachment in senile retinoschisis. Arq Bras Oftalmol. 2015;78(1):50–2. doi:10.5935/0004-2749.20150014.
16. Clemens S, Busse H, Gerding H, et al. Treatment guidelines in various stages of senile retinoschisis. Klin Monatsbl Augenheilkd. 1995;206(2):83–91. (In German)
17. Lukovskaia NG, Astakhov IS. Retinoschisis. II. Independent treatment experience in different-type retinoschisis. Vestn Oftalmol. 2004;120(4):29–31. (In Russian)
18. Ip M, Garza-Karren C, Duker JS, et al. Differentiation of degenerative retinoschisis from retinal detachment using optical coherence tomography. Ophthalmology. 1999;106(3):600–5.
19. Yeoh J, Rahman W, Chen FK, et al. Use of spectral-domain optical coherence tomography to differentiate acquired retinoschisis from retinal detachment in difficult cases. Retina. 2012;32(8):1574–80. doi:10.1097/IAE.0b013e3182411d90.
20. Shaimova VA, Pozdeeva OG, Shaimov TB, et al. Optical coherence tomography in peripheral retinal tears diagnostics. Vestn Ophthalmol. 2013;6:51–66. (In Russian)
21. Jones WL. Peripheral ocular fundus, 3rd edn. St. Louis: Butterworth-Heinemann, an imprint of Elsevier Inc.; 2007.
22. Karlin BD, Curtin BJ. Peripheral chorioretinal lesions and axial length of the myopic eye. Am J Ophthalmol. 1976;81:625–35.
23. Rutnin U, Schepens CL. Fundus appearance in normal eyes: III. Peripheral degenerations. Am J Ophthalmol. 1967;64:1063–9.
24. Fawzi AA, Nielsen JS, Mateo-Montoya A, et al. Multimodal imaging of white and dark without pressure fundus lesions. Retina. 2014;34(12):2376–87.
25. Nagpal KC, Huamonte F, Constantaras A, et al. Migratory white-without-pressure retinal lesions. Arch Ophthalmol. 1976;94(4):576–9.
26. Hunter JE. Retinal white without pressure: review and relative incidence. Am J Optom Physiol Optic. 1982;59:293–6.
27. Conart JB, Baron D, Berrod JP. Degenerative lesions of the peripheral retina. J Fr Ophthalmol. 2014;37(1):73–80. doi:10.1016/j.jfo.2013.09.001. (In French)
28. Zinn KM. Clinical atlas of peripheral retinal disorders. Berlin: Springer Science & Business Media; 1988.
29. Chhablani J, Bagdi AB. Peripheral retinal degenerations In: eye wiki. 2015. http://eyewiki.aao.org/Peripheral_Retinal_Degenerations. Accessed 17 Oct 2015.
30. Rocio I, Diaz MD. Domain optical coherence tomography characteristics of white-without-pressure. Retina. 2014;34(5):1020–1.
31. Byer NE. The peripheral retina in profile: a stereoscopic atlas. Torrance: Criterion Press; 1982.
32. Nagpal KC, Goldberg MF, Asdourian G, et al. Dark-without pressure fundus lesions. Br J Ophthalmol. 1975;59:476–9.
33. Shaimova VA (editor). Peripheral retinal degenerations. Optical coherence tomography. Retinal laser photocoagulation: atlas. St. Petersburg: Chelovek; 2015.

34. Cavallotti C, Cerulli L. Age-related changes of the human eye. Berlin: Springer Science & Business Media; 2008.
35. Foos RY, Feman SS. Reticular cystoid degeneration of the peripheral retina. Am J Ophthalmol. 1970;69(3): 392–403.
36. Robertson DM, Link TP, et al. Snowflake degeneration of the retina. Ophthalmology. 1982;89(12): 1513–7.
37. Hirose T, Lee KY, Schepens CL. Snowflake degeneration in hereditary vitreoretinal degeneration. Am J Ophthalmol. 1974;77(2):143–53.
38. Kaiser PK, Friedman NJ, Pineda R. The Massachusetts eye and ear infirmary illustrated manual of ophthalmology. Philadelphia: Saunders Elsevier; 2014.
39. Chen C, Everett TK, et al. Snowflake degeneration: an independent entity or a variant of retinitis pigmentosa? South Med J. 1986;79(1):1216–23.
40. Lee MM, Ritter III R, Hirose T, et al. Snowflake vitreoretinal degeneration: follow-up of the original family. Ophthalmology. 2003;110(12):2418–26.
41. Hirose T, Wolf E, Schepens CL. Retinal functions in snowflake degeneration. Ann Ophthalmol. 1980;12(10): 1135–46.
42. Pollack A, Uchenik D, Chemke J, et al. Prophylactic laser photocoagulation in hereditary snowflake vitreoretinal degeneration. Arch Ophthalmol. 1983;101(10): 1536–9.
43. Duke-Elder S, Dobree JH. Diseases of the retina. In: Duke-Elder S, editor. System of ophthalmology, Vol. 10. London: Henry Kimpton; 1967. p. 126–7.
44. Lonn LI, Smith TR. Ora serrata pearls: clinical and histological correlation. Arch Ophthalmol. 1967;77(6): 809–13.
45. Goldbaum MH. Retinal examination and surgery. In: Peyman GA, Saunders DR, editors. Principles and practice of ophthalmology. Philadelphia: WB Saunders; 1980. p. 988.
46. Choudhry N, Golding J, Manry MW, et al. Ultra-widefield steering-based spectral-domain optical coherence tomography imaging of the retinal periphery. Ophthalmology. 2016;23(6):1368–74. doi:10.1016/j.ophtha.2016.01.045.

Vitreoretinal Degenerations

Second Group of Peripheral Retinal Degenerations

Ruslan B. Shaimov and Venera A. Shaimova

R.B. Shaimov
Center Zreniya Medical Clinic, LLC,
Chelyabinsk, Russian Federation

Ophthalmology Department, Municipal Budgetary
Healthcare Institution, City Clinical Hospital No 6,
Chelyabinsk, Russian Federation

V.A. Shaimova (✉)
Chelyabinsk State Laser Surgery Institute,
Chelyabinsk, Russian Federation

Center Zreniya Medical Clinic, LLC,
Chelyabinsk, Russian Federation
e-mail: shaimova.v@mail.ru

© Springer International Publishing AG 2017
V.A. Shaimova (ed.), *Peripheral Retinal Degenerations*, DOI 10.1007/978-3-319-48995-7_5

Snail-Track Degeneration

Snail-track degeneration appears (Table 5.1) as a band of glistening, frost-like white dots, often oval or elongated. It is usually found closer to the equator and parallel to the ora serrata, and resembles a track left by a snail [1–3]. This degeneration is more frequently found in superotemporal and superonasal quadrants of the peripheral retina [4]. The prevalence of snail-track degeneration in general population is 10 %, it affects myopic eyes more frequently – 40 % [5].

Snail-track degeneration, as well as lattice degeneration, is characterized by retinal thinning with vitreous liquefaction (lacuna) right above the lesion, and vitreoretinal tractions [1]. According to published data, retinal tears commonly appear in the inferotemporal quadrant – 54 %, less frequently in the superotemporal – 18 %, superonasal – 16 %, and inferonasal quadrants −12 % [4].

Some experts believe that snail-track degeneration is a variation or an early stage of classic lattice degeneration [6–9]. Others classify it as a separate group [1, 3, 4, 10] given that the ultrastructural studies proved it to be an independent entity [11, 12].

Snail-track degeneration is often complicated by retinal holes, less frequently by flap tears with traction, and secondary retinal detachment [3, 13]. The indications for prophylactic laser coagulation are the same as those for lattice degeneration.

Kothari et al. (2012) were the first to publish in vivo OCT scans of snail-track degeneration as an irregular and wrinkled retinal surface without vitreous traction [10].

Shaimova et al. (2015) described the characteristic OCT features of this degeneration: irregular and jagged retinal surface, vitreous destruction, and vitreoretinal adhesions with tractions at the lesion margins [14].

In this chapter, we demonstrate different variants of OCT scans of the snail-track degeneration.

Table 5.1 Diagram of peripheral retinal degenerations

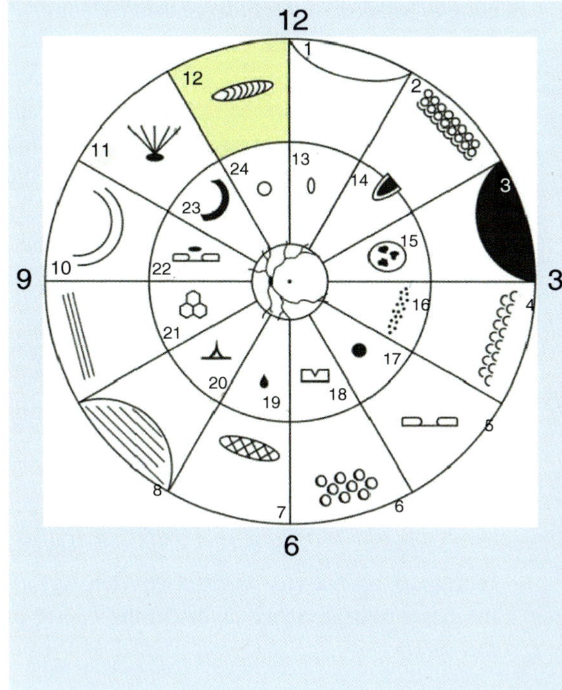

1. Retinal dialysis
2. Peripheral cystoid degeneration
3. Retinal detachment
4. Retinal drusen
5. Full-thickness tear
6. Paving-stone degeneration
7. Lattice degeneration
8. Bullous retinoschisis
9. Flat retinoschisis
10. White-without-pressure
11. Retinal tuft
12. Snail-track degeneration
13. Pearl degeneration
14. Flap tear
15. Grouped congenital hypertrophy of the retinal pigment epithelium ("bear tracks")
16. Snowflake degeneration
17. Unifocal hypertrophy of the retinal pigment epithelium
18. Atrophic retinal hole
19. Haemorrhage
20. Preretinal fibrosis
21. Honeycomb degeneration
22. Operculated retinal tear
23. Dark-without-pressure
24. Unifocal atrophy of the retinal pigment epithelium

Snail-track degeneration in sector 12 is highlighted in yellow

Case 18. Snail-Track Degeneration (Classic)

A 24-year-old male patient with moderate myopia and partial posterior vitreous detachment presented with floaters and flashes of light affecting his left eye.

Ophthalmoscopic Findings (Fig. 5.18a, b)

A bright white elongated lesion with multiple small atrophic holes is observed in the far periphery of superotemporal quadrant of the left eye. The surrounding retina is whitish, with retinal vessels poorly visualized in the area of degeneration. There are vitreous adhesions and tractions at the edges of the lesion.

OCT Scan Description (Fig. 5.18c)

Scan 1 Vitreous over the retina is considerably consolidated. The surface of the neurosensory retina is smooth. There is a locally dense area of retinal pigment epithelium.

Scan 2 The retinal surface is irregular. There are vitreoretinal adhesions with traction at the edges of the lesion. The neurosensory retina is dense and slightly elevated at the adhesion site. There is a marked density (increased reflectivity) of the inner retinal layers in the center of the image causing a "shadow" effect (decreased reflectivity) in the underlying tissues.

Scan 3 The retinal surface is irregular and jagged because of multiple areas of retinal thinning (atrophic holes). The retina is dense along the entire lesion. The photoreceptor layer is partially damaged. Retinal pigment epithelium is intact.

OCT Scan Details (Fig. 5.18c)

* Layers of medium reflectivity (increased density) in the vitreous; vitreoretinal adhesions and tractions

* Areas of retinal thinning within the lesion

* Increased reflectivity (increased density) of the inner neurosensory layers in the center of the lesion

* Areas of redistribution and increased density of the pigment epithelium

* Decreased reflectivity of the outer neurosensory layers, pigment epithelium, and choroid at the level of dense retina

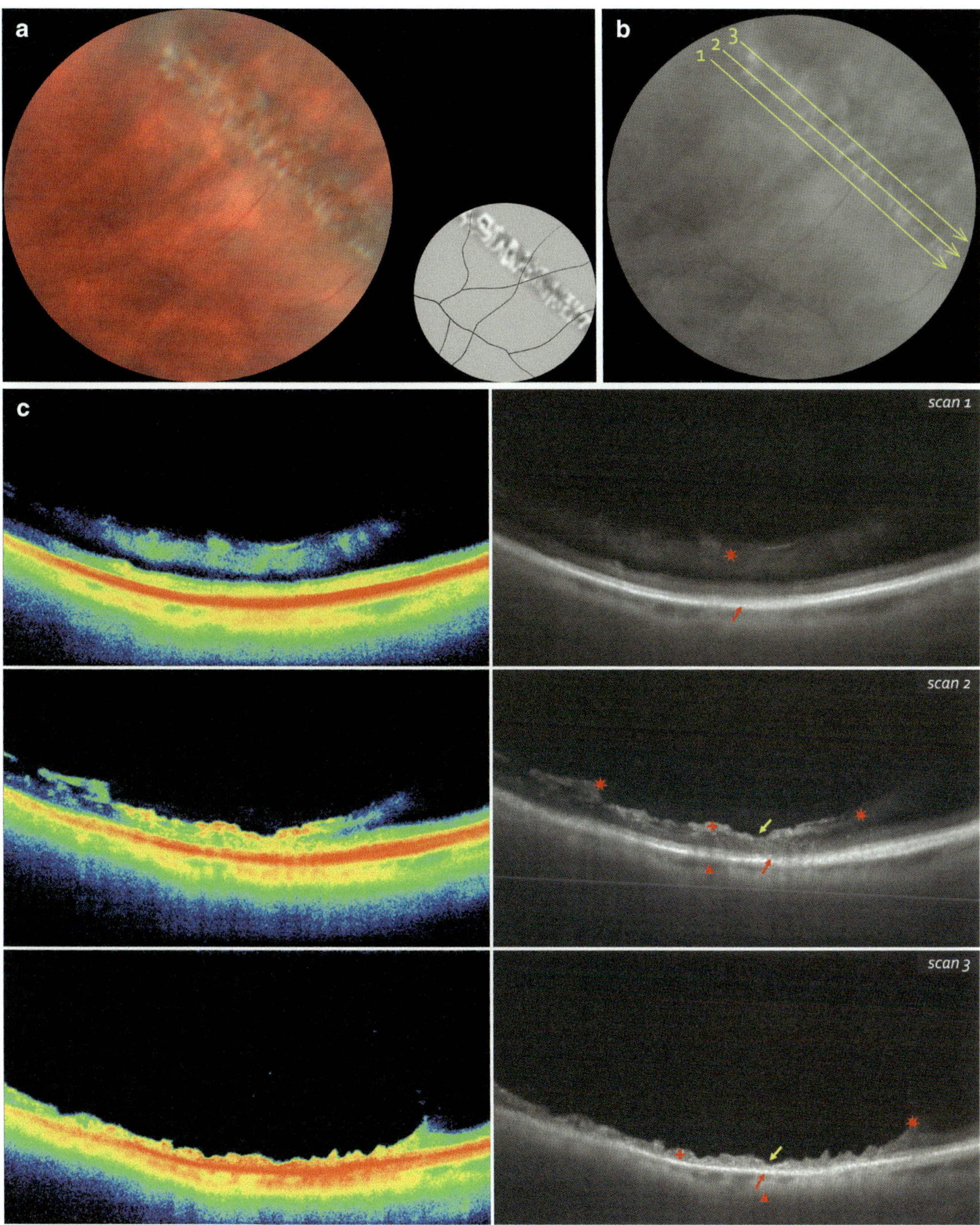

Fig. 5.18 (**a**) Snail-track degeneration. (**b**) Lines indicate OCT-scanning direction. (**c**) OCT-scanning results according to the position of the lines in (**b**)

Case 19. Snail-Track Degeneration (Double-Row)

An asymptomatic 17-year-old male patient with moderate myopia and partial posterior vitreous detachment.

Ophthalmoscopic Findings (Fig. 5.19a, b)

Two degenerative lesions are observed in the mid and far periphery of the inferotemporal quadrant of the right eye. The first lesion is at the equator with a full-thickness retinal tear in its center, shallow (subclinical) retinal detachment, and minor hyperpigmentation. The second lesion is closer to the ora serrata with hyperpigmentation and atrophic retinal holes. Vitreous traction at the edges is identified in both lesions.

OCT Scan Description (Fig. 5.19c)

Scan 1 Full-thickness tear of the neurosensory retina is seen in the center of the scan and has markedly thin and dense retina at its edge, with clear evidence of vitreoretinal adhesions and tractions. Retinal pigment epithelium is intact.

Scan 2 Multiple areas of marked retinal thinning (atrophic retinal holes) are separated by areas of increased retinal density. There are isolated vitreoretinal adhesions within the lesion and at its edges. Retinal pigment epithelium is intact.

OCT Scan Details (Fig. 5.19c)

✳ Vitreoretinal adhesions and tractions

☾ Full-thickness tear of the neurosensory retina

↙ Marked thinning of the neurosensory retina (atrophic holes)

+ Increased reflectivity (density) of the neurosensory retina along the edge of the full-thickness tear

↗ Destruction of the photoreceptor layer at the level of the thinned retina and a full-thickness tear

◆ Increased reflectivity of the choroid at the level of the dense neurosensory retina

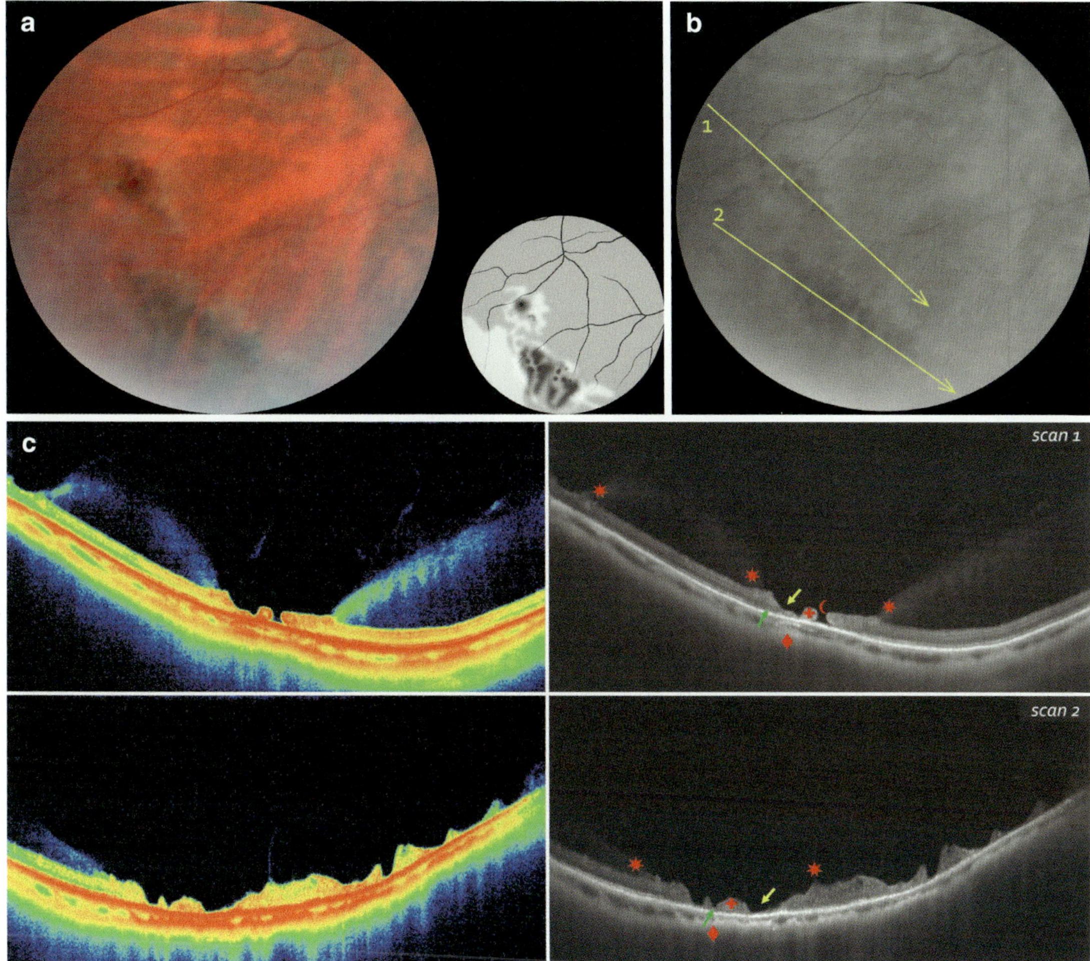

Fig. 5.19 (**a**) Snail-track degeneration (*double-row*). (**b**) Lines indicate OCT-scanning direction. (**c**) OCT-scanning results according to the position of the lines in (**b**)

Case 20. Snail-Track Degeneration with Atrophic Retinal Holes

An asymptomatic 17-year-old male patient with low myopia.

Ophthalmoscopic Findings (Fig. 5.20a, b)
A silver-white lesion with irregular surface and multiple atrophic holes is seen in the mid-periphery of the left eye at 5 o'clock position. The retinal vessel passing through the lesion is partly blurred.

OCT Scan Description (Fig. 5.20c)
Scans 1 and 2 The retinal surface is irregular and jagged. There are multiple shallow atrophic holes of different sizes in the neurosensory retina. The retina within the lesion is dense. Photoreceptor layer is partially destroyed. Retinal pigment epithelium is intact. The cross-sectional image (Scan 2) shows the area of vitreoretinal adhesion and traction.

OCT Scan Details (Fig. 5.20c)

* Vitreoretinal adhesion and traction at the edges of the lesion

* Marked thinning of the neurosensory retina (atrophic retinal holes)

* Increased reflectivity (increased density) of the neurosensory retina between the atrophic holes

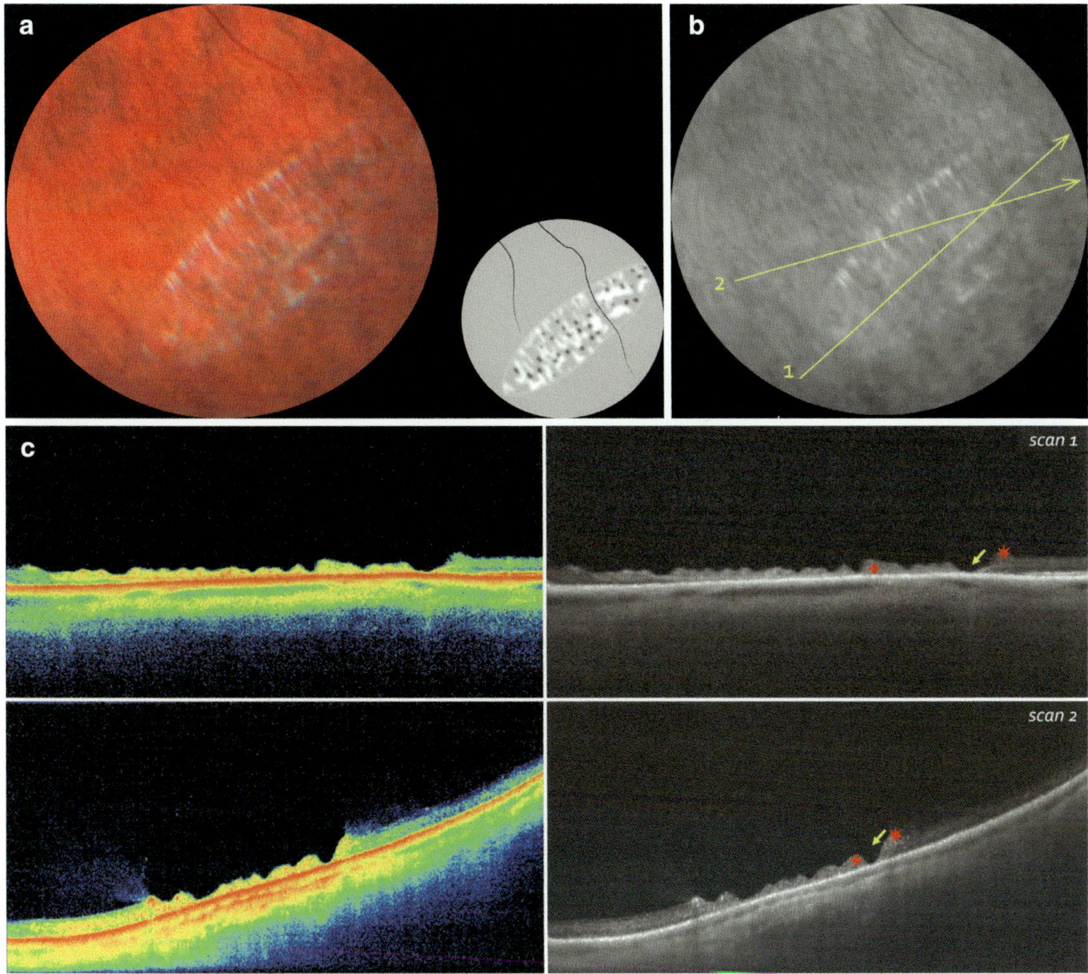

Fig. 5.20 (**a**) Snail-track degeneration with atrophic retinal holes. (**b**) Lines indicate OCT-scanning direction. (**c**) OCT-scanning results according to the position of the lines in (**b**)

Case 21. Snail-Track Degeneration with Vitreoretinal Adhesion and Retinal Tears

A 25-year-old male patient with severe myopia and partial posterior vitreous detachment presented with complaints of floaters and recurrent flashes of light affecting his right eye.

Ophthalmoscopic Findings (Fig. 5.21a, b)

A local degenerative lesion with blurred borders is observed in the mid-peripheral retina of the temporal quadrant of the left eye. The lesion is bright white, with multiple atrophic holes and full-thickness retinal tears. The vitreous is grayish, with areas of fibrosis and signs of traction. The retinal vessels passing through the lesion are hard to see.

OCT Scan Description (Fig. 5.21c)

Scan 1 There is an elevated area of the neurosensory retina with signs of increased density (increase in layers' reflectivity) caused by vitreoretinal adhesion and traction.

Scan 2 The area of vitreoretinal adhesion and traction enlarges. There is a hyporeflective band of the consolidated vitreous (preretinal fibrosis) laterally over the retina. The neuroepithelium is thick and dense in the center.

Scan 3 The scan demonstrates a marked vitreoretinal adhesion with a hyperreflective elevated band and a full-thickness tear with shallow detachment of the neurosensory retina. There is an operculum (area of medium reflectivity) detached from the retina over the tear, causing a "shadow" effect in the underlying tissues.

Scan 4 There are severe vitreoretinal adhesions and tractions, intraretinal cavities at the site of adhesion, and a shallow detachment of the neurosensory retina. The elevated part of the retina is dense. A part of the operculum is seen in the vitreous.

OCT Scan Details (Fig. 5.21c)

✹ Vitreoretinal adhesions and tractions

Area of moderate reflectivity in the vitreous (operculum) over the full-thickness tear

◖ Full-thickness tear of the neurosensory retina

+ Increased reflectivity (increased density) of the inner neurosensory layers within the degeneration

○ Shallow retinal detachment at the edges of the full-thickness tear

Dense pigment epithelium within the neurosensory detachment

▲ Hyporeflective choroid at the level of dense areas of pigment epithelium and neurosensory retina

Intraretinal hyporeflective cavity at the site of vitreoretinal adhesion

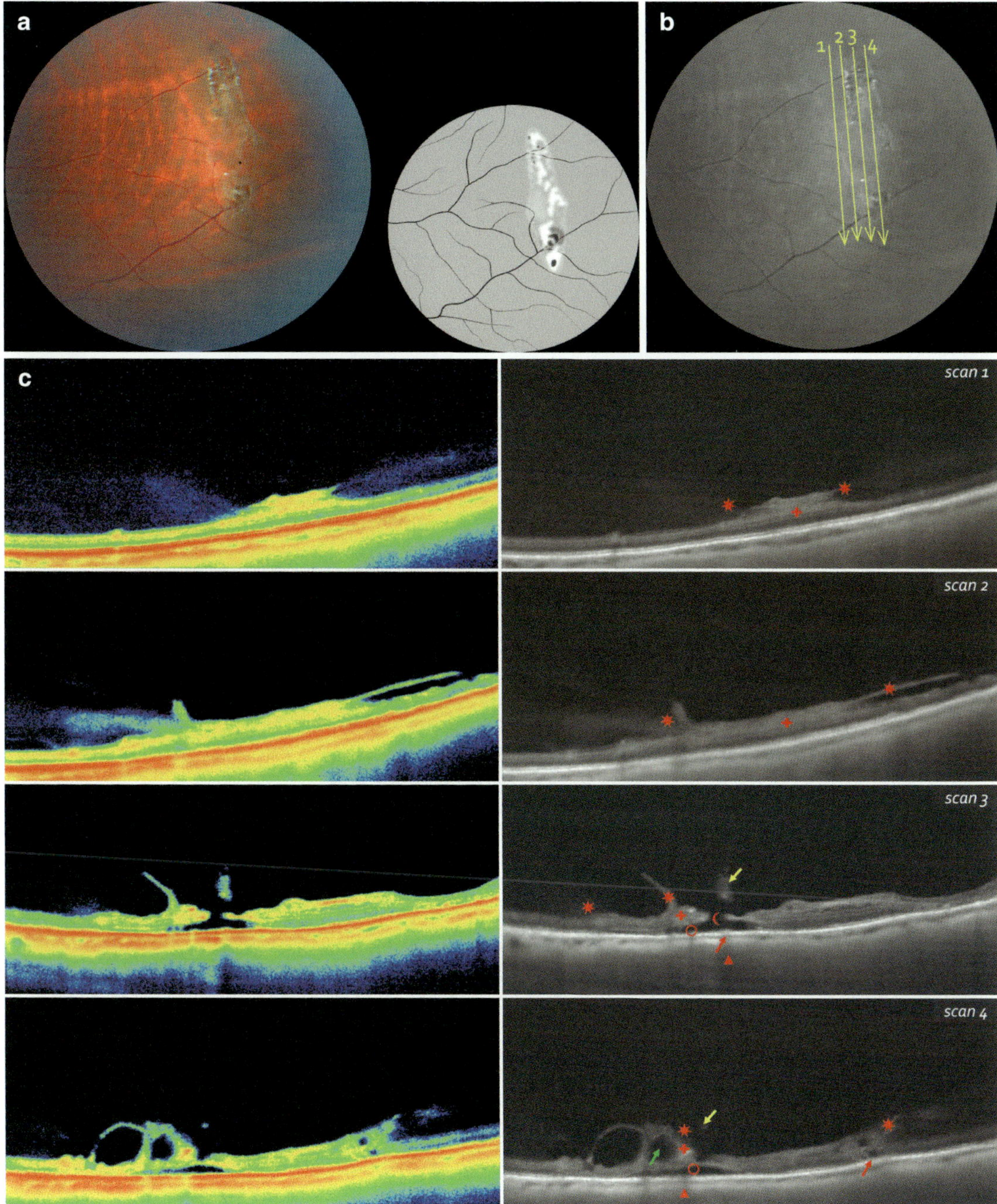

Fig. 5.21 (**a**) Snail-track degeneration with fibrosis and retinal tears. (**b**) *Lines* indicate OCT-scanning direction. (**c**) OCT-scanning results according to the position of the lines in (**b**)

Case 22. Snail-Track Degeneration with Multiple Tears and Shallow Retinal Detachment

An asymptomatic 30-year-old male patient with moderate myopia. Degeneration was diagnosed during routine fundus examination.

Ophthalmoscopic Findings (Fig. 5.22a, b)

A whitish degenerative lesion with blurred borders is observed in the far peripheral retina of the inferior quadrant of the left eye. There are multiple irregular retinal holes in the center of the lesion; and there is a single bright red full-thickness tear of the neuroepithelium surrounded by a shallow retinal detachment on the left edge of the lesion.

OCT Scan Description (Fig. 5.22c, d)

The retinal surface is jagged and irregular because of an area of vitreoretinal adhesion with traction. There are multiple atrophic holes in the neuroepithelium in the center, a full-thickness tear of the neurosensory retina with a shallow neuroepithelium detachment on the left side. Small intraretinal hyporeflective cavities are visible in the neuroepithelium. There are areas of hyperplasia of retinal pigment epithelium. Choroid is thinned.

OCT Scan Details (Fig. 5.22c, d)

✴ Vitreoretinal adhesion and traction

☾ Full-thickness tear of the neurosensory retina

◤ Marked thinning of the neurosensory retina (atrophic holes)

✚ Increased reflectivity (increased density) of the neurosensory retina within the lesion

○ Shallow retinal detachment at the edges of the full-thickness tear

↗ Dense areas of pigment epithelium at the sides of retinal detachment

▲ Decreased reflectivity of the choroid at the level of dense pigment epithelium

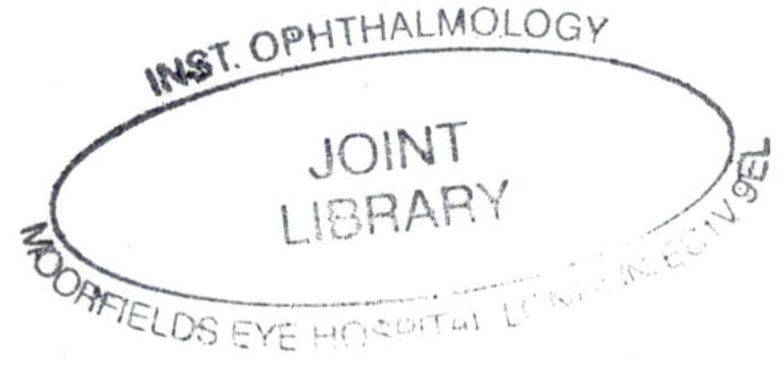

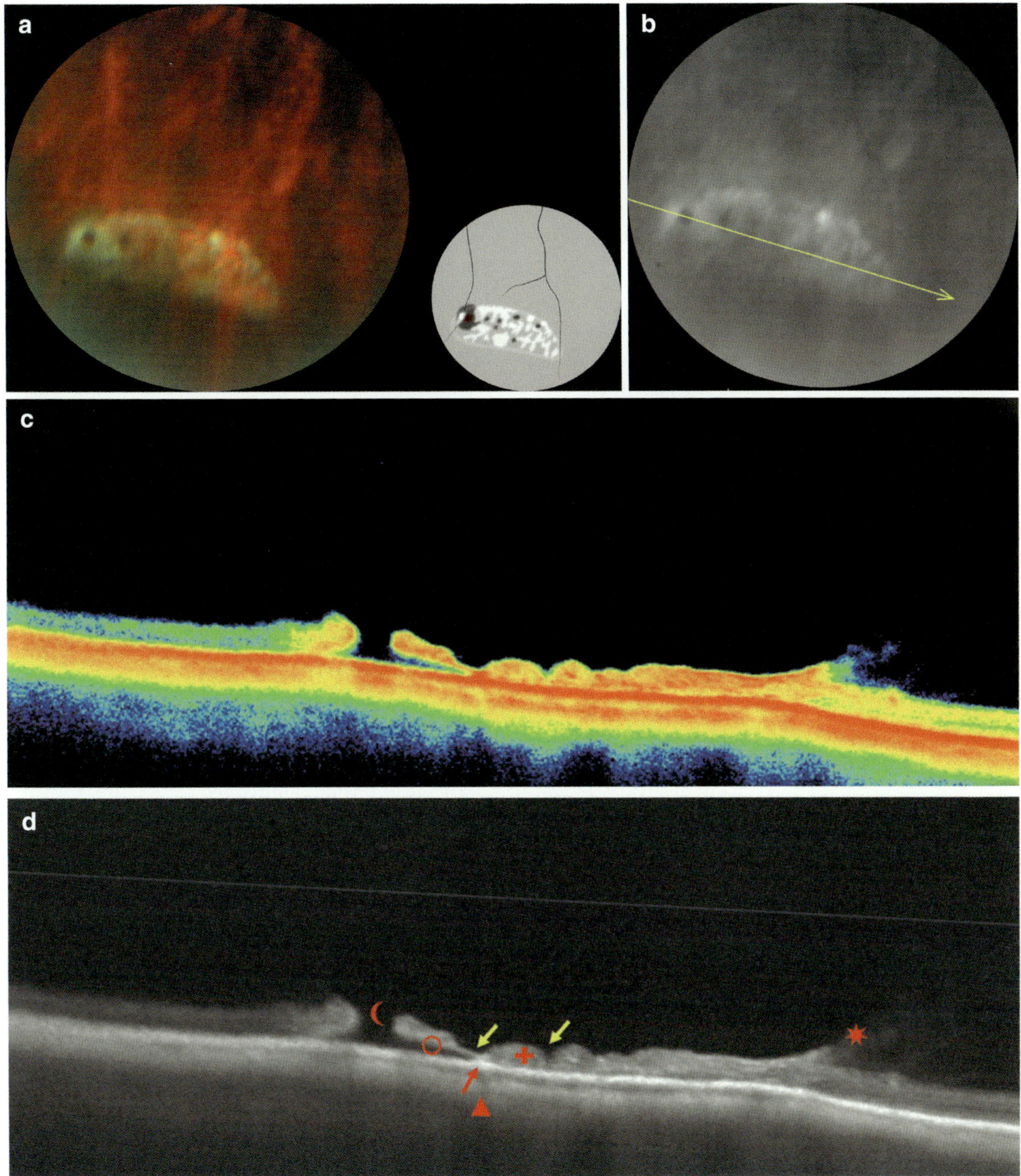

Fig. 5.22 (**a**) Snail-track degeneration with multiple tears. (**b**) *Line* indicates OCT-scanning direction. (**c, d**) OCT-scanning results according to the position of the line in Fig. (**b**)

Case 23. Snail-Track Degeneration with Retinal Detachment and Vitreous Fibrosis with Traction

A 45-year-old female patient with moderate myopia and partial posterior vitreous detachment presented with a 10-day history of floaters affecting her right eye.

Ophthalmoscopic Findings (Fig. 5.23a, b)

Two degenerative lesions are observed. The first lesion is located in the mid-periphery of the right eye at 7 o'clock position and has a spongy appearance, grayish cast, blurred borders (shallow retinal detachment), and red full-thickness tears. The vitreous is gray and dense with marked retinal adhesions producing tractions. The second lesion with atrophic holes and vitreoretinal adhesion is located at 8 o'clock position.

OCT Scan Description (Fig. 5.23c)

Scan 1 There is a marked vitreoretinal adhesion with dense (increasingly reflective) neurosensory retina. The vitreous has multiple layers of high and moderate reflectivity and multiple fibrotic bands. A shallow retinal detachment of the neurosensory retina is observed along the whole area of degeneration.

Scan 2 Layers of fibrosis in the vitreous are connected with vitreoretinal adhesions at the borders of the lesion. There is a single large intraretinal cavity at the adhesion site. The shallow retinal detachment is irregular and more elevated in the adhesion area.

Scan 3 Vitreoretinal adhesions become larger and occupy half of the lesion. Multiple intraretinal cavities of different forms and sizes are observed at the level of these adhesions and the shallow neurosensory retinal detachment there looks irregular and more elevated.

Scan 4 At the sites of adhesions, the retina appears dense and elevated, with isolated intraretinal cavities. The intraretinal reflectivity increases casting a "shadow" (reflectivity decrease) over the choroid. The neurosensory retinal detachment in this scan is large, and it enlarges even more in the area of adhesions. Medially, there is a full-thickness tear of the neuroepithelium.

OCT Scan Details (Fig. 5.23c)

* Vitreoretinal adhesions and tractions with layers of moderate and high reflectivity (fibrosis) in the vitreous

+ Increased reflectivity (increased density) of the neurosensory inner retinal layers at the site of vitreoretinal adhesions

↗ Intraretinal hyporeflective cavities within marked vitreoretinal adhesions

○ Neurosensory retinal detachment within the lesion

▲ Hyporeflective inner retinal layers, pigment epithelium, and choroid at the dense retina level

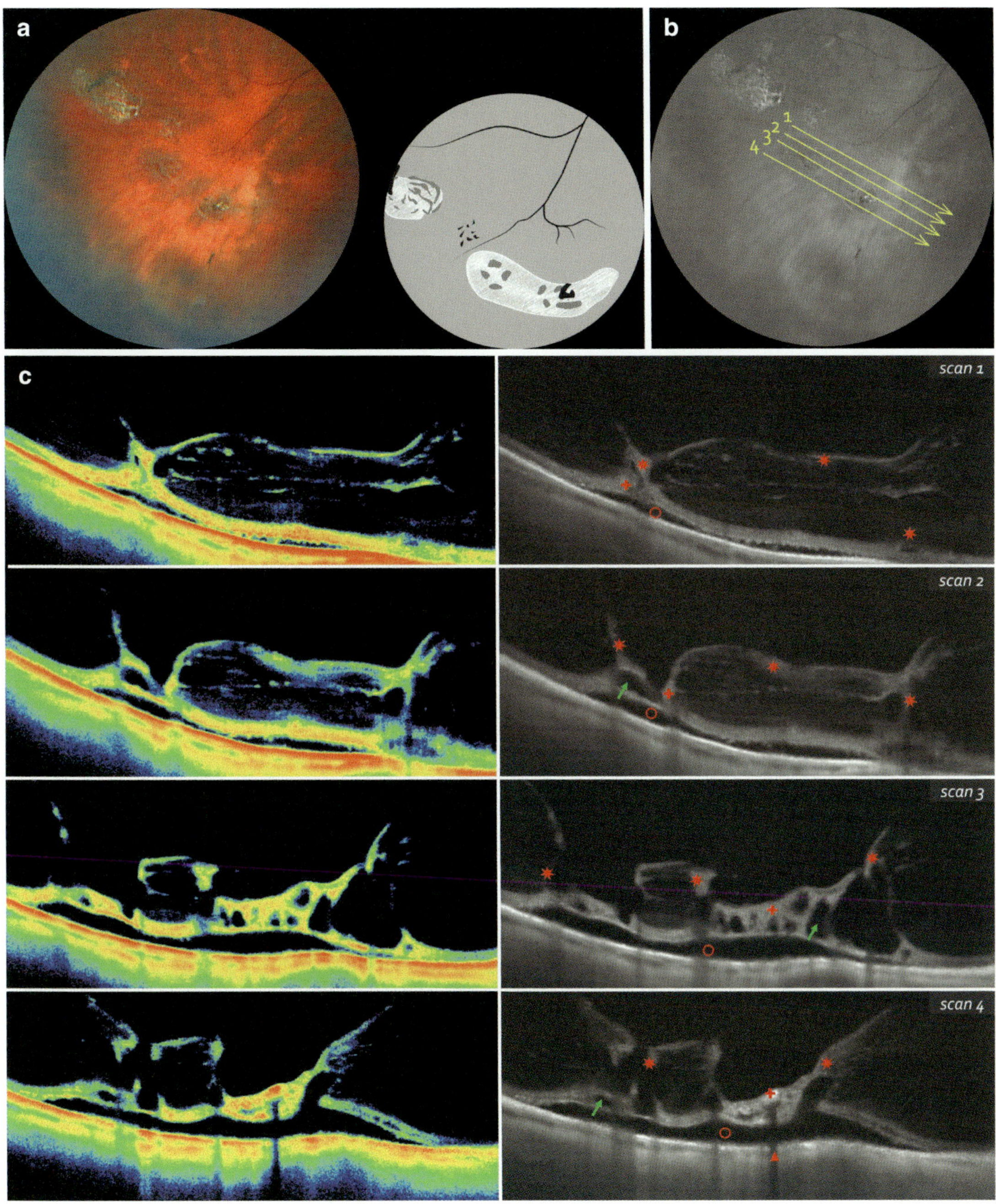

Fig. 5.23 (**a**) Snail-track degeneration with shallow neuroepithelium detachment and vitreous fibrosis. (**b**) *Lines* indicate OCT-scanning direction. (**c**) OCT-scanning results according to the position of the lines in (**b**)

Case 24. Snail-Track Degeneration with Multiple Tears

A 35-year-old highly myopic female patient with partial posterior vitreous detachment presented with complaints of floaters affecting her left eye.

Ophthalmoscopic Findings (Fig. 5.24a, b)

A dark gray lesion with three round, full-thickness tears of different sizes is observed in the mid-periphery of the inferior quadrant of the left eye. The retina is elevated and looks spongy (shallow detachment).

OCT Scan Description (Fig. 5.24c, d)

The retinal surface is irregular because of vitreoretinal adhesion with traction. There are three full-thickness tears of the neuroepithelium with shallow retinal detachment and several small hyperreflective deposits in the neuroepithelium. The photoreceptor layer is partially destroyed. Destructive changes are seen in retinal pigment epithelium.

OCT Scan Details (Fig. 5.24c, d)

* Vitreoretinal adhesion and traction

* Full-thickness tears of the neurosensory retina

* Areas of marked thinning of the neurosensory retina

* Increased reflectivity (increased density) of the neurosensory retina within the area of degeneration

* Shallow retinal detachment at the edges of full-thickness tears

* Pigment epithelium destruction

* Hyperreflective choroid in the area of pigment epithelium destruction

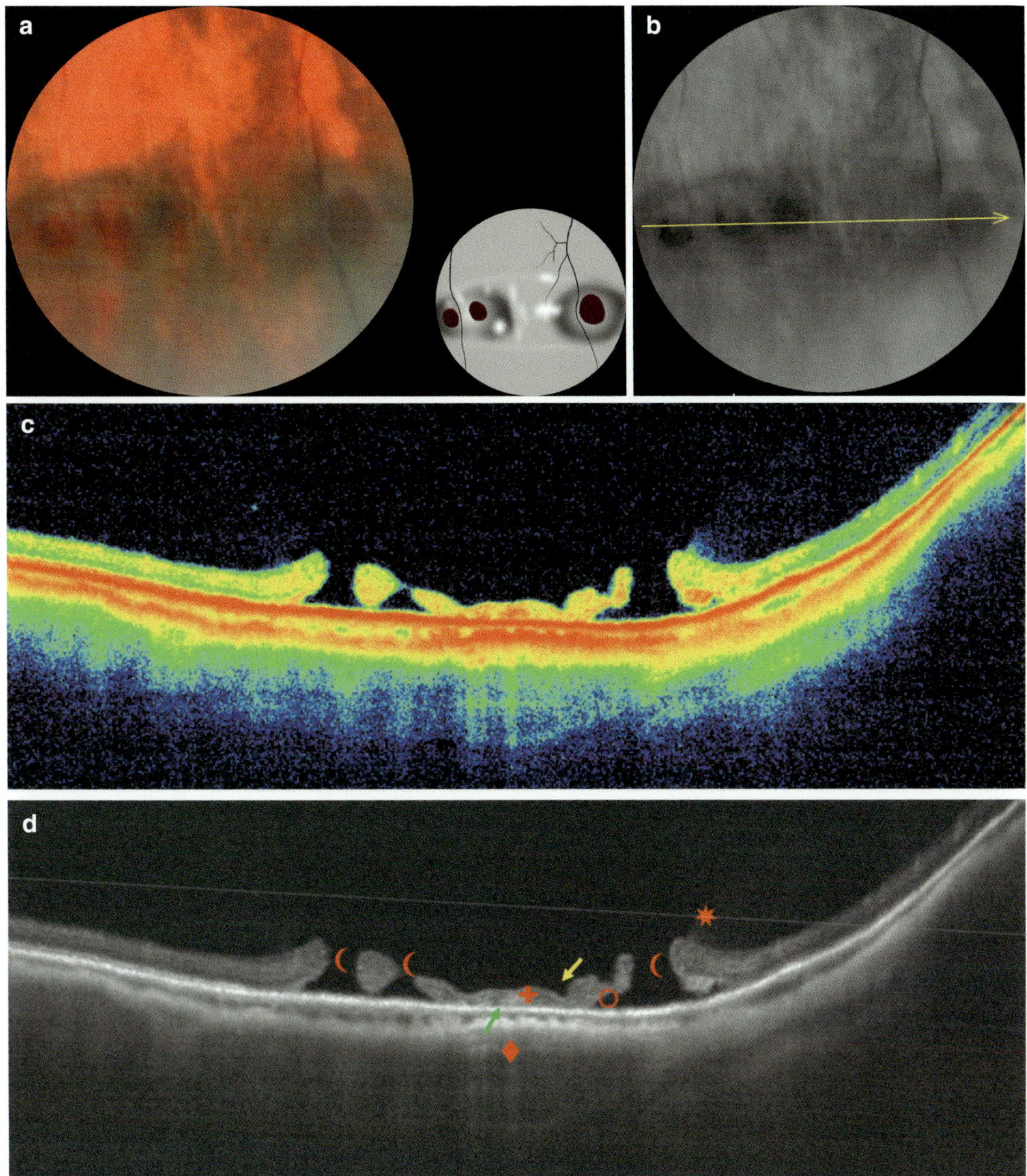

Fig. 5.24 (**a**) Snail-track degeneration with multiple tears. (**b**) *Line* indicates OCT-scanning direction. (**c, d**) OCT-scanning results according to the position of the line in (**b**)

Case 25. Snail-Track Degeneration with Retinal Tear and Pigment Epithelium Atrophy

A 19-year-old male patient with partial posterior vitreous detachment and no symptomatic complaints.

Ophthalmoscopic Findings (Fig. 5.25a, b)

A degenerative lesion with multiple whitish deposits, retinal thinning, and atrophic retinal holes is observed in the far-peripheral retina of the inferior quadrant of the right eye. Two well-defined oval lesions at the borders of degeneration correspond to a retinal tear (red lesion on the left) and pigment epithelium atrophy (white lesion on the right).

OCT Scan Description (Fig. 5.25c)

Scan 1 The retinal surface is smooth. Layers of neuroepithelium are well visualized. Retinal pigment epithelium is intact. The hyperreflective (consolidated) layer of the vitreous forms an adhesion with the retinal surface. Overlying vitreous layers are hyporeflective.

Scan 2 The retinal surface is irregular and slightly elevated by the site of vitreoretinal adhesion with traction at its borders. In the middle of adhesion, there are multiple hyperreflective deposits in the neuroepithelium.

Scan 3 The retinal surface is irregular because of the site of vitreoretinal adhesion with traction at its borders. Laterally, there is an atrophic hole

in the neuroepithelium and medially – an area of the pigment epithelium atrophy with a hyperreflective "shadow" in the choroid (comet-tail). The neuroepithelium in the center of the scan is thinned and hyperreflective with no distinguishable layers.

Scan 4 Transverse scan through the area of degeneration. The center of the scan shows an atrophic hole in the neuroepithelium with a hyperreflective "shadow" in the underlying tissues. The neuroepithelium is thinned and consolidated. There are vitreoretinal adhesions with marked traction at the edges of the lesion.

OCT Scan Details (Fig. 5.25c)

Layers of moderate reflectivity in the vitreous (consolidation)

Vitreoretinal adhesion and traction at the edges of degeneration

Hyperreflective (dense) neurosensory retina at the edges of degeneration, at the sites of vitreoretinal adhesions

Full-thickness tear of the neurosensory retina

Dense and thin neurosensory retina in the center of degeneration

Pigment epithelium destruction

Increased reflectivity of the choroid in the areas of pigment epithelium destruction.

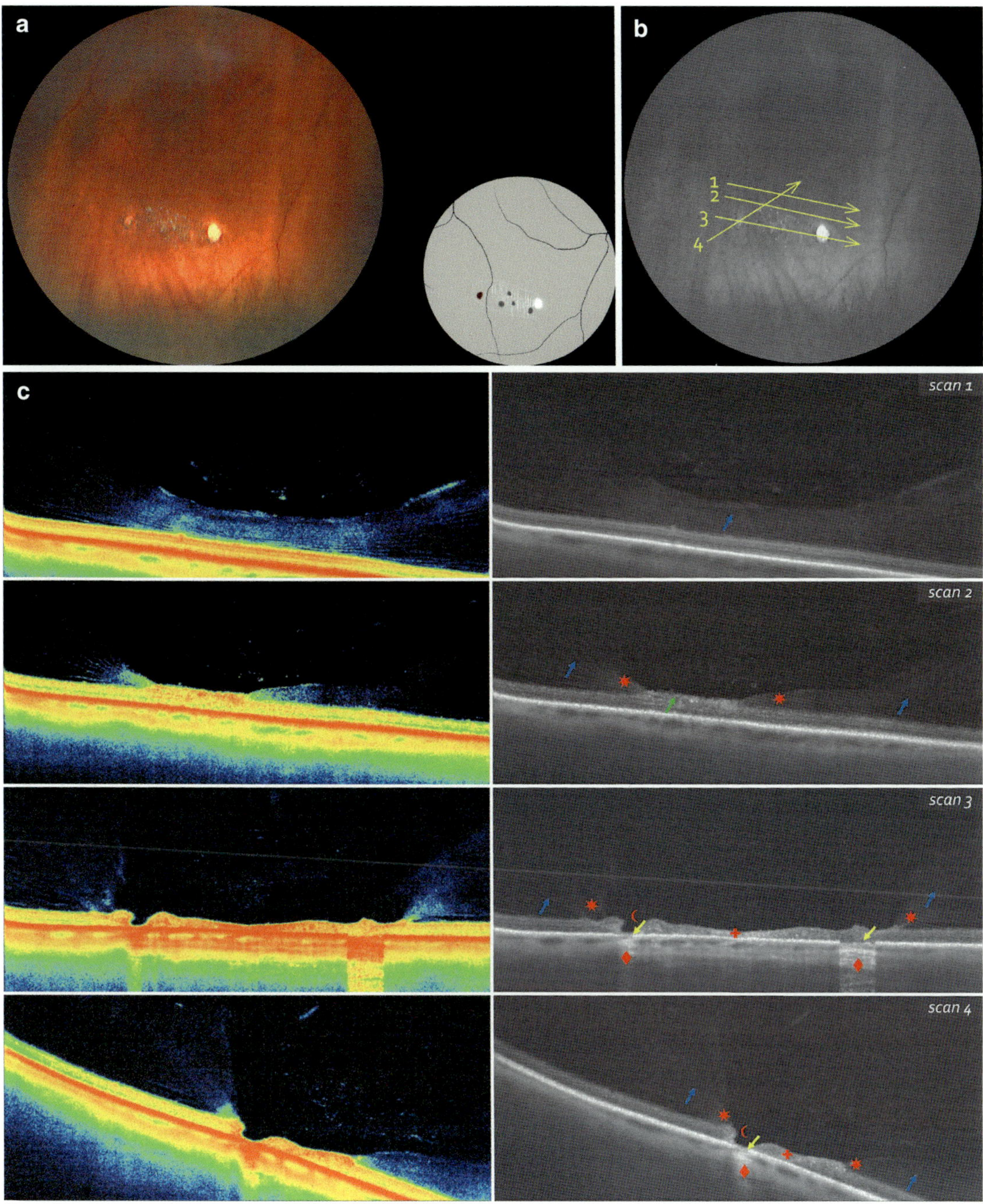

Fig. 5.25 (**a**) Snail-track degeneration with retinal tear and pigment epithelium atrophy. (**b**) *Lines* indicate OCT-scanning direction. (**c**) OCT-scanning results according to the position of the *lines* in (**b**)

Case 26. Snail-Track Degeneration with Retinal Tear and Pigment Epithelium Destruction

A 21-year-old male patient with low myopia presented with no complaints. Retinal degeneration was diagnosed during routine examination.

Ophthalmoscopic Findings (Fig. 5.26a, b)

A white oval degenerative lesion with blurred borders is observed in the mid-periphery of the superotemporal quadrant of the right eye. Retina in the center of the lesion is lighter and has whitish deposits. There is a wide band of hyperpigmentation in the far retinal periphery.

OCT Scan Description (Fig. 5.26c)

Scan 1 The retinal surface is irregular and jagged because of multiple atrophic lesions in the neuroepithelium. There is an atrophic area of retinal pigment epithelium with destructed photoreceptor layer in the center of the scan. This atrophic area casts a "shadow" over the choroid making it look hyperreflective. The vitreous at the edges of the lesion is consolidated, it attaches to the retinal surface and causes tractions. There is a hyporeflective cavity over the lesion – lacuna (optically void area). Choroid in the area of degeneration is thinned.

Scan 2 There are multiple atrophic lesions in the neuroepithelium and a full-thickness tear in the center of the scan. Neuroepithelium at the tear margins is dense. There are signs of vitreoretinal adhesion and traction over the lesion surface.

OCT Scan Details (Fig. 5.26c)

✳ Vitreoretinal adhesions

☾ Full-thickness tear of the neurosensory retina

◤ Marked thinning of the neurosensory retina (atrophic hole)

✚ Hyperreflective (dense) neurosensory retina at the tear margins

➶ Destructed photoreceptor layer in the area of retinal thinning and the full-thickness tear

◆ Hyperreflective choroid in the area of dense neurosensory retina

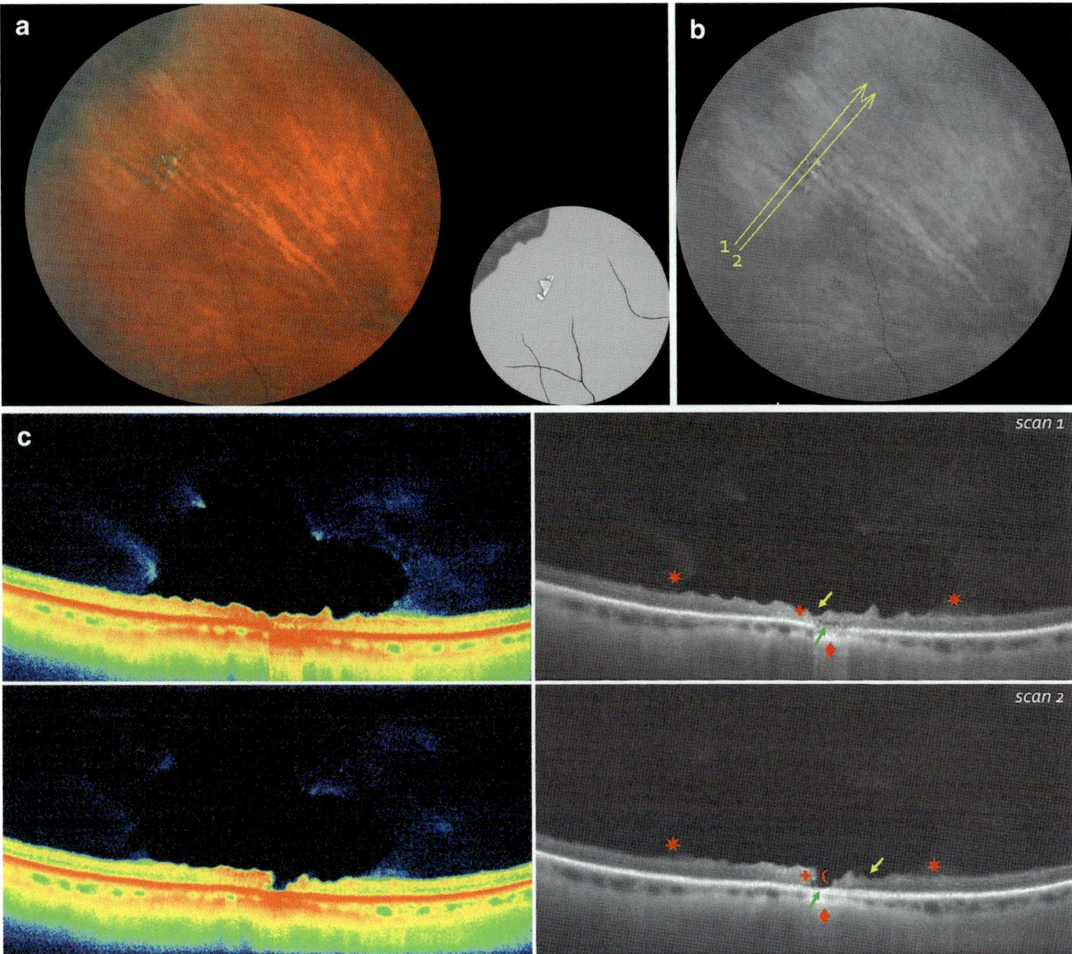

Fig. 5.26 (**a**) Snail-track degeneration with retinal tear and pigment epithelium destruction. (**b**) *Lines* indicate OCT-scanning direction. (**c**) OCT-scanning results according to the position of the *lines* in (**b**)

Lattice Degeneration

Lattice degeneration (Table 5.3) appears as retinal thinning with the loss of neurosensory layer and marked vitreoretinal adhesion at the margins of the lesion [15]. Lattice degeneration is found in 6–8 % of eyes in general population [7, 16, 17]. This condition affects both retina and vitreous, and is considered a severe peripheral vitreochoreoretinal degeneration with risk of retinal tears and rhegmatogenous retinal detachment caused by vitreous traction [15, 18, 19]. The degenerative changes comprise retinal thinning with subsequent fibrosis and vitreous liquefaction over the lesion (lacuna). Vitreoretinal adhesions at the margins of the lesion are a common finding [13, 20, 21]. This degeneration can have an oval or linear pattern of lesions with either single or grouped distribution [19]. Lesions may be isolated or multiple, with radial or circumferential crisscrossing lines, and in some cases have tiny white or yellowish deposits, pigment clumps, atrophic holes, or retinal tears [17, 19, 22–24].

Two types of lattice degeneration are distinguished: typical and atypical. Typical lattice degeneration appears as well-outlined, spindle-like areas of retinal thinning, with white crisscrossing lines between the equator and the posterior margin of the vitreous base. Atypical lesions usually have radial perivascular distribution. Lattice degeneration can cause tractional retinal tears along its posterior edge because of tight vitreoretinal adhesions with resulting rhegmatogenous retinal detachment [13].

The frequency of lattice degeneration in eyes with retinal detachment is reported to be 13.9–35 % [25, 26]. Furthermore, this degeneration is found in 14.5–26.18 % of fellow eyes [8, 27]. In eyes with acute posterior vitreous detachment associated with lattice degeneration, flap tears are found in 1.5–2 %, and operculated tears in 16–24 % of cases [3, 21, 28]. However, lattice degeneration itself seldom causes retinal detachment, accounting for 1 % [23], 2–4 % of patients [7].

To date, no universally accepted indications for the prophylactic laser coagulation of lattice degeneration have been proposed. Some experts believe that prophylactic treatment is indicated for clinically significant symptoms, flap tears, retinal detachment in the fellow eye, aphakia, or family history [29]. Other authors recommend laser treatment only in case of retinal detachment in the fellow eye associated with lattice degeneration [15, 17]. Laser surgery does not always prevent the retinal detachment because new retinal tears can occur in seemingly healthy retina. It is thought that one should not always seek medical care in case of lattice degeneration with atrophic holes [17]. Alternatively, prophylactic laser photocoagulation is advocated in any type of lattice degeneration by some researchers [3].

Some authors emphasize that lattice degeneration without retinal tears or with retinal holes should be treated individually according to the guidelines of the American Academy of Ophthalmology (see Table 7.1 in Chap. 7). Prophylactic laser treatment is indicated in flap tears with persistent vitreous traction. According to Brinton and Wilkinson (Table 5.2), laser photocoagulation should be performed around the lesion and at the base of the vitreous body to decrease the risk of post-operative retinal detachment due to insufficient scarring around the tear [6].

The review by Wilkinson (2014) found no randomized controlled trials showing clinical benefits of prophylactic laser surgery for asymptomatic tears and lattice degeneration. The author concluded that prophylactic treatment is only justified in managing vitreous traction and retinal tears associated with symptoms of flashes and floaters [30].

Table 5.2 Guidelines for prophylactic laser photocoagulation in lattice degeneration with or without retinal holes

Type of break	With symptoms	Asymptomatic			
		No risk factors	High myopia	Fellow eye[a]	Pseudophakia[b]
Lattice degeneration with/without retinal holes	Sometimes	No	Rarely	Sometimes	Rarely

Adapted version of table from [6]. Reproduced with the permission of Oxford University Press. Taken from original version in *Precursors of Rhegmatogenous Retinal Detachment in Adults*. San Francisco, CA: American Academy of Ophthalmology; 2008, by Permission of American Academy of Ophthalmology Retina Panel. Preferred Practice Pattern®Guidelines. Available at: www.aao.org/ppp
[a]Applies to patients who have had a retinal detachment in the other eye
[b]Applies to pseudophakes, aphakes, and patients prior to cataract surgery

Table 5.3 Diagram of peripheral retinal degenerations

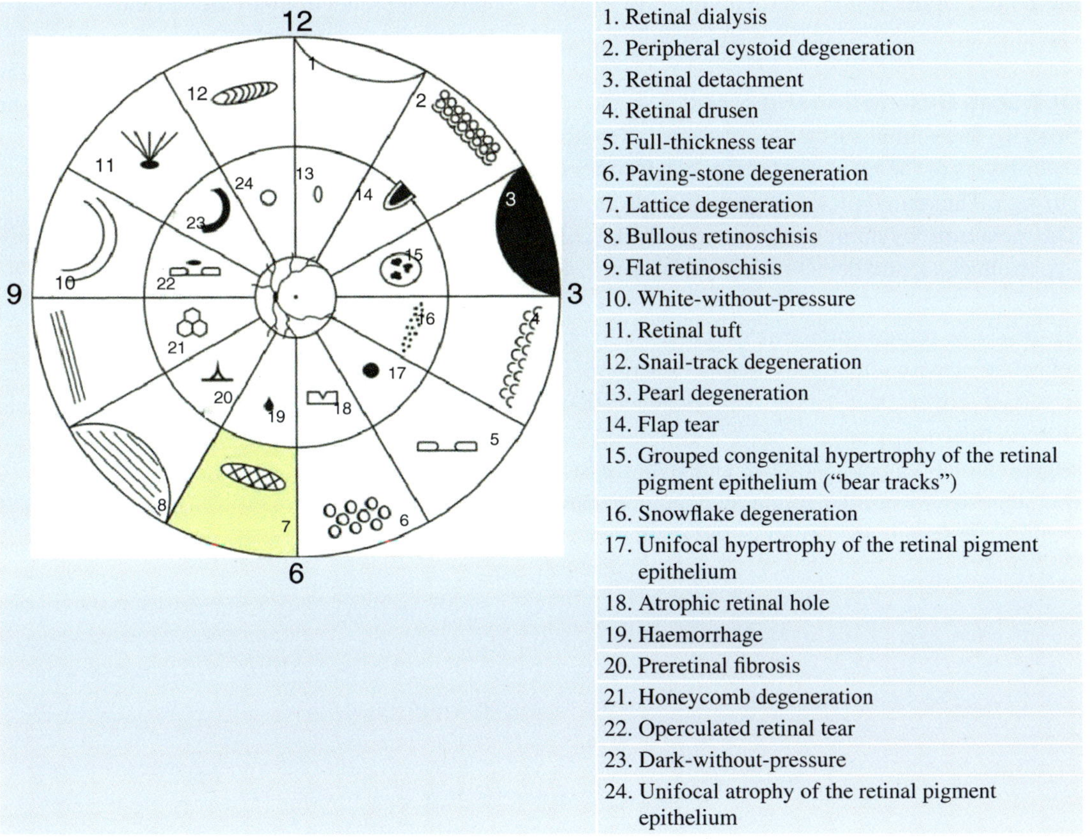

1. Retinal dialysis
2. Peripheral cystoid degeneration
3. Retinal detachment
4. Retinal drusen
5. Full-thickness tear
6. Paving-stone degeneration
7. Lattice degeneration
8. Bullous retinoschisis
9. Flat retinoschisis
10. White-without-pressure
11. Retinal tuft
12. Snail-track degeneration
13. Pearl degeneration
14. Flap tear
15. Grouped congenital hypertrophy of the retinal pigment epithelium ("bear tracks")
16. Snowflake degeneration
17. Unifocal hypertrophy of the retinal pigment epithelium
18. Atrophic retinal hole
19. Haemorrhage
20. Preretinal fibrosis
21. Honeycomb degeneration
22. Operculated retinal tear
23. Dark-without-pressure
24. Unifocal atrophy of the retinal pigment epithelium

Lattice degeneration in sector 7 is highlighted in yellow

Case 27. Lattice Degeneration (Classic)

A 59-year old female patient with moderate myopia and partial posterior vitreous detachment presented with complaints of floaters affecting her left eye.

Ophthalmoscopic Findings (Fig. 5.27a, b)

A hyperpigmented degenerative lesion with blurred borders and a white retinal vessel in the center is observed in the mid-periphery of the inferotemporal quadrant of the left eye. Vitreoretinal adhesions with traction are seen at the border of the lesion. Retinal structure in the center of the lesion is changed and atrophic.

OCT Scan Description (Fig. 5.27c)

Scan 1 The retinal surface is smooth. Inner and outer layers of the neuroepithelium can be distinguished. The retinal pigment epithelium is intact. The posterior hyaloid membrane is thickened, hyperreflective, and detached from the retina.

Scan 2 The retinal surface is irregular. A hyporeflective cavity in the vitreous (lacuna) is observed over the area of degeneration. Vitreoretinal adhesions are present at the edge of degeneration. Marked thinning and hyperreflective deposits within the retina and pigment epithelium are seen in the center of the scan.

Scan 3 The retinal surface is irregular because of vitreoretinal adhesions and traction at the borders of the lesion. A hyperreflective sclerosed blood vessel is observed within the neuroepithelium. Hyperplasia of the pigment epithelium is seen at the sides.

Scan 4 The retinal surface is irregular because of three areas of neuroepithelium thinning. Vitreous traction is moderate.

OCT Scan Details

* Vitreoretinal adhesion and traction; layers of moderate reflectivity in the vitreous

* Thin and dense neurosensory retina within the lesion. Marked retinal thinning closer to the center of the lesion

* Dense pigment epithelium in the center of the lesion and at the level of the vitreoretinal tractions

* Decreased choroid reflectivity at the level of the dense pigment epithelium

* Cross-section image of the sclerosed retinal vessel with tough walls

* Photoreceptor layer destruction at the border of the lesion

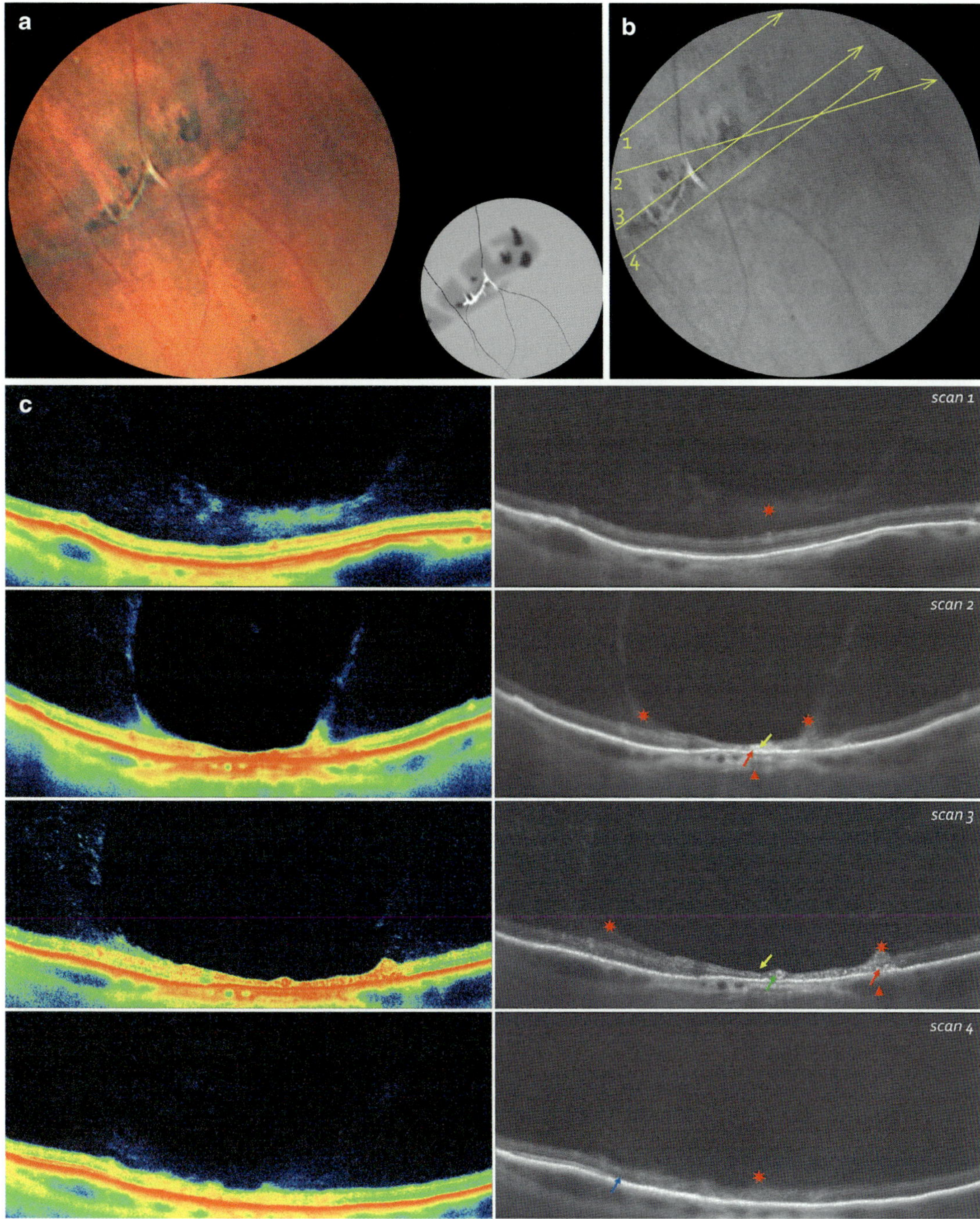

Fig. 5.27 (**a**) Classic lattice degeneration. (**b**) *Lines* indicate OCT-scanning direction. (**c**) OCT-scanning results according to the position of the lines in (**b**)

Case 28. Lattice Degeneration with Retinal Tears and Sclerosed Retinal Vessels

A 64-year old male patient with pseudophakia of his right eye presented with floaters affecting his right eye and incidental flashes of light during eye movements.

Ophthalmoscopic Findings (Fig. 5.28a, b)

A large lesion with multiple full-thickness tears of various forms and sizes is observed in the mid-periphery of the superior quadrant of the right eye. Multiple sclerosed retinal vessels (branching white lines) and atrophic areas of the retinal pigment epithelium with various pigmented deposits are seen within the area of degeneration.

OCT Scan Description (Fig. 5.28c, d)

The retinal surface is irregular because of three full-thickness tears with shallow retinal detachment at the edges. The intact neuroepithelium has small hyporeflective cavities and areas of increased density in the pigment epithelium.

OCT Scan Details (Fig. 5.28c, d)

- Full-thickness tears of the neurosensory retina

- Areas of marked thinning and consolidation of the neurosensory retina between the tears

- Isolated intraretinal hyporeflective cavities in the margin of the full-thickness tear

- Increased density of the pigment epithelium

- Decreased reflectivity of the choroid at the level of the dense pigment epithelium

- Destroyed pigment epithelium

- Increased choroid reflectivity at the level of the pigment epithelium destruction

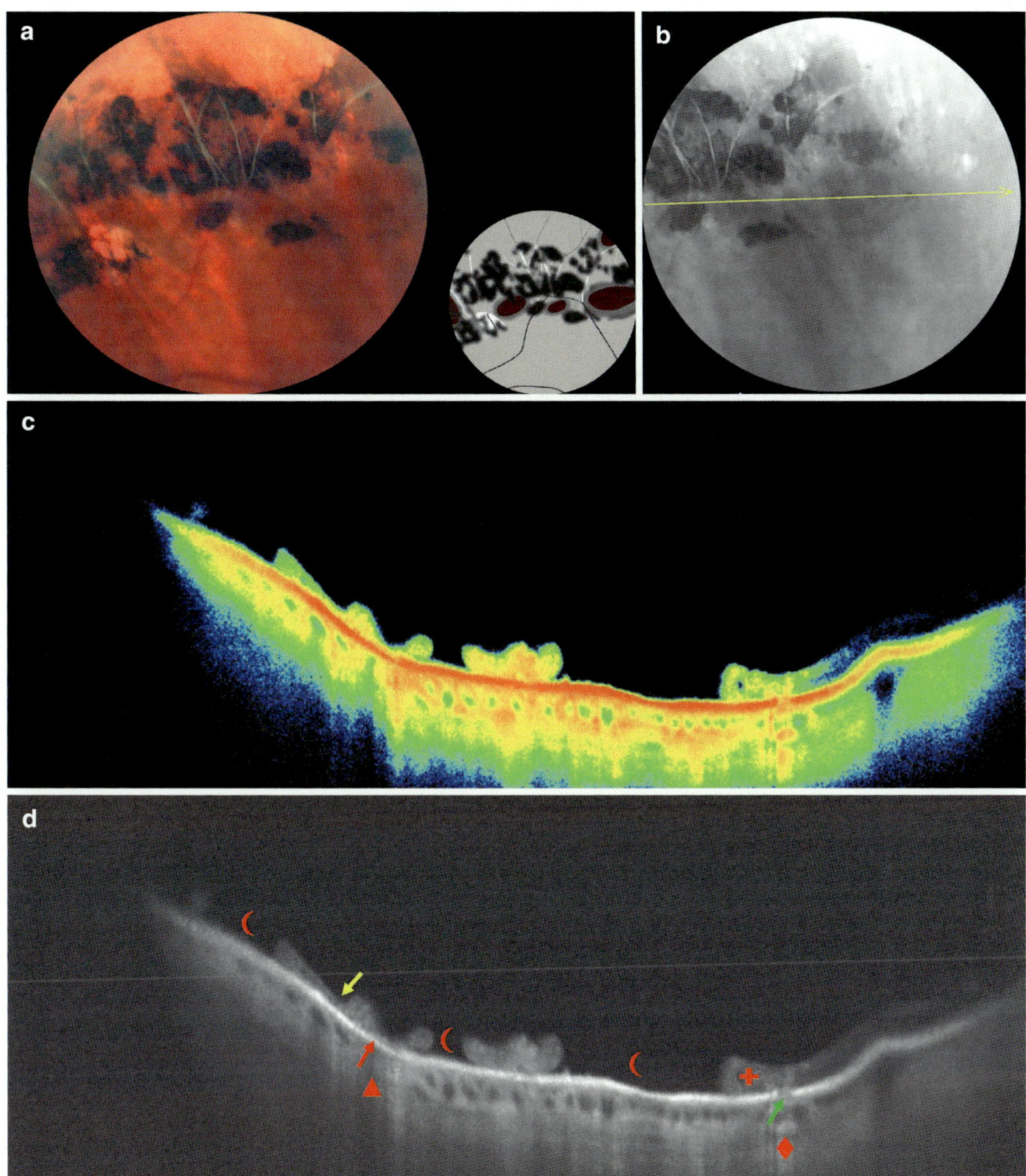

Fig. 5.28 (**a**) Lattice degeneration with retinal tears, hyperpigmentation, and sclerosed vessels. (**b**) Line indicates OCT-scanning direction. (**c, d**) OCT-scanning results according to the position of the line in (**b**)

Case 29. Lattice Degeneration with Hyperpigmentation and Pigment Epithelium Atrophy

An asymptomatic 27-year old male patient with moderate myopia and lattice degeneration in his left eye presented with complaints of decreased vision in his left eye.

Ophthalmoscopic Findings (Fig. 5.29a, b)

An elongated irregular lesion with blurred borders is observed in the mid-periphery of the inferior quadrant of the left eye. All through the lesion, there are whitish areas of pigment epithelium atrophy with choroid showing through. In the center and at the sides of the lesion there are dark pigment clumps. The gray line along the border of the lesion indicates vitreous traction.

OCT Scan Description (Fig. 5.29c)

Scan 1 The retinal surface is irregular and wavy because of vitreous adhesion and two areas of pigment epithelium atrophy. The neurosensory retina in the center of the atrophic region is thinned. The comet-tail effect is observed in the choroid.

Scan 2 Vitreoretinal adhesions with traction at the borders enlarge. Atrophic lesions and pigment epithelium hyperplasia are seen in the center.

Scan 3 Vitreoretinal adhesion enlarges sharply. Neuroepithelium is thinned at the edges, thickened and hyperreflective in the center.

Scan 4 Vitreous traction at the edges of the degenerative lesion persists. Thin areas of neuroepithelium at the edges of the area of degeneration interchange with thick areas in the center. Hyperplasia of the pigment epithelium is observed in the center of the scan.

OCT Scan Details (Fig. 5.29c)

Vitreoretinal adhesion and traction

Marked thinning of the neurosensory retina at the edge of the lesion

Increased density of the neurosensory retina, more pronounced in the center of the lesion

Pigment epithelium destruction

Increased density of the pigment epithelium

Increased reflectivity of the choroid in the area of pigment epithelium destruction

Decreased reflectivity of the choroid in the area of dense pigment epithelium

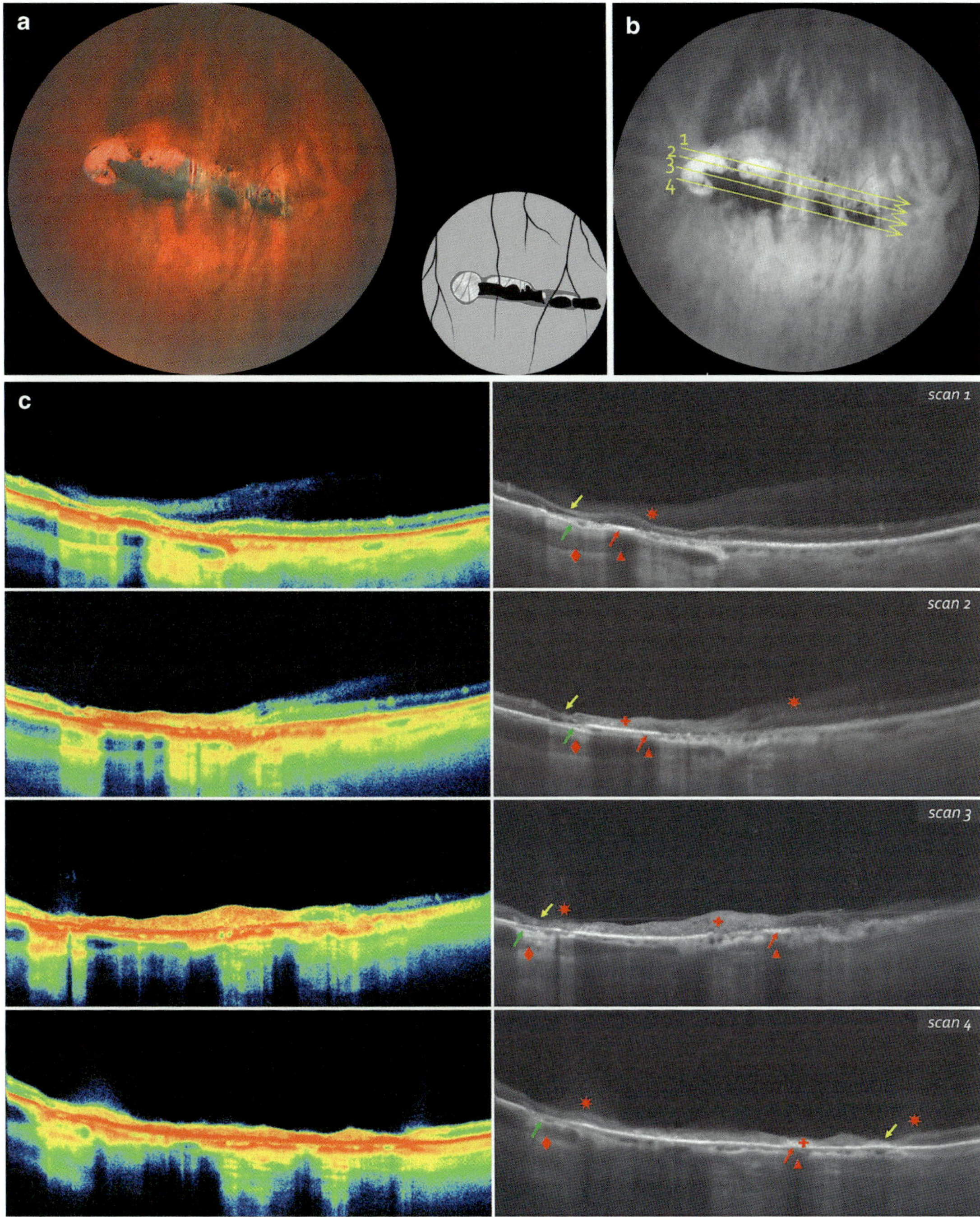

Fig. 5.29 (**a**) Lattice degeneration with hyperpigmentation and areas of pigment epithelium atrophy. (**b**) *Lines* indicate OCT-scanning direction. (**c**) OCT-scanning results according to the position of the lines in (**b**)

Case 30. Lattice Degeneration with Linear Hyperpigmentation

A 77-year old male patient with low hyperopia and early stage cortical cataract presented with the main complaint of decreased vision.

Ophthalmoscopic Findings (Fig. 5.30a, b)

Multiple pigment deposits are observed along the retinal vessel in the mid-periphery of the supero-temporal quadrant of the right eye. Pigment deposits are arranged in parallel lines. The retina in the affected region is dark and grayish.

OCT Scan Description (Fig. 5.30c)

Scans 1 and 2 The retinal surface is irregular. There are multiple hyperreflective deposits of various shapes in the area of thinned neuroepithelium, shadowing the underlying tissues. A vitreoretinal adhesion with traction is seen at the edge of the area of degeneration.

OCT Scan Details (Fig. 5.30c)

✳ Vitreoretinal adhesion and traction

◤ Thinned and dense neurosensory retina within the lesion, with more prominent thinning in the central part

↗ Increased density of the pigment epithelium

✚ Intraretinal hyperreflective deposits within the whole area of degeneration

▲ Decreased reflectivity of the choroid at the level of the intraretinal deposits

↗ Destructed pigment epithelium between the intraretinal deposits

◆ Increased reflectivity of the choroid in the area of pigment epithelium destruction

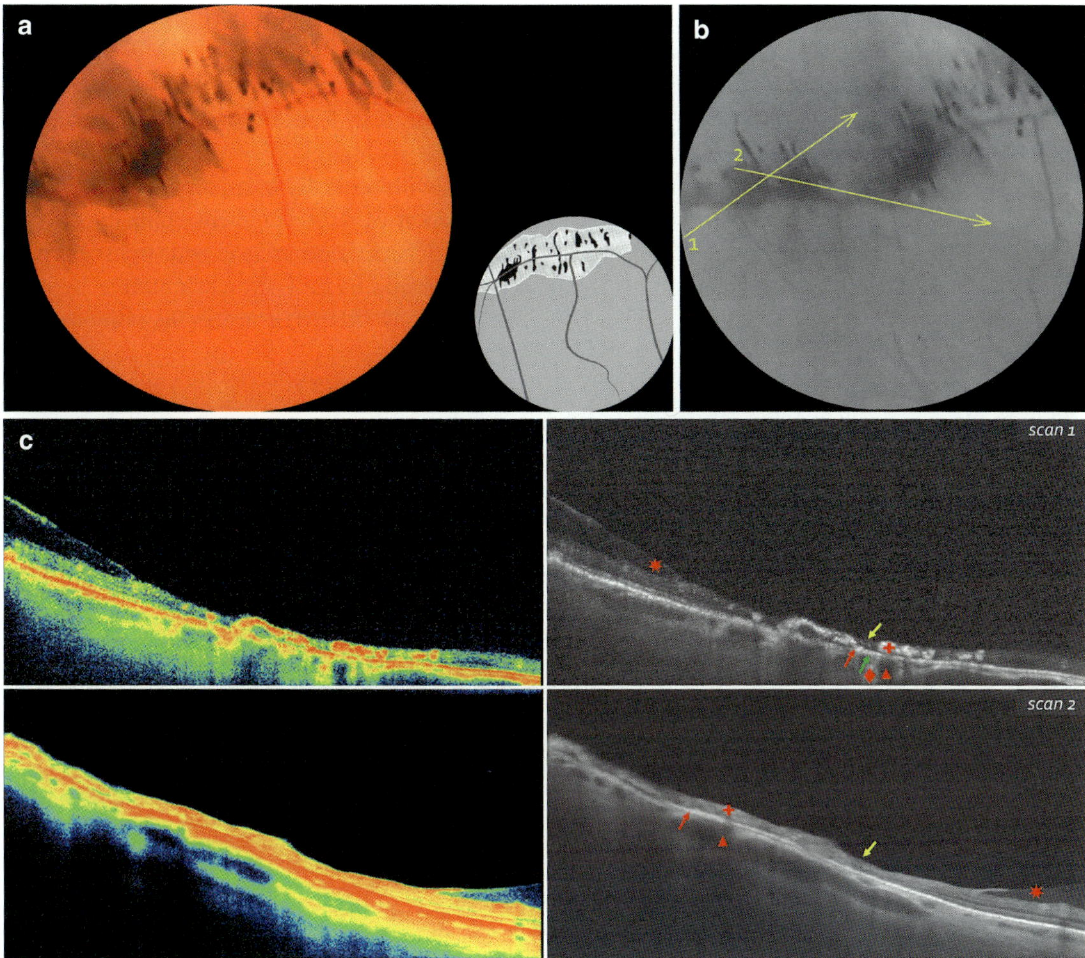

Fig. 5.30 (**a**) Lattice degeneration with linear hyperpigmentation along the retinal vessel. (**b**) *Lines* indicate OCT-scanning direction **c** OCT-scanning results according to the position of the lines in (**b**)

Case 31. Lattice Degeneration with Flap Tear and Shallow Retinal Detachment

A 50-year-old female patient presented with a 3-day history of flashes of light, sparkles, and floaters affecting her right eye after physical exercises. Her ophthalmic history included preventive retinal laser photocoagulation of her right eye 4 years ago.

Ophthalmoscopic Findings (Fig. 5.31a, b)

An area of vaguely delineated lattice degeneration with a horseshoe tear and shallow retinal detachment is observed in the mid-periphery of the superotemporal quadrant of the right eye. White sclerosed vessels, hyperpigmented zones, light silvery lines, and a dark-brown haemorrhage along the edge of the retinal tear are observed in the area of degeneration. There are several laser burns under the shallow retinal detachment along the border of degeneration.

OCT Scan Description (Fig. 5.31c, d)

There is a full-thickness retinal tear in the left part of the scan. The neurosensory retina is detached around the tear. There are marked vitreoretinal adhesions with traction and multiple intraretinal cavities with optically transparent content. There is a section of dense pigment epithelium in the area of degeneration and the neurosensory retina stays attached to it. There are multiple hyperreflective (consolidated) layers in the vitreous.

OCT Scan Details

- Full-thickness tear of the neurosensory retina

- Neurosensory retinal detachment cavity

- Multiple intraretinal cavities in the detached retina

- An elevated dense flap of the detached neurosensory retina

- A section of dense pigment epithelium the retina stays attached to

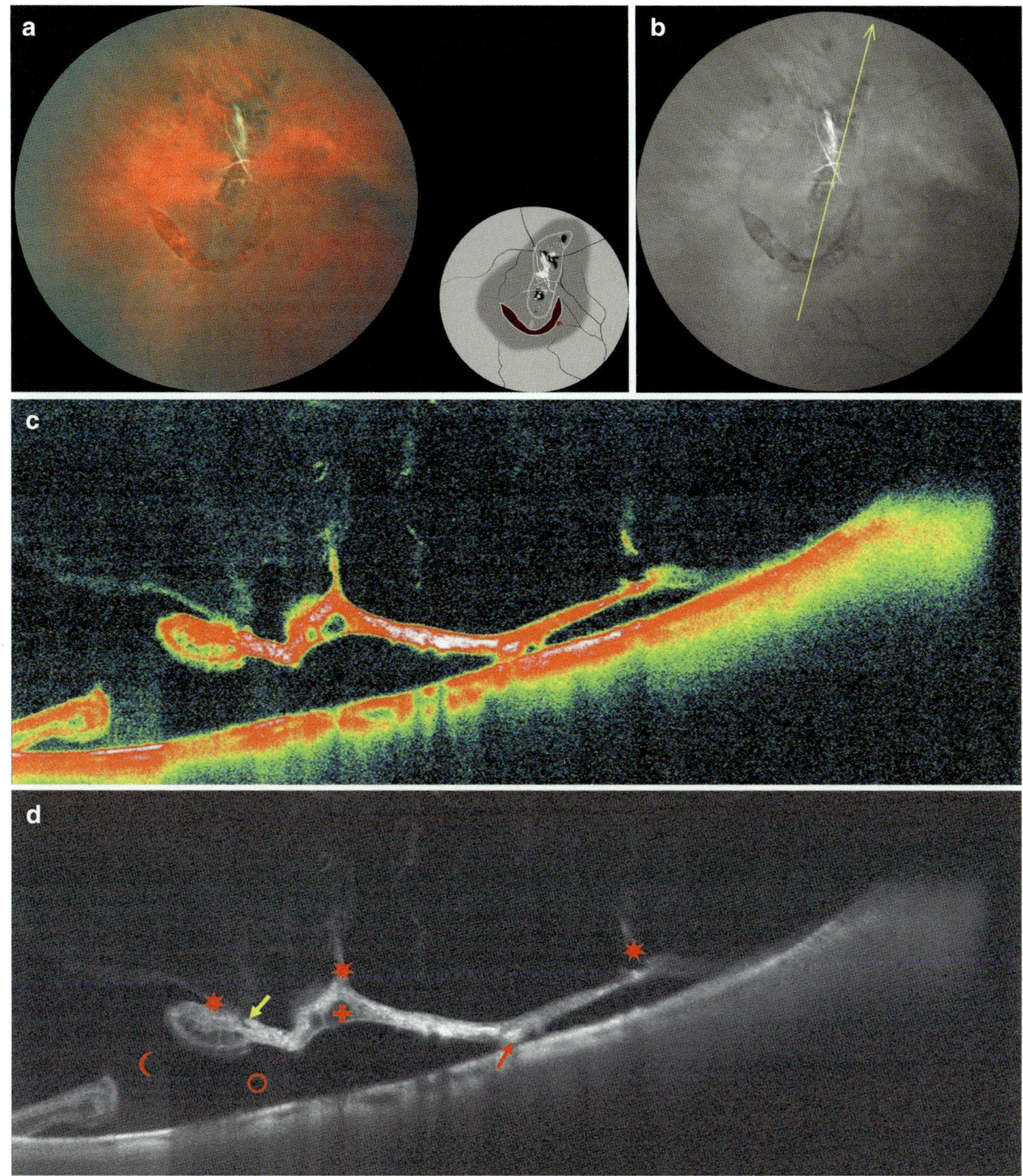

Fig. 5.31 (**a**) Full-thickness retinal tear with shallow retinal detachment associated with lattice degeneration. (**b**) *Line* indicates OCT-scanning direction. (**c, d**) OCT-scanning results according to the line direction in (**b**)

Case 32. "Silvery" Lattice Degeneration

A 29-year-old male patient presented with the main complaint of flashes of light after physical exercises.

Ophthalmoscopic Findings

A large area of degeneration along the retinal vessel is observed in the mid-periphery of the superior quadrant of the right eye. The lesion has clear borders, silvery luster, multiple pigment clumps of various sizes and multiple sclerosed vessels (Fig. 5.32a, b).

OCT Scan Description (Fig. 5.32c, d)

The retinal surface is irregular, excavated, because of vitreoretinal adhesion with traction at the sides of the lesion. There are areas of pigment epithelium hyperplasia. The retina along the blood vessel is hyperreflective. The layers of the neuroepithelium are dense and undistinguished. The neurosensory retina is thinned.

OCT Scan Details

✳ Vitreoretinal adhesion and traction

✚ Increased density of the neurosensory retina. Density increases closer to the central part of degeneration

◤ Sclerosed retinal vessel in the center of the lesion

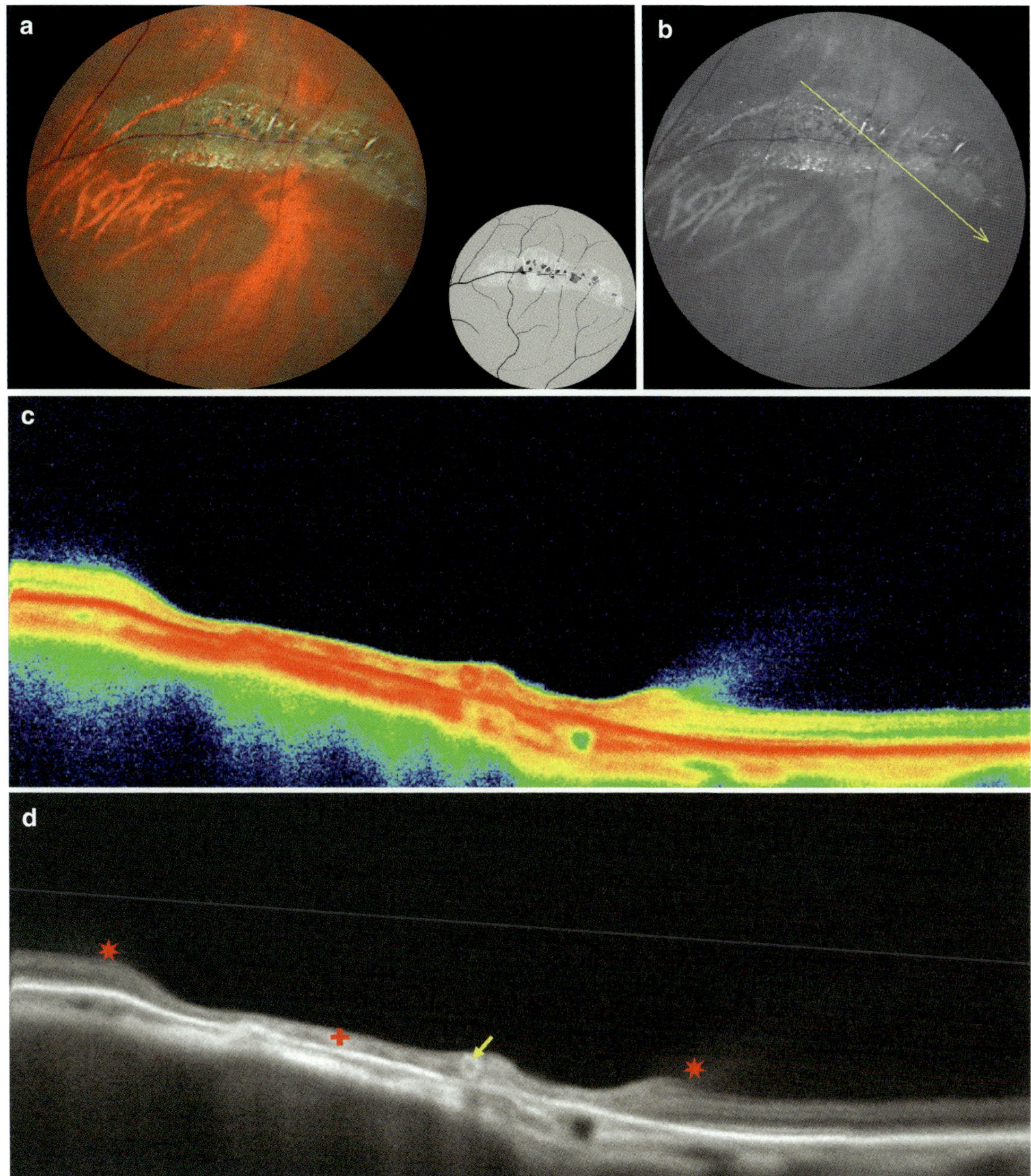

Fig. 5.32 (**a**) Lattice degeneration. (**b**) *Line* indicates OCT-scanning direction. (**c**, **d**) OCT-scanning results according to the line direction in (**b**)

Case 33. Lattice Degeneration with "Snow Clumps"

A 24-year old moderately myopic female patient with partial posterior vitreous detachment presented with the main complaint of floaters affecting her right eye.

Ophthalmoscopic Findings (Fig. 5.33a, b)

Whitish, thinned area with blurred borders is observed in the equatorial retina of the superotemporal quadrant of the right eye. There is a white "snow clump" in the center of the lesion. Along the edges of the lesion vitreous is changed and produces tractions. A brunch of retinal vessel passing through the white clump is poorly visualized.

OCT Scan Description (Fig. 5.33c, d)

The retinal surface is irregular because of vitreoretinal adhesion with traction. There is a retinal vessel in the center of degeneration with thinned neuroepithelium around it. The photoreceptor layer is partially destroyed. The retinal pigment epithelium is intact.

OCT Scan Details (Fig. 5.33c, d)

✳ Vitreoretinal adhesion and traction

⬐ Marked thinning of the retina

✚ Increased reflectivity (increased density) of the neurosensory retina

⬈ Destructed photoreceptor layer within the area of degeneration

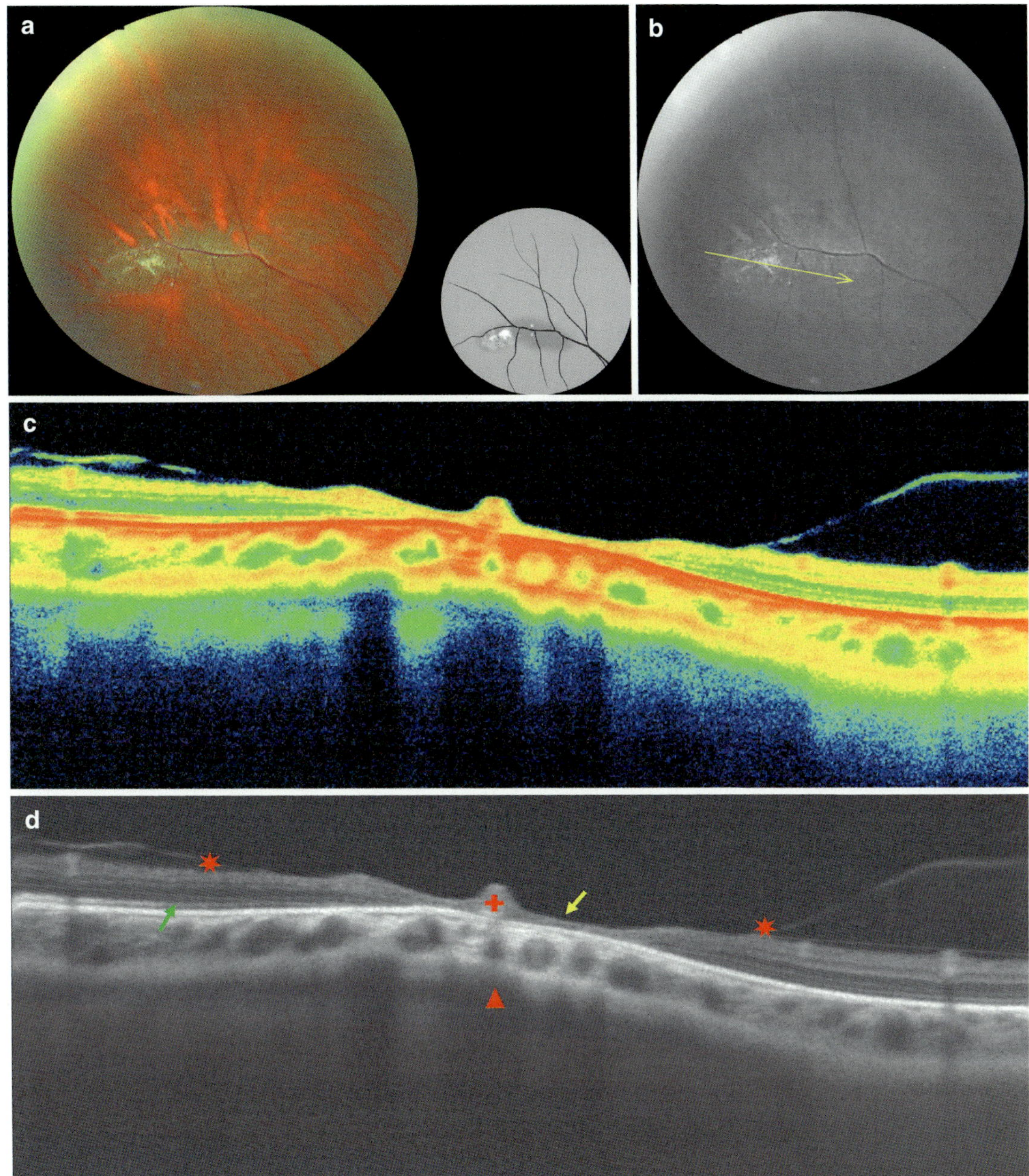

Fig. 5.33 (**a**) Lattice degeneration with "snow clumps" along the retinal vessel. (**b**) *Line* indicates OCT-scanning direction. (**c, d**) OCT-scanning results according to the *line* direction in (**b**)

Case 34. Round-Shaped Lattice Degeneration

A 27-year old emmetropic male patient presented with a 3-days history of floaters and flashes of light affecting his left eye after physical exercises.

Ophthalmoscopic Findings (Fig. 5.34a, b)

A round area of retinal thinning with clearly outlined borders is observed in the mid-periphery of the temporal quadrant of the left eye. Along the borders of the lesion vitreous is grayish, with marked traction. In the center of the lesion, the retina is dense, with areas of hyperpigmentation.

OCT Scan Description (Fig. 5.34c)

Scan 1 The retinal surface is irregular because of a local area of vitreoretinal adhesion with traction at the sides. Neurosensory retina layers are destructively changed and can not be distinguished. There are isolated intraretinal hypore-flective cavities. Pigment epithelium is dense. The IS/OS line of photoreceptors is not visualized.

Scan 2 The retinal profile is irregular, with slightly elevated inner retinal surface and marked vitreo-retinal traction. Neuroepithelial and photoreceptor layers are destructed. Hyporeflective cavities are enlarged. Pigment epithelium is partially dense.

OCT Scan Details (Fig. 5.34c)

* Vitreoretinal adhesions and tractions

+ Increased reflectivity (increased density) of the neurosensory retina

Intraretinal hyporeflective cavities at the level of vitreoretinal adhesions

Dense pigment epithelium within the lesion

Decreased reflectivity of choroid in the area of dense parts of pigment epithelium

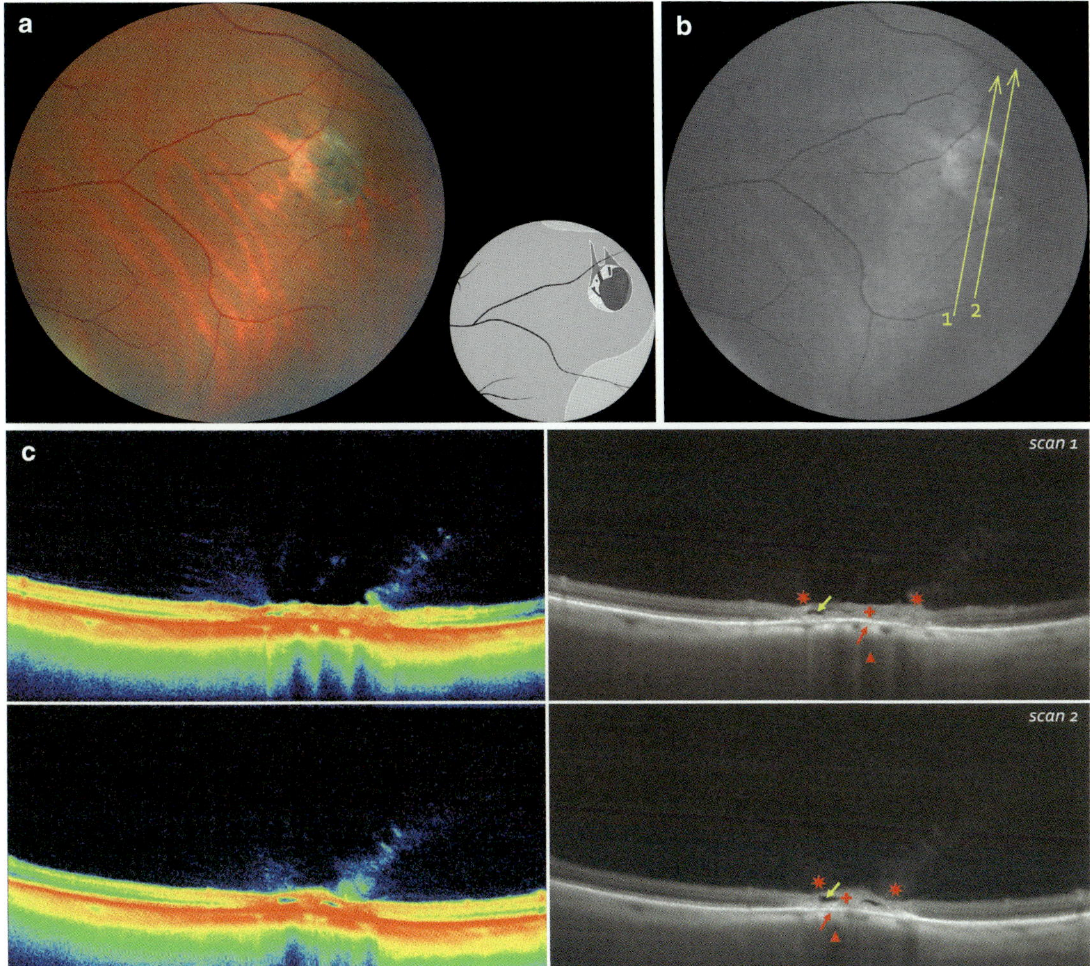

Fig. 5.34 (**a**) Round-shaped lattice degeneration. (**b**) *Lines* indicate OCT-scanning direction. (**c**) OCT-scanning results according to the *lines* direction in (**b**)

Case 35. Lattice Degeneration with Retinal Tears and Vitreoretinal Traction

A 46-year old female patient with moderate myopia and partial posterior vitreous detachment presented with a 1-week history of flashes of light and floaters affecting her left eye.

Ophthalmoscopic Findings (Fig. 5.35a, b)
An oval lesion with marked hyperpigmentation is seen in the mid-periphery of the superior quadrant of the left eye. Vitreous traction is observed as grayish bands of dense vitreous humor at the sides of degeneration. The retina in the center of the lesion is thinned, with multiple tiny red defects. Small whitish deposits on the retinal surface represent snowflake degeneration.

OCT Scan Description (Fig. 5.35c)
Scans 1 and 2 The retinal surface is irregular. There are multiple defects in the neuroepithelium with vitreoretinal adhesions and traction. Retinal thinning and focal hyperplasia of the pigment epithelium are observed in the center of the scan.

Scan 3 The retinal surface is slightly elevated because of vitreoretinal traction. The posterior hyaloid membrane is thickened, hyperreflective, and tightly adherent to the retinal surface. The neuroepithelium in traction area is hyperreflective and thickened. Hyperreflective deposits are seen in the inner retinal layers.

Scan 4 The retinal surface is smooth. Multiple hyperreflective deposits in the inner retinal layers are observed in the center of the scan. The neuroepithelium is thinned, posterior hyaloid membrane - thickened and adherent to the retinal surface.

OCT Scan Details (Fig. 5.35c)

✱ Vitreoretinal adhesions and tractions

◤ Marked thinning of the neurosensory retina (atrophic holes)

+ Increased density of the neurosensory retina, with marked consolidation in areas of vitreoretinal adhesions

↗ Areas of consolidation and redistribution of pigment epithelium

▲ Decreased reflectivity of the choroid corresponding to the dense areas of pigment epithelium and marked vitreoretinal adhesion

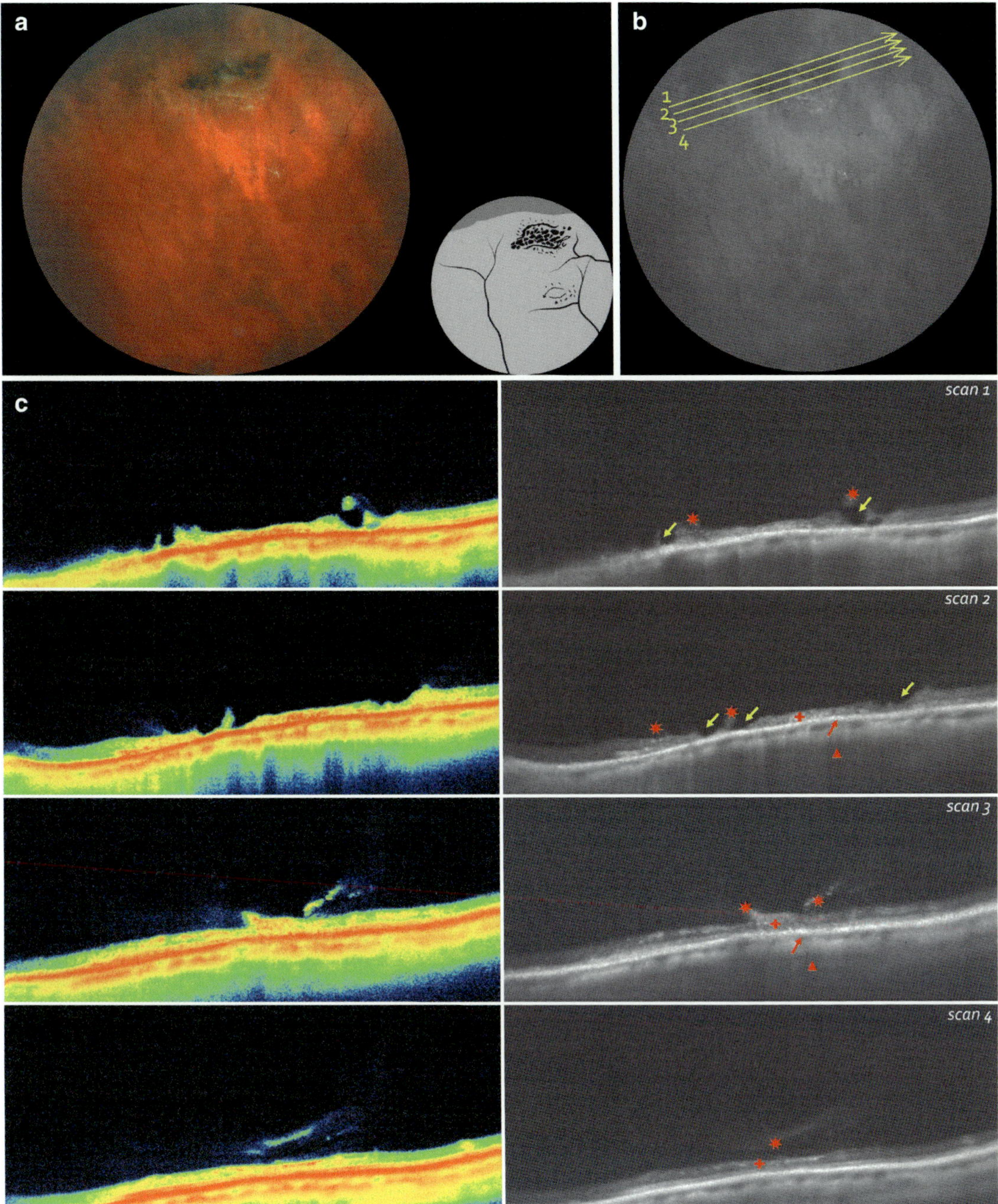

Fig. 5.35 (**a**) Lattice degeneration with retinal tears and vitreoretinal traction. (**b**) *Lines* indicate OCT-scanning directions. (**c**) OCT-scanning results according to the *lines* direction in (b)

Case 36. "Tortuous" Lattice Degeneration

A 47-year old male patient with moderate myopia and mild cortical cataract presented with decreased vision and floaters affecting his left eye.

Ophthalmoscopic Findings (Fig. 5.36a, b)

A clearly outlined whitish area of degeneration is seen in the mid-periphery of the inferior quadrant of the left eye. The lesion is elongated and tortuous. Sclerosed vessels and coarse pigment clumps are seen within the lesion.

OCT Scan Description (Fig. 5.36c)

Scan 1 The retinal surface is irregular. The center is elevated because of posterior hyaloid membrane traction. Neuroepithelium is denser in the center; vitreoretinal tractions are seen on both sides.

Scan 2 Vitreoretinal adhesion and traction sites are elongated. Posterior hyaloid membrane in traction area is thickened and tightly adherent to the retinal surface in the center. Neuroepithelium is slightly thickened.

Scan 3 Vitreoretinal adhesion site is even longer. Neuroepithelium in the center is thinned and contains multiple hyperreflective deposits. There are areas of destructive changes in the pigment epithelium.

Scan 4 The scanning was performed across the degenerative lesion. At the edges of the lesion, intense vitreous traction and areas of vitreoretinal adhesion are seen. In the area of degeneration there are multiple hyperreflective neuroepithelium deposits, pigment epithelium is destructed.

OCT Scan Details (Fig. 5.36c)

✳ Vitreoretinal adhesion and traction

✚ Increased density of the neurosensory retina at the site of vitreoretinal adhesion

◤ Thinned and dense areas of neurosensory retina

➶ Intraretinal hyperreflective deposits

○ Cross-section image of sclerosed vessels with thickened walls

➶ Pigment epithelium destruction

◆ Increased reflectivity of the choroid at the level of the pigment epithelium destruction

▲ Decreased reflectivity of the choroid at the level of the intraretinal deposits

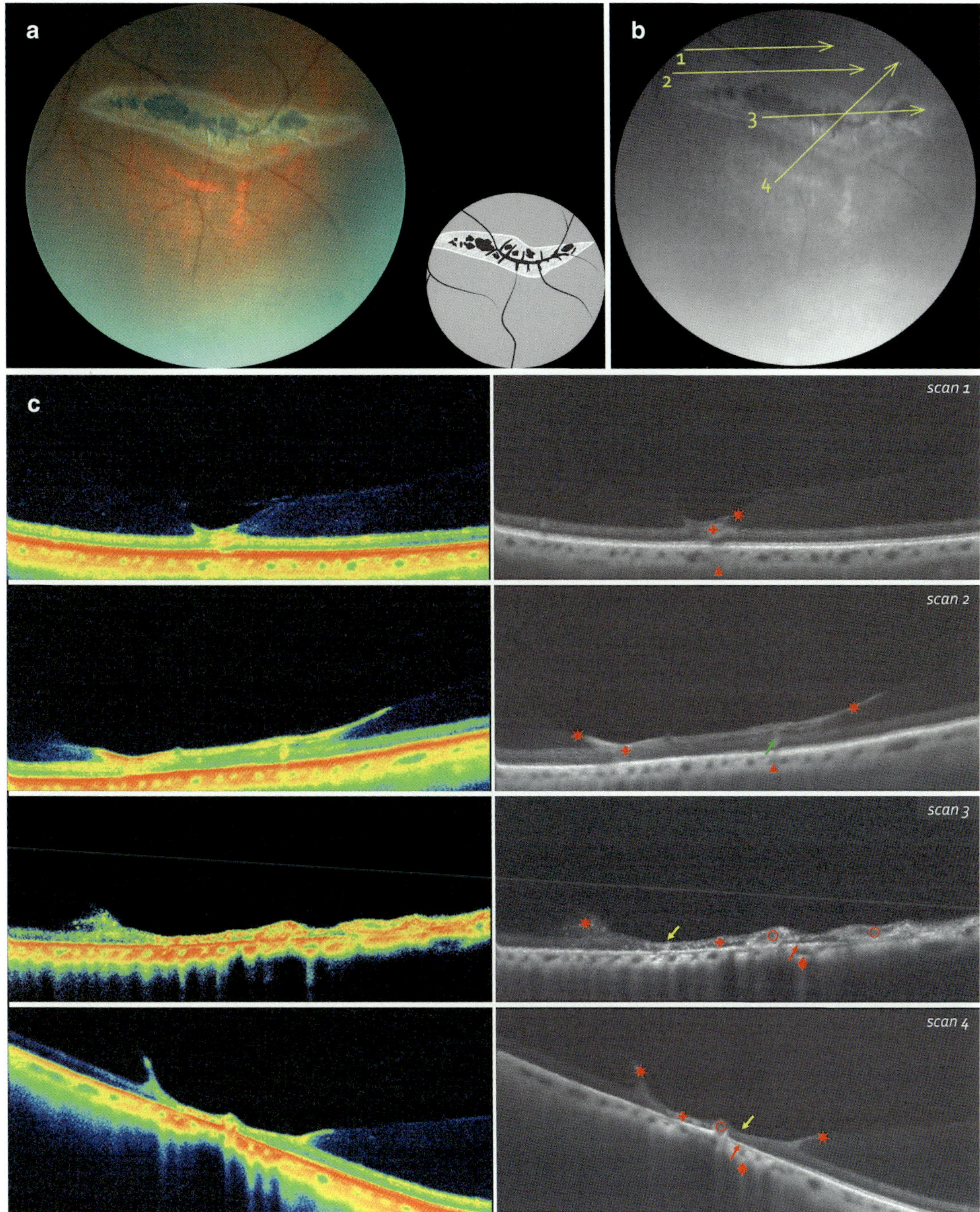

Fig. 5.36 (**a**) Tortuous lattice degeneration. (**b**) *Lines* indicate OCT-scanning direction. (**c**) OCT-scanning results according to the *lines* direction in (**b**)

Case 37. Lattice Degeneration with Retinoschisis

A 54-year old female patient with moderate myopia and partial posterior vitreous detachment presented with a 15-day history of flashes of light and floaters affecting her right eye.

Ophthalmoscopic Findings (Fig. 5.37a, b)

An elongated lesion with marked hyperpigmentation and blurred borders is seen in the midperiphery of the inferotemporal quadrant of the right eye. The vitreous humor over the degenerative lesion is gray, cloudy and dense; therefore, it is difficult to see the degeneration in details. There is an oval full-thickness retinal tear in the upper part of the lesion.

OCT Scan Description (Fig. 5.37c)

Scan 1 The retinal surface is smooth. In the center of the scan, there are multiple hyperreflective deposits in the neuroepithelium. On the right side of the scan (bottom of the lesion) retinal layers separate forming retinoschisis. Posterior hyaloid membrane is thickened and hyperreflective, tightly adherent to the retinal surface. No vitreoretinal traction is apparent.

Scan 2 The retinal surface is irregular because of vitreoretinal adhesion site, with traction at the edges of the lesion, and a full-thickness tear on the upper edge of degeneration. Intraretinal hyporeflective cavities, retinoschisis, and hyperplasia of the retinal pigment epithelium

are observed in the center and at the bottom of the lesion.

Scan 3 Vitreoretinal adhesion and traction persists. Multiple hyporeflective cavities are observed on the left side of the scan (upper part of the lesion). Retinal cavities merge and separate the retina on the right side of the scan.

OCT Scan Details (Fig. 5.37c)

✳ Vitreoretinal adhesion and traction

☾ Full-thickness tear of the neurosensory retina

✛ Dense neurosensory retina at the sites of vitreoretinal adhesion

◯ Cross-section image of a sclerosed vessel with thickened walls

↗ Intraretinal hyporeflective cavities within the lesion

↗ Separation of the neurosensory retina layers by multiple intraretinal hyporeflective cavities

↗ Dense pigment epithelium

▲ Decreased reflectivity of the choroid

◆ Increased reflectivity of choroid at the level of the pigment epithelium destruction and blood vessel sclerosis

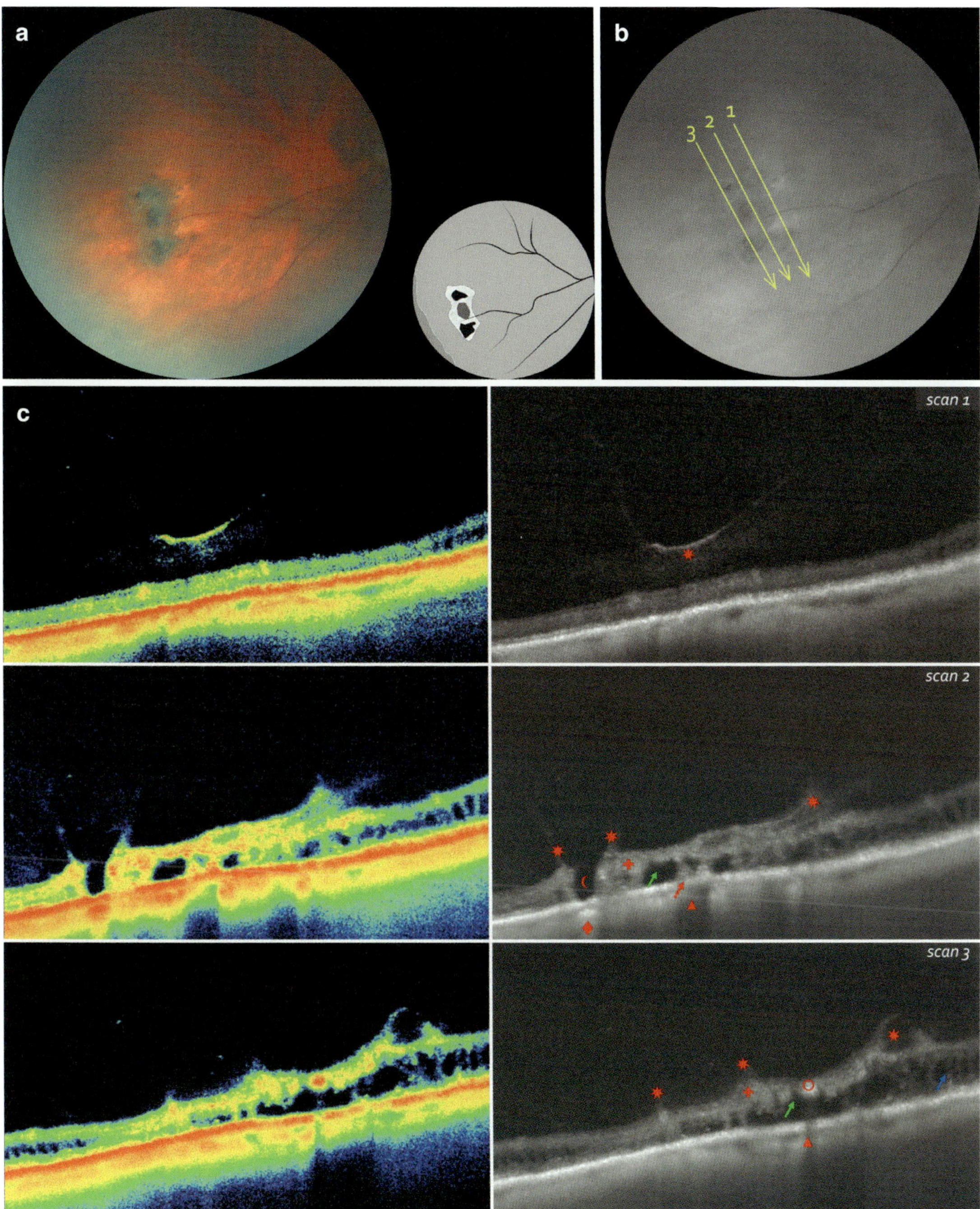

Fig. 5.37 (**a**) Lattice degeneration with hyperpigmentation and spongy retina around. (**b**) *Lines* indicate OCT-scanning direction. (**c**) OCT-scanning results according to the *lines* direction in (**b**)

Case 38. Atypical Lattice Degeneration

A 41-year old male patient presented with a 1-week history of floaters affecting his right eye.

Ophthalmoscopic Findings (Fig. 5.38a, b)

An elongated lesion with areas of spongy pigmentation, irregular surface and blurred borders is observed in the mid-periphery of the inferotemporal quadrant of the right eye. The lesion has atypical localization: perpendicular to the equator, along the retinal vessel.

OCT Scan Description (Fig. 5.38c, d)

The retinal surface is irregular because of vitreoretinal adhesion site with traction at the edges. Areas of dense neuroepithelium, hyperplasia of the pigment epithelium, and a retinal vessel with thickened walls are observed in the center of the lesion. On the left side of the scan, there is a full-thickness tear with an operculum, which is fixed by vitreoretinal adhesion.

OCT Scan Details (Fig. 5.38c, d)

✴ Vitreoretinal adhesion and traction

✚ Intraretinal hyporeflective cavities

☾ Full-thickness tear of the neurosensory retina

○ Cross-section image of the vessels with thickened walls

↗ Dense pigment epithelium

▲ Decreased reflectivity of the choroid at the level of dense pigment epithelium

↗ Pigment epithelium destruction

◆ Increased choroidal reflectivity

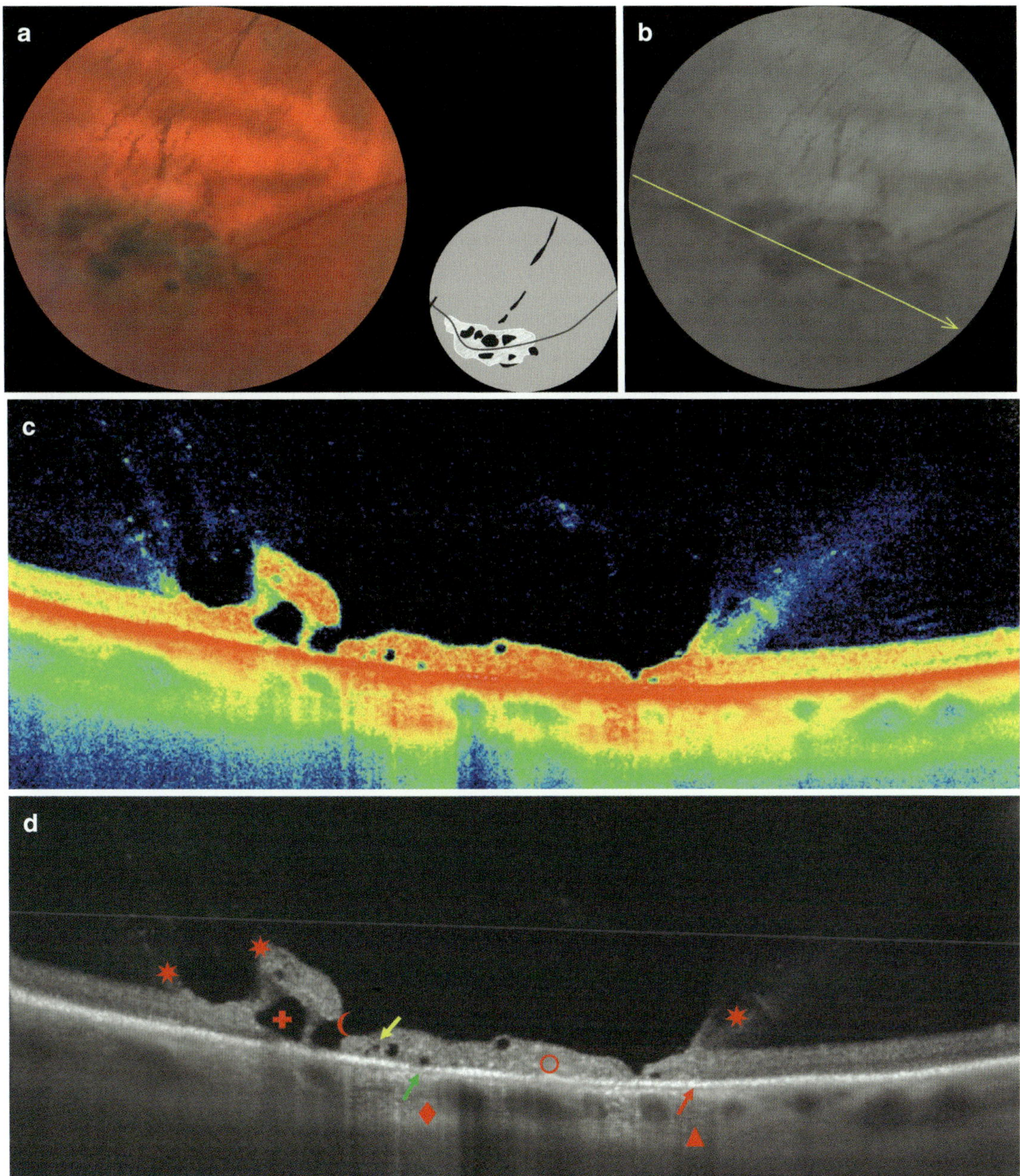

Fig. 5.38 (**a**) Atypical lattice degeneration. (**b**) *Line* indicates OCT-scanning direction. (**c, d**) OCT-scanning results according to the *line* direction in (**b**)

Retinal Tufts

Retinal tuft (vitreoretinal fibrous band) is a small area of retinal degeneration, in which retina is attached to and pulled by the vitreous (Table 5.4). This process causes significant vitreous traction [1, 31]. Various authors distinguish several types of retinal tufts: cystic, noncystic, and zonular traction tufts [32–35]. Noncystic retinal tufts are as a rule less than 0.1 mm in size, are not associated with vitreous traction, and are more commonly found in the far-peripheral, or less commonly, in the pre-equatorial retina. Cystic tufts are larger than 0.1 mm, and can be found in any part of the retina, with mainly equatorial distribution [1].

Noncystic tufts are present in up to 72 % of adults, and are bilateral in nearly half of the cases. Cystic tufts are present in 5 % of adult patients and are bilateral in only 6 % of cases. Zonular traction tufts occur in 15 % of adults, and 15 % of cases have bilateral distribution [34].

Persistent vitreous traction associated with retinal tufts can result in retinal tears and detachment. Cystic retinal tufts are reported to be found in 10 % of patients with retinal detachment; however, this degeneration accounts for less than 1 % of rhegmatogenous retinal detachment [15].

The need for prophylactic laser treatment for retinal tufts remains controversial. Given the low risk of retinal detachment, prophylactic laser treatment is not recommended by the majority of experts; however, patients should be routinely examined [29].

Table 5.4 Diagram of peripheral retinal degenerations

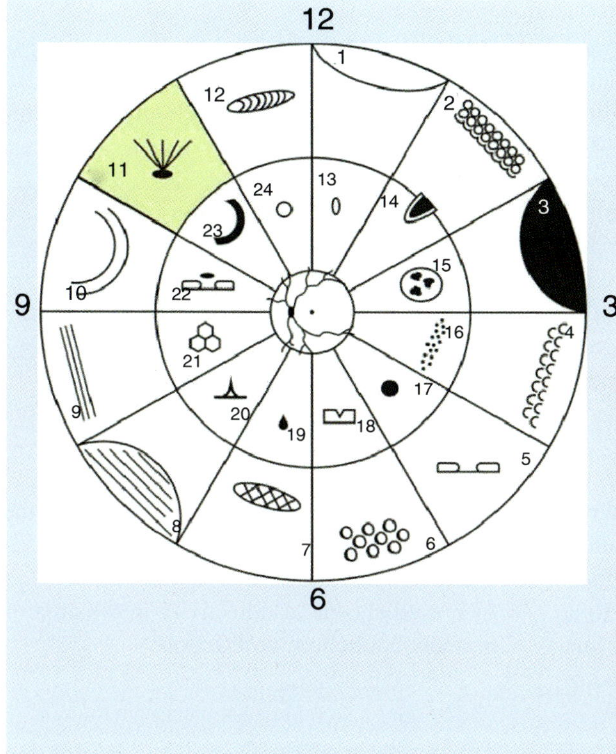

1. Retinal dialysis
2. Peripheral cystoid degeneration
3. Retinal detachment
4. Retinal drusen
5. Full-thickness tear
6. Paving-stone degeneration
7. Lattice degeneration
8. Bullous retinoschisis
9. Flat retinoschisis
10. White-without-pressure
11. Retinal tuft
12. Snail-track degeneration
13. Pearl degeneration
14. Flap tear
15. Grouped congenital hypertrophy of the retinal pigment epithelium ("bear tracks")
16. Snowflake degeneration
17. Unifocal hypertrophy of the retinal pigment epithelium
18. Atrophic retinal hole
19. Haemorrhage
20. Preretinal fibrosis
21. Honeycomb degeneration
22. Operculated retinal tear
23. Dark-without-pressure
24. Unifocal atrophy of the retinal pigment epithelium

Retinal tuft in sector 11 is highlighted in yellow

Case 39. Noncystic Retinal Tuft

An asymptomatic 28-year-old male patient presented with mild myopia. Retinal degeneration was diagnosed during ophthalmoscopic examination with a 60.0 D lens.

Ophthalmoscopic Findings (Fig. 5.39a, b)

A well-outlined irregular atrophic lesion of the pigment epithelium is observed along a retinal vessel in the mid-periphery of the temporal quadrant of the left eye. The lesion is surrounded by black pigment clumps. The retina in the center of degeneration is grayish and elevated into the vitreous.

OCT Scan Description (Fig. 5.39c, d)

The retina is locally elevated. Neurosensory retina is thickened; there is an early-stage shallow detachment, and small hyporeflective cavities. Vitreous traction is observed. Two areas of retinal thinning and pigment epithelium atrophy are seen on both sides of the lesion, causing a shadow effect on the underlying tissues.

OCT Scan Details (Fig. 5.39c, d)

✳ Vitreoretinal adhesion and tractions

✚ Dense neurosensory retina elevated by vitreous traction

◣ Marked retinal thinning along the adhesion site

↗ Pigment epithelium destruction along the adhesion site

↗ Dense pigment epithelium along the borders of destruction

▲ Decreased choroidal reflectivity at the level of the elevated retina and dense pigment epithelium

◆ Increased choroidal reflectivity in the area of pigment epithelium destruction

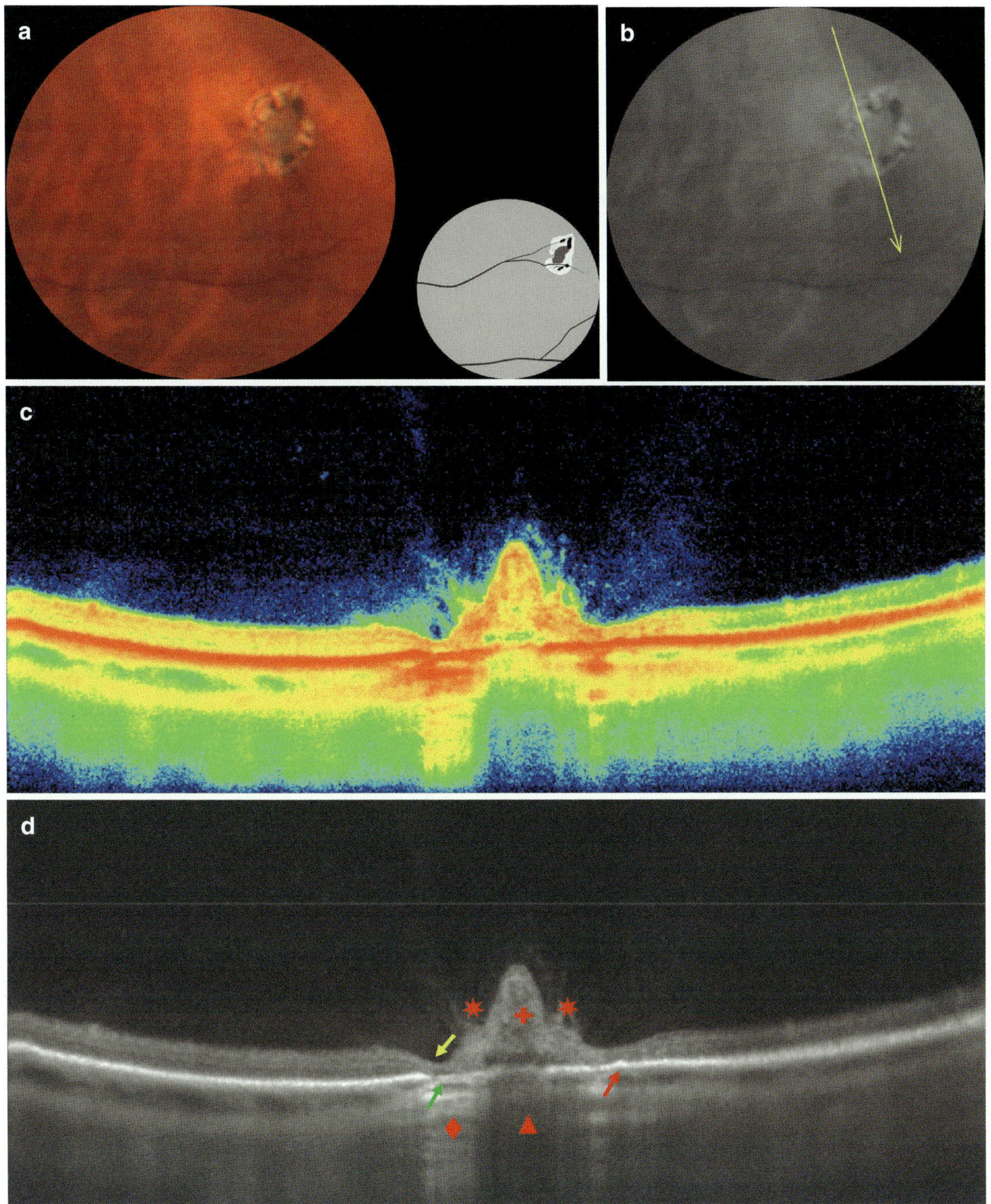

Fig. 5.39 (**a**) Noncystic retinal tuft. (**b**) *Line* indicates OCT-scanning direction. (**c, d**) OCT-scanning results according to the *line* direction in (**b**)

Case 40. Retinal Tuft with Focal Pigment Epithelium Atrophy

A 21-year-old female patient with moderate myopia presented with a 1-month history of floaters affecting her right eye during eye movements.

Ophthalmoscopic Findings (Fig. 5.40a, b)

An oval atrophic lesion is observed in the mid-periphery of the inferior quadrant of the right eye. Its inferotemporal border is marked with a gray spongy line that deepens into the atrophic cavity. Pigment clumps are seen at the edges of the area of degeneration. The choroid is clearly visible through the lesion.

OCT Scan Description (Fig. 5.40c)

Scan 1 The retinal surface is slightly changed because the neuroepithelium layer is thinned. The IS/OS line cannot be visualized. The pigment epithelium appears atrophic. The choroid is more transparent. Vitreous is condensed, its reflectivity is irregular.

Scan 2 Retina is more incurvated, because its neurosensory layer became thinner. Destructive changes are observed in the pigment epithelium.

Scan 3 Vitreoretinal adhesion and traction are clearly seen. The retinal incurvation is seen in the center, and IS/OS line is not observed. Pigment epithelium destruction casts a hyperreflective shadow over the choroid. Vitreous over the degenerative lesion is radically destructed, and an area of vitreous liquefaction is seen in the center of the scan.

OCT Scan Details (Fig. 5.40c)

✳ Dense vitreous at the sites of vitreoretinal adhesion

↙ Retinal thinning in the atrophic region

↗ Destroyed pigment epithelium and the photo-receptor layer

◆ Increased choroidal reflectivity at the level of the pigment epithelium destruction

✚ Dense elevation of the neurosensory retina with vitreoretinal adhesion

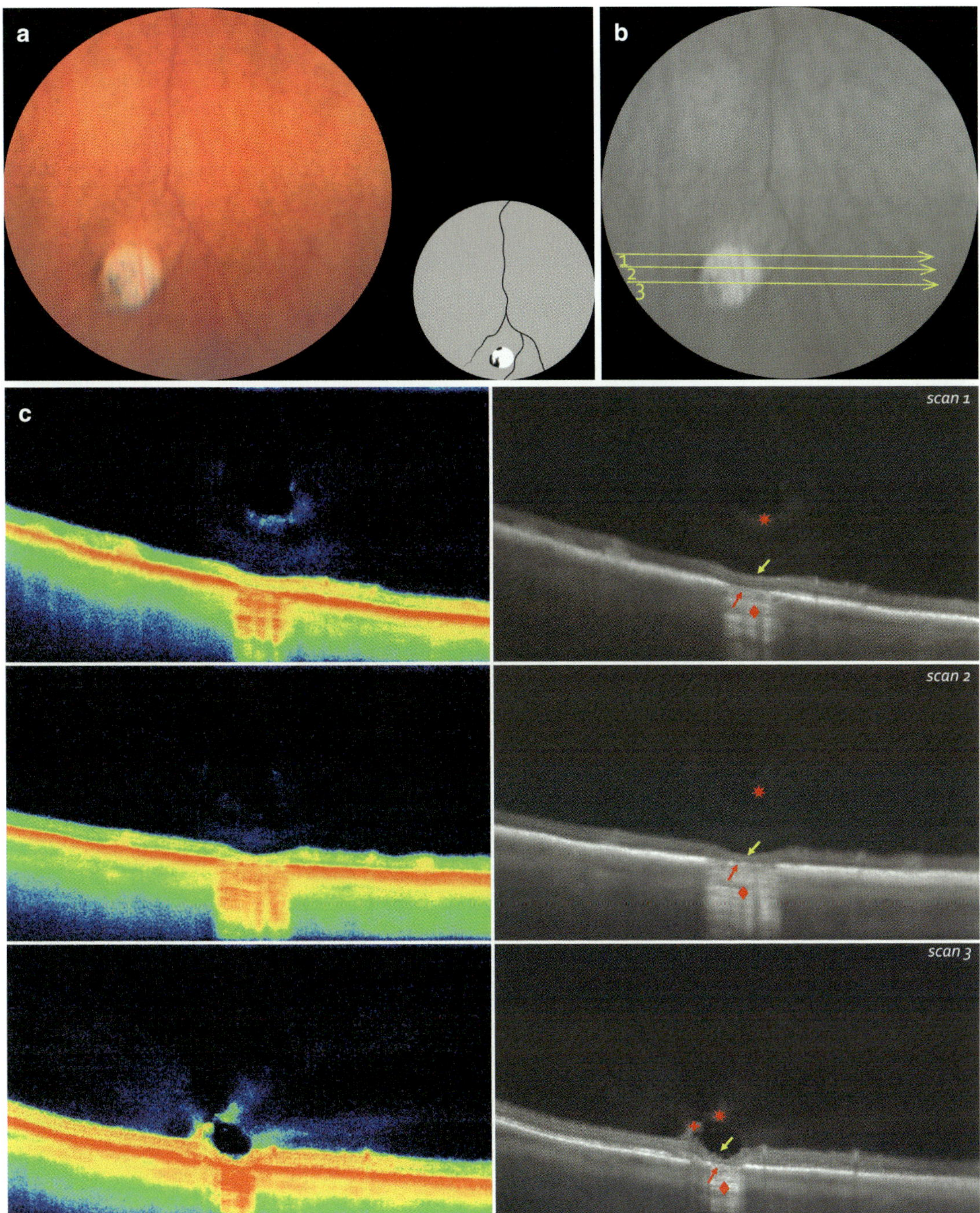

Fig. 5.40 (**a**) Vitreoretinal tuft with focal pigment epithelium atrophy. (**b**) Lines indicate OCT-scanning direction. (**c**) OCT-scanning results according to the *lines* direction in (**b**)

Case 41. Cystic Retinal Tuft

A 37-year-old female patient with low hyperopia presented with a 1-month history of floaters affecting her left eye.

Ophthalmoscopic Findings (Fig. 5.41a, b)

Two focal areas of hyperpigmentation are observed in the mid-periphery of the temporal quadrant of the left eye. The lesions are gray and elongated.

OCT Scan Description (Fig. 5.41c)

Scan 1 The retinal surface is smooth, the layers of neurosensory retina are well distinguished. Pigment epithelium is dense and has increased reflectivity.

Scan 2 Vitreoretinal adhesions change the retinal surface. There is a hyporeflective cavity in the neurosensory retina. The reflectivity of the pigment epithelium and choroid is decreased.

Scan 3 Retinal surface remains irregular because of dense and elevated area of neuroepithelium with dense pigment epithelium at the sides.

Scan 4 Retinal surface is irregular because of traction area with a hyporeflective cavity. The neuroepithelial layers are indistinguishable. Multiple intraretinal hyporeflective cavities on both sides of the elevation separate the neurosensory retina into the inner and outer layers.

OCT Scan Details (Fig. 5.41c)

✹ Vitreoretinal adhesion and traction site

⬏ Elevated and dense neurosensory retina

⬈ Dense area of pigment epithelium

▲ Decreased reflectivity of the choroid at the level of vitreoretinal adhesion

○ Intraretinal hyporeflective cavity in the outer neurosensory layers at the level of vitreoretinal adhesion

✚ Multiple intraretinal hyporeflective cavities between the inner and outer layers of the neurosensory retina

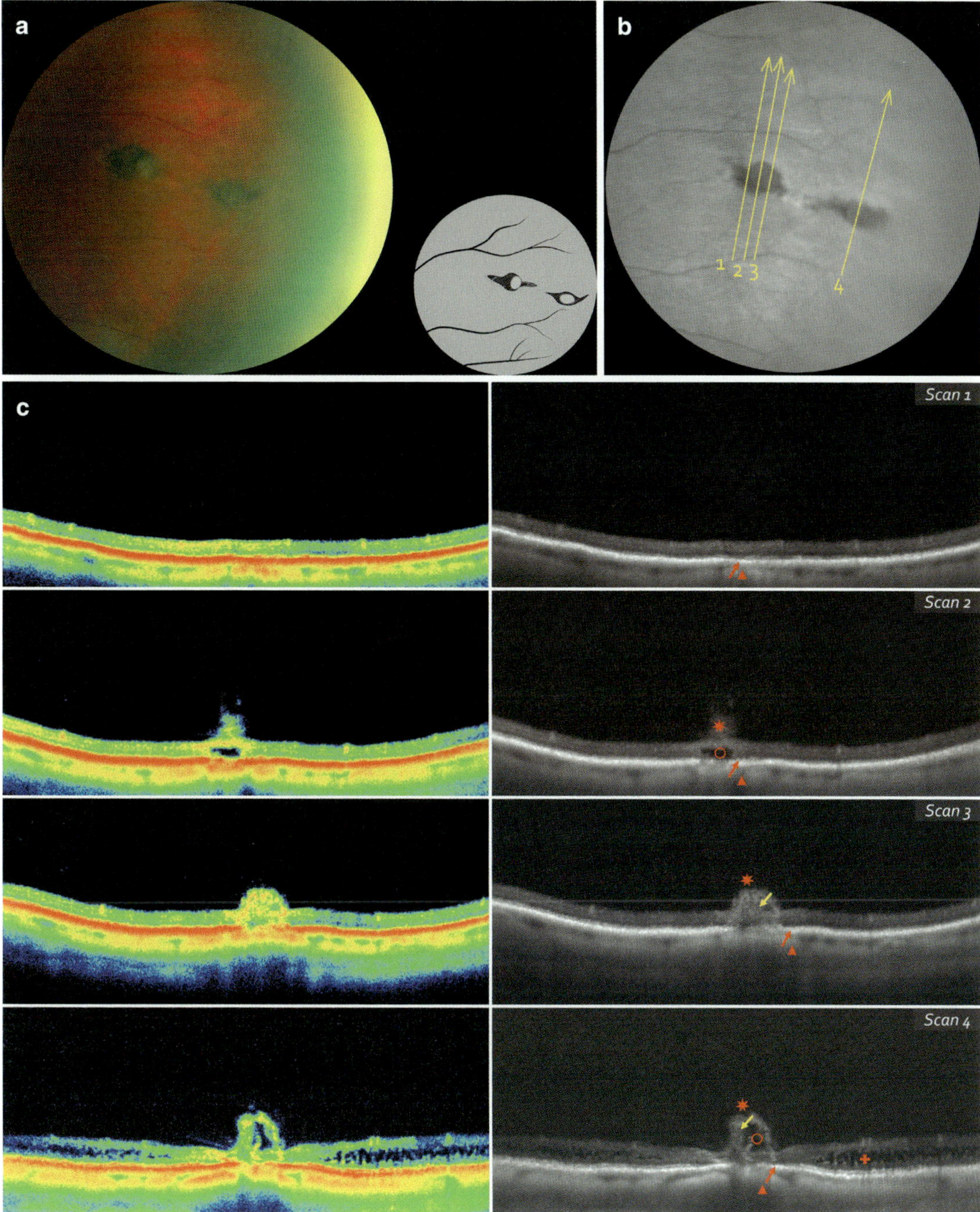

Fig. 5.41 (**a**) Cystic vitreoretinal tufts. (**b**) *Lines* indicate OCT-scanning direction. (**c**) OCT-scanning results according to the *lines* direction in (**b**)

Case 42. Retinal Tuft with Shallow Retinal Detachment

A 61-year-old female patient with moderate myopia and partial posterior vitreous detachment presented with a 1-week history of floaters affecting her left eye.

Ophthalmoscopic Findings (Fig. 5.42a, b)

An irregular hyperpigmented area of pigment epithelium with blurred borders is observed between two retinal vessels in the mid-periphery of the inferotemporal quadrant of the left eye. The retina in the center and at the edges of the lesion is gray and elevated.

OCT Scan Description (Fig. 5.42c, d)

The retinal profile is elevated by traction of the posterior hyaloid membrane. There is a shallow retinal detachment with hyporeflective content and large, merging hyporeflective cavities within the elevation. The elevated area of dense retina decreases choroidal reflectivity. The pigment epithelium is partially destroyed along the degeneration border, which makes the choroid hyperreflective.

OCT Scan Details (Fig. 5.42c, d)

✳ Vitreoretinal adhesion and traction

◣ Elevated dense inner layers of the neurosensory retina with irregular reflectivity

✚ Large intraretinal cavity filled with hyporeflective fluid separating the inner and outer neurosensory layers

○ Shallow detachment of the neurosensory retina

➚ Pigment epithelium and photoreceptor layer destruction

◆ Increased choroidal reflectivity at the level of the pigment epithelium destruction

▲ Decreased choroidal reflectivity at the level of the retinal elevation

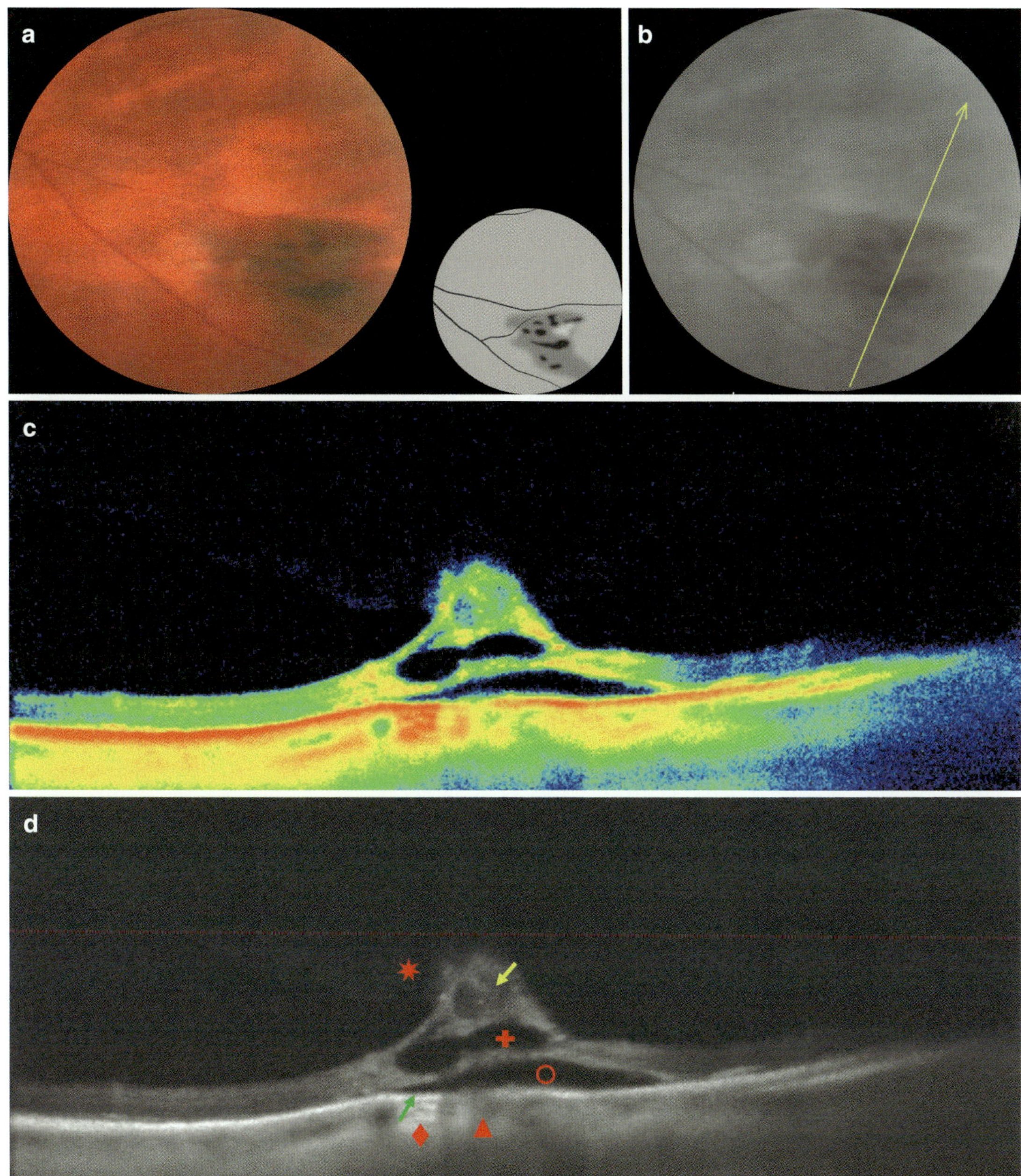

Fig. 5.42 (**a**) Retinal tuft with shallow retinal detachment. (**b**) *Line* indicates OCT-scanning direction. (**c, d**) OCT-scanning results according to the *line* direction in (**b**)

Case 43. Granular Retinal Tuft ("Granular Tails")

A 45-year-old mildly myopic female patient presented with a 3-month history of flashes of light affecting her right eye. The patient had a car accident 1 year prior to this presentation but was not referred to an ophthalmologist.

Ophthalmoscopic Findings (Fig. 5.43a, b)

A large area of preretinal fibrosis closely adherent to the retina is observed in the midperiphery of the inferior quadrant of the right eye. The lesion is gray, irregular, and clearly outlined.

OCT Scan Description (Fig. 5.43c, d)

The retinal profile is altered by elevated area of neuroepithelium with vitreoretinal adhesion. A hyporeflective intraretinal cavity is observed within the lesion, causing a decrease in choroidal reflectivity. Layers of the neuroepithelium and pigment epithelium cannot be distinguished. The pigment epithelium is destructed, and choroid is hyperreflective along the edge of the lesion.

OCT Scan Details (Fig. 5.43c, d)

- Elevated and dense neurosensory retina

- Vitreoretinal adhesion and traction

- A large intraretinal hyporeflective cavity separating the inner and outer neurosensory layers

- Pigment epithelium and photoreceptor layer destruction

- Increased choroidal reflectivity at the level of the pigment epithelium destruction

- Decreased choroidal reflectivity at level of the dense elevation of the neurosensory retina

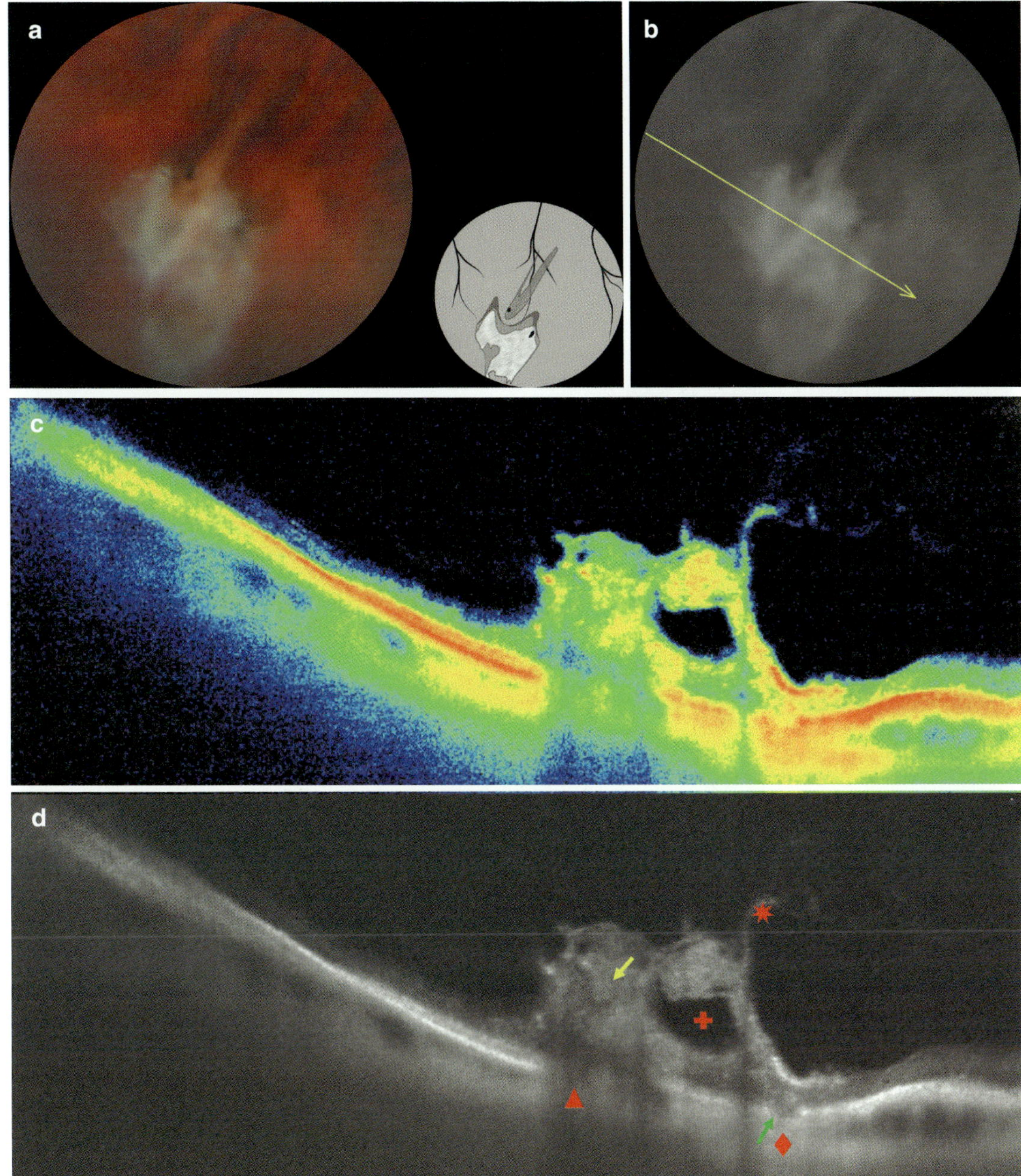

Fig. 5.43 (**a**) Granular retinal tuft. (**b**) *Line* indicates OCT-scanning direction. (**c, d**) OCT-scanning results according to the *line* direction in (**b**)

Case 44. Retinal Tuft with Areas of Chorioretinal Atrophy

An asymptomatic emmetropic 50-year-old male patient came for a routine examination.

Ophthalmoscopic Findings (Fig. 5.44a, b)

Three irregular whitish areas of pigment epithelium atrophy are observed in the mid-periphery of the superotemporal quadrant of the right eye. The lesions are clearly outlined, with retinal vessels observed within them. An irregular gray area of fibrosis with blurry borders is seen between the lesions.

OCT Scan Description (Fig. 5.44c, d)

The retinal surface is irregular because of the large elevated area of vitreoretinal adhesion. In the center of the adhesion there are multiple irregular intraretinal cavities filled with hyporeflective fluid, and multiple hyperreflective deposits. Vitreous adhesions are seen at the borders of the elevated area. Laterally, there is an atrophic area of pigment epithelium that casts a hyperreflective comet-tail shadow and an area of thinned neuroepithelium.

OCT Scan Details (Fig. 5.44c, d)

* Elevated neurosensory retina at the site of vitreoretinal adhesion

* Intraretinal hyporeflective cavities in the elevated neurosensory retina

* Pigment epithelium destruction

* Dense areas of the pigment epithelium

* Increased choroidal reflectivity at the level of the pigment epithelium destruction

* Decreased choroidal reflectivity at the level of dense areas of the pigment epithelium

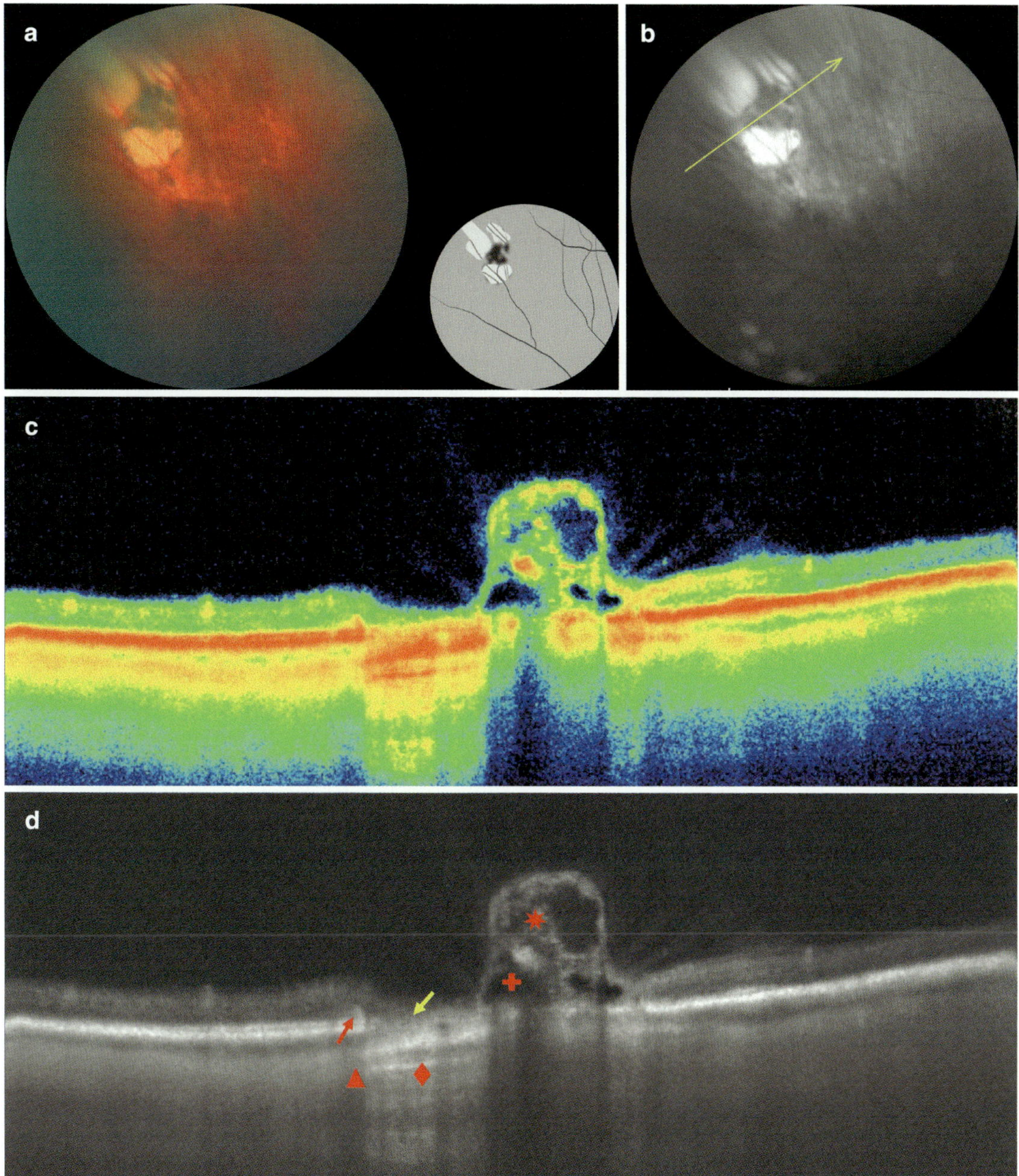

Fig. 5.44 (**a**) Retinal tuft surrounded by areas of chorioretinal atrophy. (**b**) *Line* indicates OCT-scanning direction. (**c, d**) OCT-scanning results according to the *line* direction in (**b**)

Peripheral Retinal Tears

Isolated peripheral retinal tear (Table 5.6) is a deep defect in the sensory retina. Isolated tears are considered the most severe retinal degeneration because of a high risk of rhegmatogenous retinal detachment (2.9–18 %) [8, 36, 37]. The prevalence of isolated retinal tears is 9–12 % in general population [38, 39]. Flap tears with vitreous traction are associated with retinal detachment in 33–55 % of cases [6].

Isolated peripheral lesions are subdivided into retinal tears or retinal holes [13]. Round retinal hole is a result of atrophic changes in the neurosensory retina, whereas retinal tear is secondary to vitreous traction [3, 17, 30]. Retinal tears are caused by traction at the sites of vitreoretinal adhesion that often occurs in acute posterior vitreous detachment. Retinal tears are reported to occur in eyes with PVD in 8.2–47.6 % of cases [40]. There are several types of isolated peripheral retinal tears: retinal holes, flap tears, operculated tears, and ora tears [8, 13, 41]. The frequency of flap tears in idiopathic intraocular haemorrhage and in PVD was reported to be 70 % and 15 %, respectively [3].

Prophylactic laser treatment is indicated in all cases of retinal dialysis and flap tears, less frequently performed in operculated tears, and is usually not performed for atrophic retinal holes [17]. According to some experts, symptomatic tears are associated with the highest risk of rhegmatogenous retinal detachment and should always be treated surgically [39, 42, 43].

Symptomatic retinal tears include tears with persistent vitreous traction (horseshoe or flap tears), which are an indication for immediate prophylactic treatment, and tears without traction (operculated tears), which do not require immediate prophylactic treatment [6]. We would recommend to follow recommendations of the American Academy of Ophthalmology for laser coagulation in retinal tears adapted by Brinton and Wilkinson in Table 5.5 [6].

The most common prophylactic treatment is transpupillary retinopexy, in which two to five rows of confluent laser burns are placed around the lesion. The pulse energy depends on the retinal pigmentation around the tear [13, 39, 44]. The recommended spot size is 200 μm, with exposure time 0.1–0.2 s [13].

Saurabh et al. proposed a different approach in treating retinal tears with large confluent laser spots (up to 3 mm) to ensure complete closure of the tear. The following parameters were proposed: power – 800–1,200 mW, spot size – 1.2–3.0 mm, exposure time – 5–10 sec. It is noteworthy that the size of the chorioretinal scar did not correlate with the pigmentation [45].

Table 5.5 Guidelines for prophylactic laser photocoagulation

Type of break	With symptoms	Asymptomatic			
		No risk factors	High myopia	Fellow eye[a]	Pseudophakia[b]
Dialysis	Always[c]	Always[c]	Always[c]	Always[c]	Always[c]
Subclinical retinal detachment	Always[c]	Sometimes	Frequently	Frequently	Frequently
Horseshoe tear	Always[c]	Sometimes	Sometimes	Frequently	Frequently
Operculated tear	Sometimes	No	Rarely	Rarely	Rarely
Atrophic break	Rarely	Rarely	Rarely	Rarely	Rarely

Adapted version of table from Brinton and Wilkinson [6]. Reproduced with the permission of Oxford University Press. Taken from original version in *Precursors of Rhegmatogenous Retinal Detachment in Adults*. San Francisco, CA: American Academy of Ophthalmology; 2008, by Permission of American Academy of Ophthalmology Retina Panel. Preferred Practice Pattern®Guidelines. Available at: www.aao.org/ppp
[a]Applies to patients who have had a retinal detachment in the other eye
[b]Patients with pseudophakia, aphakia, and prior to cataract surgery
[c]Exceptions may apply

Table 5.6 Diagram of peripheral retinal degenerations

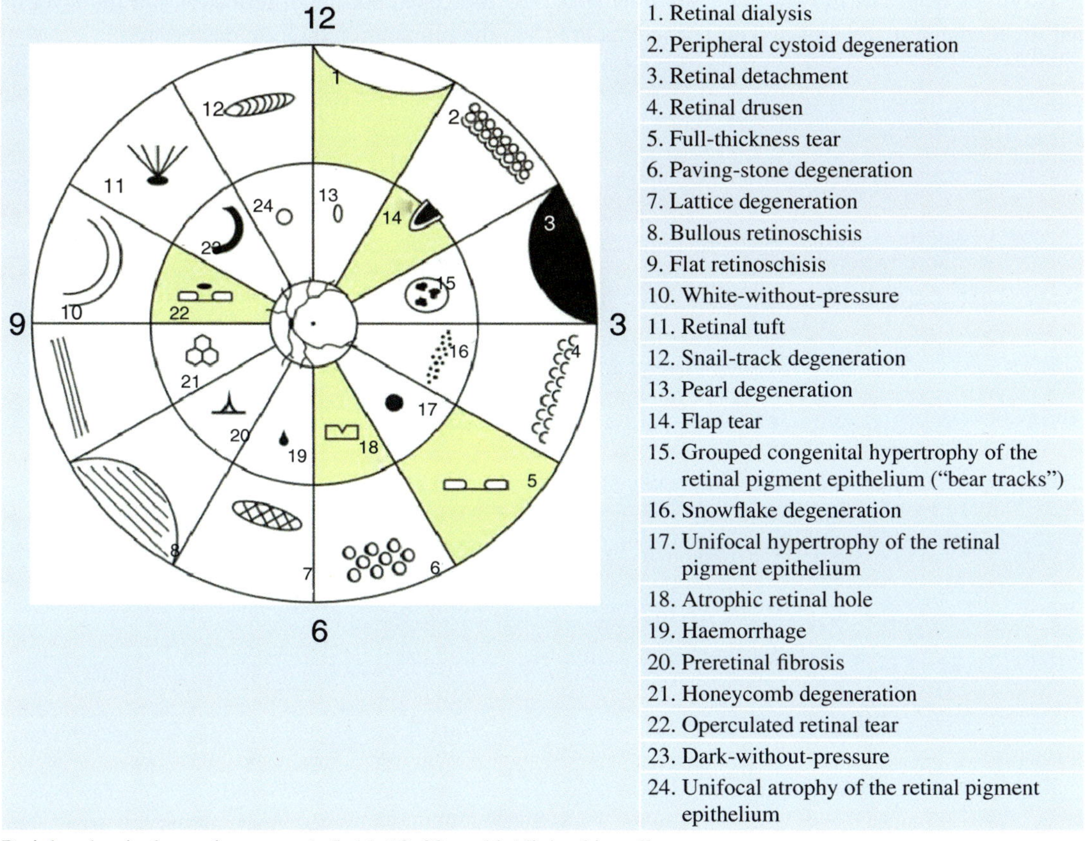

1. Retinal dialysis
2. Peripheral cystoid degeneration
3. Retinal detachment
4. Retinal drusen
5. Full-thickness tear
6. Paving-stone degeneration
7. Lattice degeneration
8. Bullous retinoschisis
9. Flat retinoschisis
10. White-without-pressure
11. Retinal tuft
12. Snail-track degeneration
13. Pearl degeneration
14. Flap tear
15. Grouped congenital hypertrophy of the retinal pigment epithelium ("bear tracks")
16. Snowflake degeneration
17. Unifocal hypertrophy of the retinal pigment epithelium
18. Atrophic retinal hole
19. Haemorrhage
20. Preretinal fibrosis
21. Honeycomb degeneration
22. Operculated retinal tear
23. Dark-without-pressure
24. Unifocal atrophy of the retinal pigment epithelium

Peripheral retinal tears in sectors 1, 5, 14, 18, 22 are highlighted in yellow

Case 45. Isolated Tear with Shallow Retinal Detachment

A 22-year-old male patient with moderate myopia presented with low vision in his right eye.

Ophthalmoscopic Findings (Fig. 5.45a, b)

A round, bright red full-thickness tear with clear borders is observed in the far-periphery of the inferior quadrant of the right eye. The surrounding retina is gray and elevated by shallow (subclinical) retinal detachment.

OCT Scan Description (Fig. 5.45c, d)

There is a full-thickness tear of the neurosensory retina in the center of the scan with shallow retinal detachment at the edges. The tear edges are thickened, with multiple small intraretinal hyporeflective cavities.

OCT Scan Details (Fig. 5.45c, d)

◖ Full-thickness tear of the neurosensory retina

✚ Detached neurosensory retina at the tear edges, with multiple hyporeflective cavities

◯ Hyporeflective space of the shallow neurosensory detachment

◤ Pigment epithelium destruction within the tear

◆ Increased choroidal reflectivity at the level of the pigment epithelium destruction

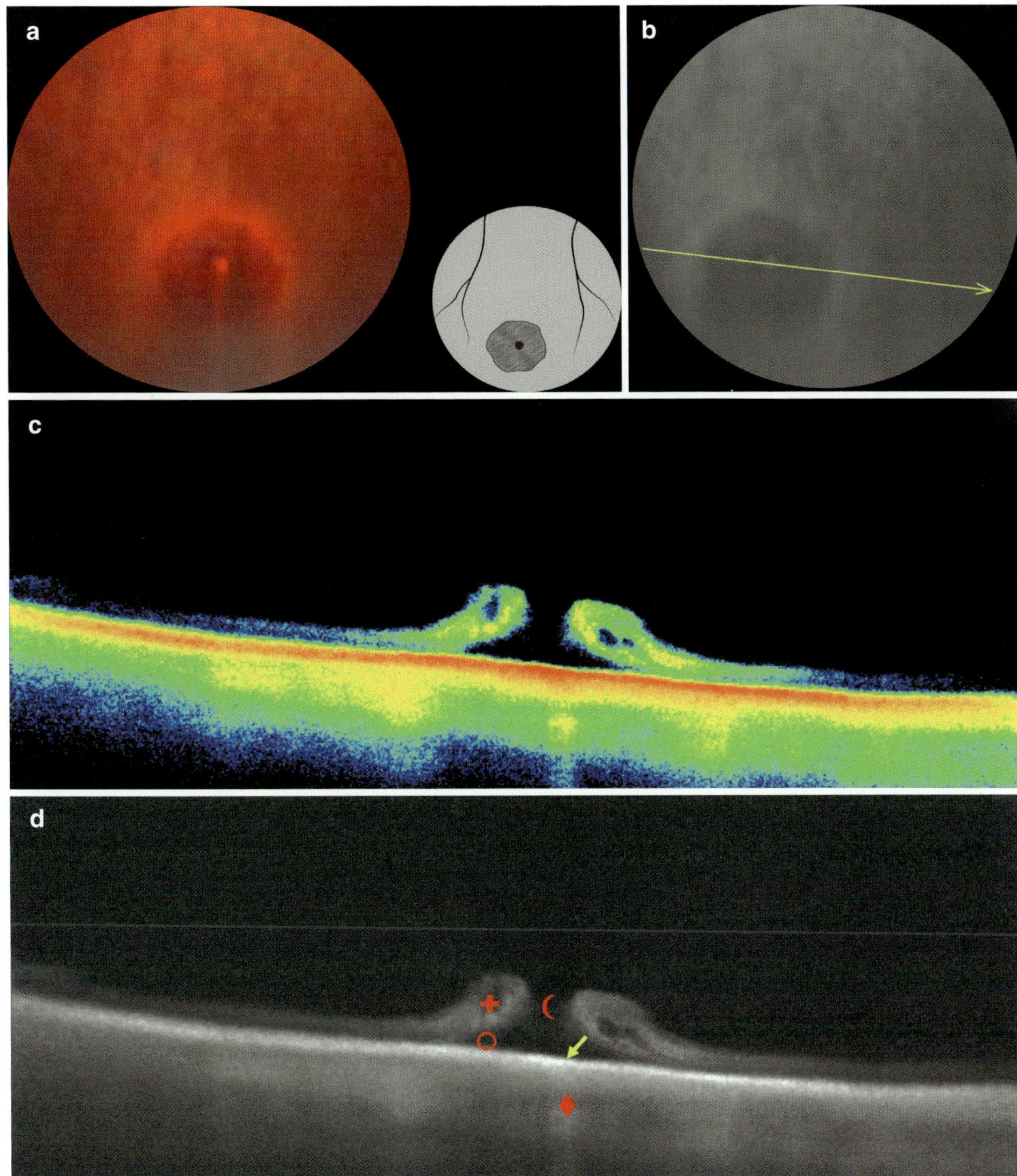

Fig. 5.45 (**a**) Isolated retinal tear with shallow detachment. (**b**) *Line* indicates OCT-scanning direction. (**c, d**) OCT-scanning results according to the *line* direction in (**b**)

Case 46. Isolated Retinal Tear with a Demarcation Line

A 69-year-old female patient with low hyperopia, early-stage cataract and partial posterior vitreous detachment presented with a 1-month history of floaters affecting her right eye.

Ophthalmoscopic Findings (Fig. 5.46a, b)
A round-shaped, full-thickness tear with well-defined borders is observed in the superotemporal segment of the mid-peripheral retina of the right eye. The retina in the center of the tear is bright red, with whitish deposits. The surrounding retina is gray and spongy, with a hyperpigmented demarcation ring. Gray operculum is seen in the vitreous.

OCT Scan Description (Fig. 5.46c, d)
The retinal surface is irregular because of the full-thickness tear. The pigment epithelium is thickened at the tear margins, and there is a shallow neurosensory detachment with multiple hyporeflective intraretinal cavities.

OCT Scan Details (Fig. 5.46c, d)

(Full-thickness tear of the neurosensory retina

+ Hyporeflective intraretinal cavities in the tear margins

O Shallow neurosensory detachment at the edges of the tear

Pigment epithelium destruction at the tear edges

Increased choroidal reflectivity at the level of the pigment epithelium destruction

Dense areas of pigment epithelium along the borders of its destruction

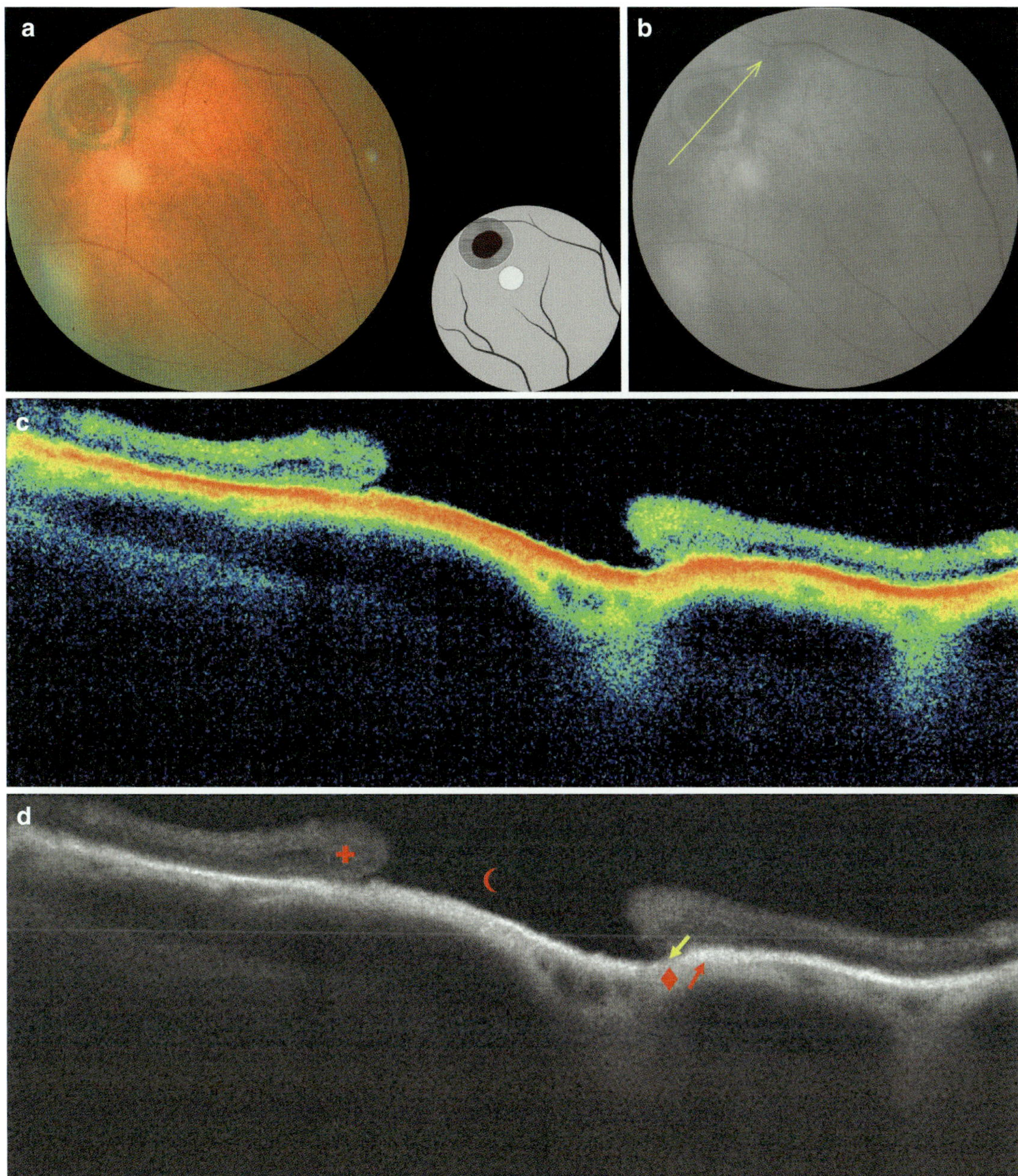

Fig. 5.46 (**a**) Demarcated retinal tear with an operculum in the vitreous. (**b**) *Line* indicates OCT-scanning direction. (**c, d**) OCT-scanning results according to the *line* direction in (**b**)

Case 47. Operculated Retinal Tear with Shallow Retinal Detachment

A 77-year-old female patient with mild hyperopia and early-stage cataract of her left eye presented with complaints of flashes of light and floaters affecting her left eye.

Ophthalmoscopic Findings (Fig. 5.47a, b)

A bright red full-thickness tear is observed in the mid-periphery of the inferotemporal quadrant of the left eye. There is a grayish operculum in the vitreous over the tear. The tear is surrounded by the atrophic pigment epithelium, with pigment clumps of various shapes. The retina around the tear has a spongy appearance.

OCT Scan Description (Fig. 5.47c, d)

The retinal surface is irregular because of the full-thickness tear. There is a hyperreflective operculum adherent to the posterior hyaloid membrane at the vitreous level. At the edges of the tear, the pigment epithelium is dense, and there is a shallow neurosensory detachment.

OCT Scan Details (Fig. 5.47c, d)

✳ Vitreoretinal adhesion and traction

➶ A moderately reflective operculum floating in the vitreous, with a shadow effect on the choroid

☾ Full-thickness tear of the neurosensory retina

✛ Detached neurosensory retina at the tear margin

◯ Hyporeflective space under the shallow neurosensory detachment

➶ Areas of thick and spongy pigment epithelium at the edges of the shallow neurosensory detachment

◆ Increased choroidal reflectivity at the level of the spongy pigment epithelium

▲ Decreased choroidal reflectivity at the level of the floating operculum

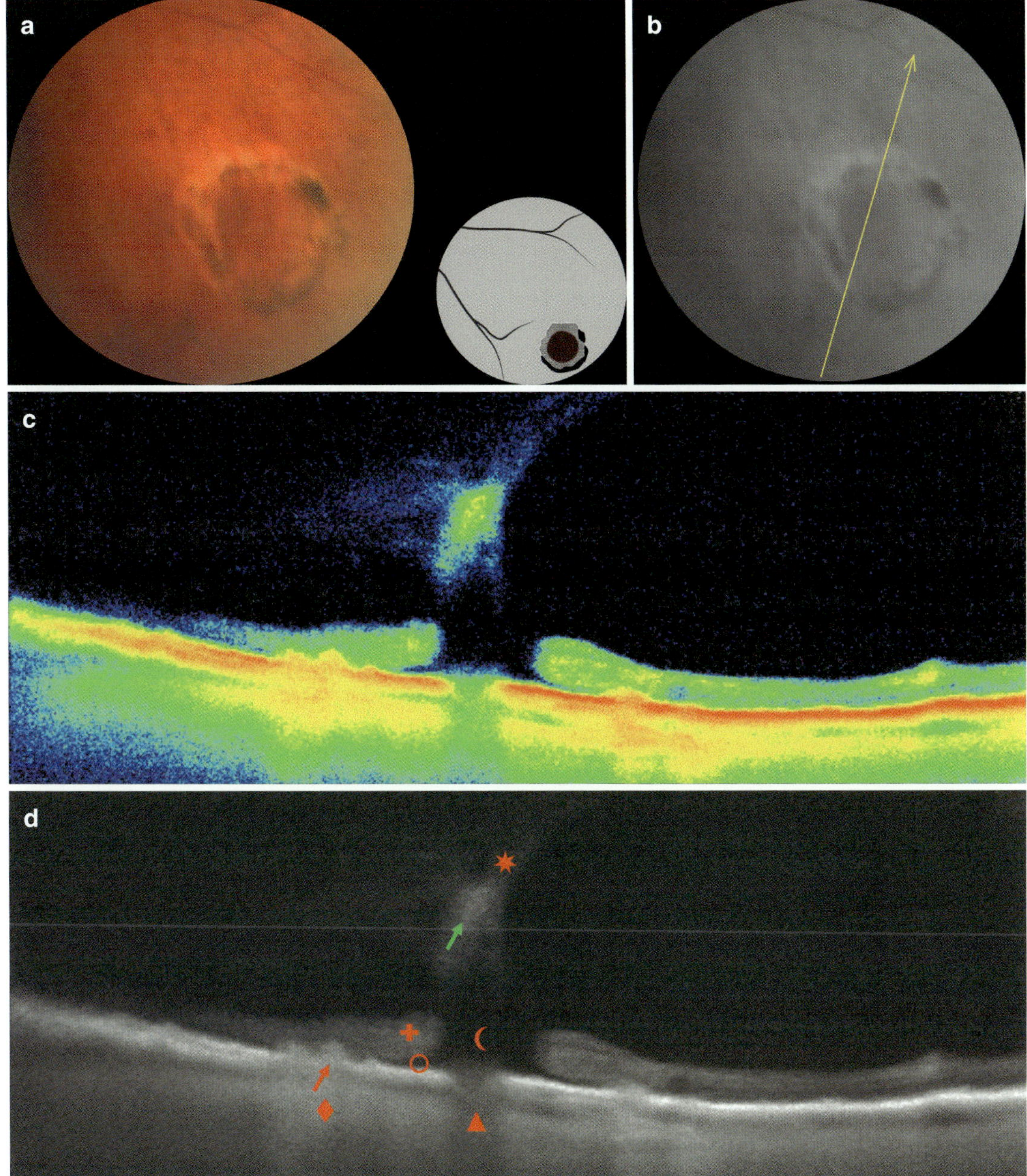

Fig. 5.47 (**a**) Operculated retinal tear with shallow retinal detachment. (**b**) *Line* indicates OCT-scanning direction. (**c, d**) OCT-scanning results according to the *line* direction in (**b**)

Case 48. Double Tear with Shallow Retinal Detachment

A 29-year-old male patient with moderate hyperopia and posterior vitreous detachment presented with complaints of sudden floaters in his right eye.

Ophthalmoscopic Findings (Fig. 5.48a, b)

Two well-defined bright red full-thickness retinal tears are observed along the retinal vessel in the mid-periphery of the inferior quadrant of the right eye. Both tears are surrounded by clearly outlined elevated grayish areas with subretinal fluid, i.e. shallow (subclinical) retinal detachment.

OCT Scan Description (Fig. 5.48c, d)

The retinal surface is irregular because of two full-thickness neurosensory tears. A retinal vessel is seen between the tears in the intact neuroepithelium. A shallow neuroepithelium detachment surrounds the tears. There are two vitreous fibrotic folds of moderate reflectivity at the edges of the lesion, that cause traction. The neuroepithelium contains small cylindrical cavities with hyporeflective content in the traction area. The pigment epithelium is intact.

OCT Scan Details (Fig. 5.48c, d)

✳ Vitreoretinal adhesion and traction

☾ Full-thickness tear of the neurosensory retina

✛ Small intraretinal cavities with hyporeflective content

◯ Shallow detachment of the neurosensory retina

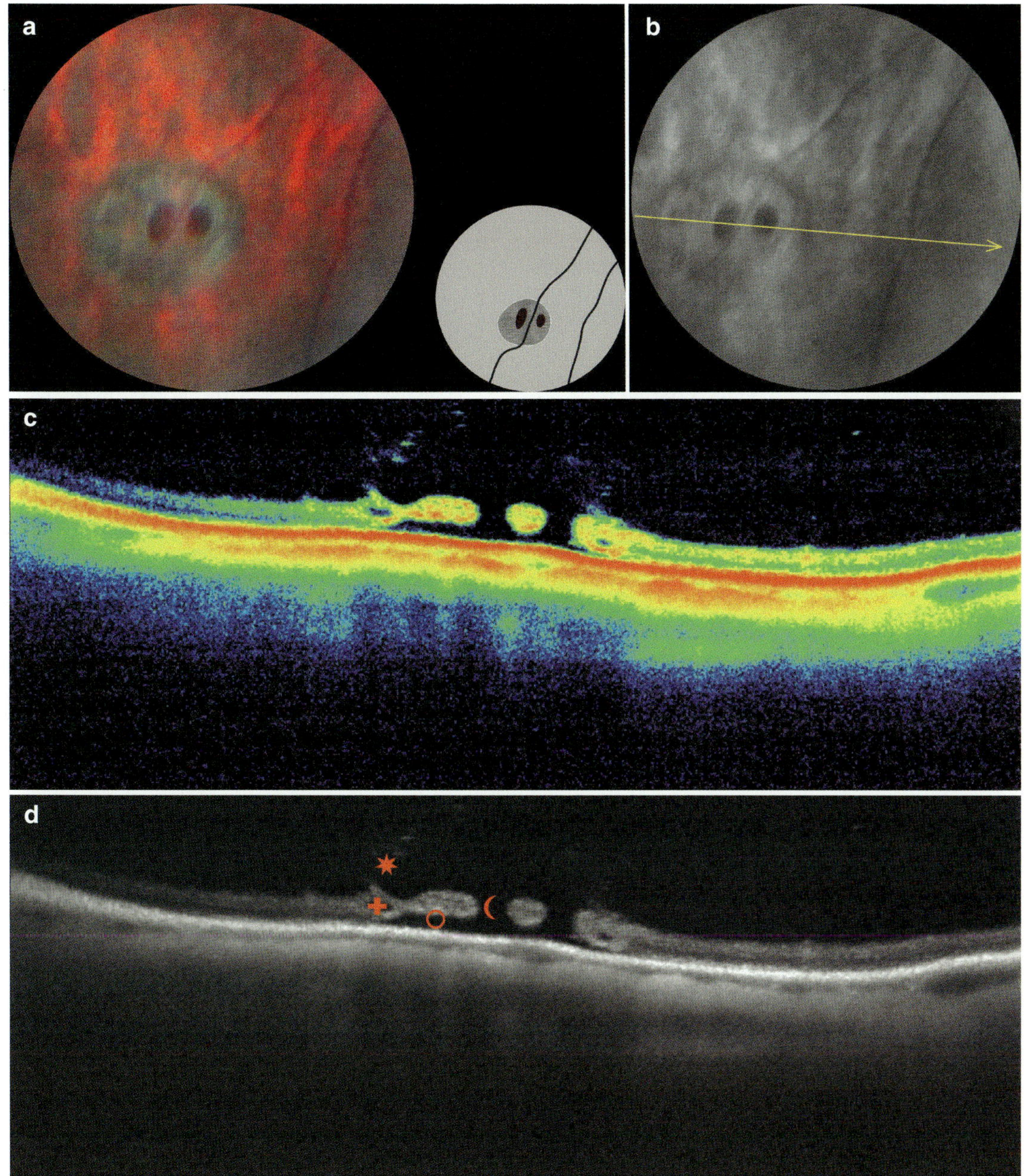

Fig. 5.48 (**a**) Double tear with shallow retinal detachment. (**b**) *Line* indicates OCT-scanning direction. (**c, d**) OCT-scanning results according to the *line* direction in (**b**)

Case 49. Multiple Tears with Shallow Retinal Detachment

A 24-year-old male patient with moderate myopia, incomplete posterior vitreous detachment, presented with a 1-year history of lightnings and floaters affecting his left eye and complaints about low vision. Examination revealed multiple tears with shallow retinal detachment. The patient's condition improved after laser photocoagulation.

Ophthalmoscopic Findings (Fig. 5.49a, b)

Four full-thickness round-shaped retinal tears are observed over a shallow retinal detachment in the far-periphery of the inferotemporal quadrant of the left eye. The retina is spongy and gray at the detachment level. All retinal tears with shallow detachment are limited by three to four rows of pigmented laser spots. The laser spots are clearly seen.

OCT Scan Description (Fig. 5.49c)

Scan 1 The neurosensory retina is detached. Vitreoretinal adhesion with traction is observed at the apex of detachment.

Scan 2 Shallow neuroepithelium detachment, a full-thickness retinal tear, and isolated areas of vitreoretinal adhesions and tractions are observed. Areas of pigment epithelium are destructed and cause hyperreflectivity of the underlying tissues with the scanning beam easily passing through.

OCT Scan Details (Fig. 5.49c)

✳ Vitreoretinal adhesion and traction, with layers of moderate reflectivity in the vitreous

➕ Detached neurosensory retina around the tear, with isolated vitreoretinal adhesions

☾ Full-thickness tear of the neurosensory retina

○ Hyporeflective space of the detached neurosensory retina

◤ Areas of pigment epithelium destruction within the detached neurosensory retina

◆ Increased choroidal reflectivity at the pigment epithelium destruction level

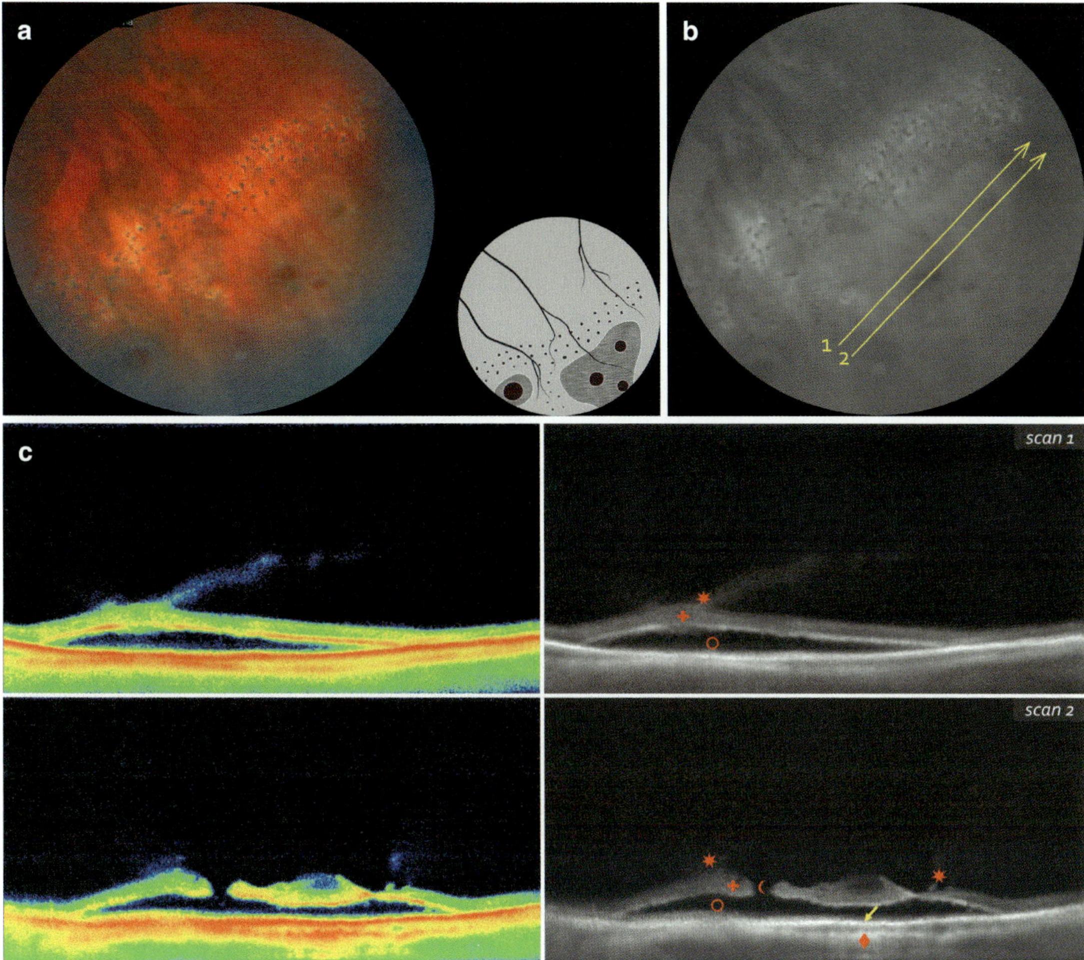

Fig. 5.49 (**a**) Multiple tears with shallow neuroepithelium detachment. (**b**) *Lines* indicate OCT-scanning direction. (**c**) OCT-scanning results according to the *lines* direction in (**b**)

Case 50. Multiple Isolated Retinal Tears

An 18-year-old male patient with mild myopia and partial posterior vitreous detachment presented with a 1-week history of floaters and flashes of light during eye movements.

Ophthalmoscopic Findings (Fig. 5.50a, b)

Three round-shaped full-thickness retinal tears with well-defined borders are observed in the far-periphery of the inferotemporal quadrant of the left eye. The retina around the tears is gray and elevated because of shallow (subclinical) retinal detachment.

OCT Scan Description (Fig. 5.50c)

Scan 1 A full-thickness tear of the neurosensory retina is observed in the center of the scan. There is a shallow retinal detachment at the edges of the tear with the retina elevated by vitreous adhesion and traction. Hyporeflective cavities are observed in the detached retinal tissue. At the level of the tear, there is an isolated hyperreflective zone, with adjacent area of pigment epithelium destruction that makes choroid hyperreflective.

Scan 2 Another full-thickness neurosensory retina tear is observed, with mild vitreoretinal adhesions at the side. Area of pigment epithelium is destructed at the level of the tear, and the choroid is hyperreflective.

Scan 3 A third full-thickness tear with flat retinal detachment and vitreoretinal adhesion with traction at the edge is observed. The neurosensory retina is dense and hyperreflective at the site of adhesion. Area of pigment epithelium is destructed at the level of the tear, and choroid is hyperreflective.

OCT Scan Details (Fig. 5.50c)

✳ Vitreoretinal adhesions and tractions

☾ Full-thickness tear of the neurosensory retina

↗ Area of dense neurosensory retina elevated by vitreoretinal traction

○ Hyporeflective space of the shallow retinal detachment

+ Isolated hyporeflective cavities at the base of the shallow detachment and at the border of the full-thickness tear

↙ Isolated hyperreflective area on the pigment epithelium

↗ Pigment epithelium destruction in the area of the full-thickness tear

◆ Increased choroidal reflectivity at the level of the pigment epithelium destruction

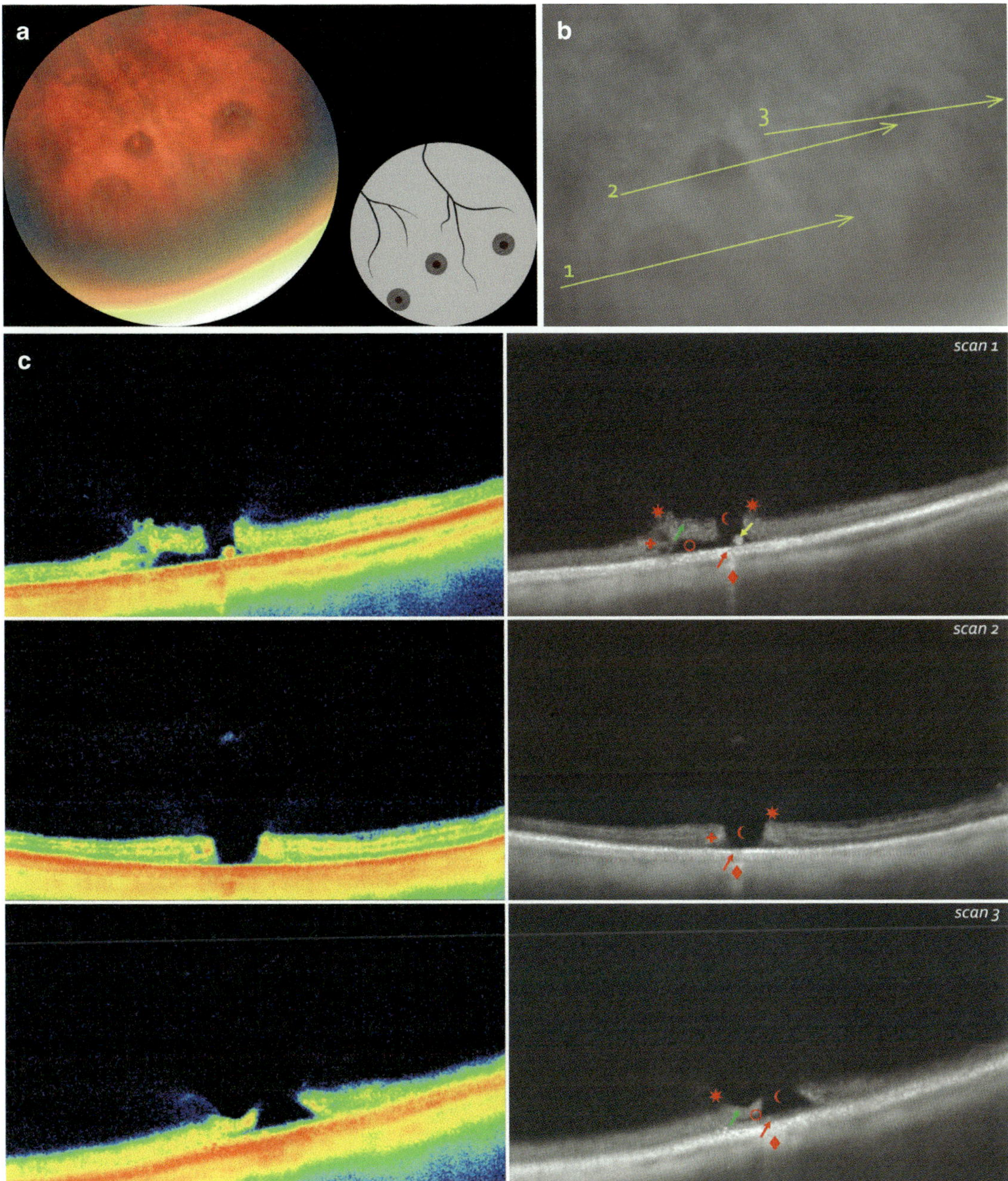

Fig. 5.50 (**a**) Multiple isolated retinal tears. (**b**) *Lines* indicate OCT-scanning direction. (**c**) OCT-scanning results according to the *lines* direction in (**b**)

Case 51. Operculated Retinal Tear and Complete Posterior Vitreous Detachment

A 62-year-old female patient with moderate myopia and complete posterior vitreous detachment presented with an 8-day history of floaters affecting her right eye.

Ophthalmoscopic Findings (Fig. 5.51a, b)

An elongated, cylindrical full-thickness retinal tear with irregular inner borders is observed in the far-periphery of the inferior quadrant of the right eye. The retina around the tear is gray-colored and spongy. A gray operculum is seen floating in the vitreous over the tear. An area of hyperpigmented pigment epithelium is on the left side of the retinal tear with no details visible (See OCT image).

OCT Scan Description (Fig. 5.51c)

Scan 1 The retinal surface is irregular because of the full-thickness tear. A hyporeflective operculum adheres to the posterior hyaloid membrane and casts a shadow over the underlying structures. There is a shallow retinal detachment at the edges of the tear. Isolated areas of dense pigment epithelium are seen within the tear. The posterior hyaloid membrane is wrinkled and detached all along the scan.

Scan 2 A large, full-thickness retinal tear with dense margins is observed. There are isolated areas of dense pigment epithelium within the tear. The posterior hyaloid membrane is wrinkled and detached all along the scan.

OCT Scan Details (Fig. 5.51c)

✳ Vitreoretinal adhesion and traction, with layers of increased reflectivity in the vitreous

↗ An operculum floating in the vitreous over the tear (a small area of neurosensory retina adhering to the vitreous)

☾ Full-thickness tear of the neurosensory retina

✚ Dense and detached neurosensory retina at the tear margins

○ Shallow neurosensory detachment at the tear margins

↗ Areas of pigment epithelium destruction within the tear and shallow detachment

◆ Increased choroidal reflectivity at the level of the pigment epithelium destruction

▲ Decreased choroidal reflectivity at the level of the floating operculum and vitreoretinal adhesion

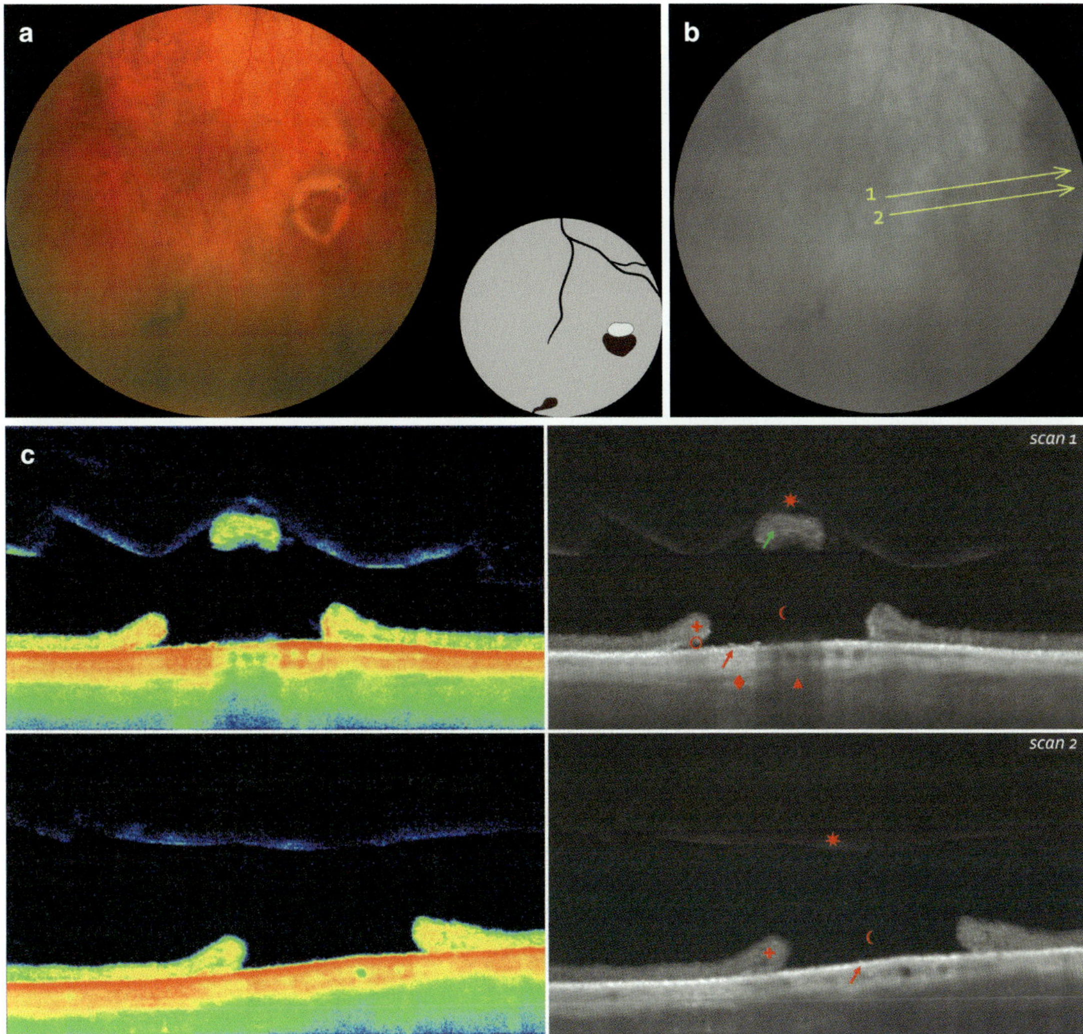

Fig. 5.51 (a) Operculated retinal tear. (b) *Lines* indicate OCT-scanning direction. (c) OCT-scanning results according to the *lines* direction in (b)

Case 52. Operculated Retinal Tear in Chorioretinal Atrophic Focus

A 78-year-old male patient with moderate myopia and early-stage cortical cataract presented with complaints of decreased visual acuity in his left eye. Differential diagnosis excluded toxoplasmosis.

Ophthalmoscopic Findings (Fig. 5.52a, b)

A large round area of pigment epithelium atrophy with well-defined borders is observed in the mid-periphery of the inferotemporal segment of the left eye. Black pigment clumps are seen in the center and along the borders of the lesion. There is a bright red, round retinal tear in the center of the lesion. An operculum is seen floating freely in the vitreous over the tear. Choroidal vessels are clearly visible through the atrophic lesion. The ocular media are opaque because of cortical cataract.

OCT Scan Description (Fig. 5.52c, d)

The retinal surface is irregular, as neuroepithelium is partially thinned and thickened, and there is a large full-thickness retinal tear. A hyperreflective operculum at the level of the tear causes a shadow effect in the underlying tissues. There is a large area of pigment epithelium atrophy with hyperreflective zones around and at the edges of the tear. Vitreoretinal adhesion and traction is observed at the tear edges.

OCT Scan Details (Fig. 5.52c, d)

Moderately reflective operculum floating in the vitreous, and shadowing the underlying tissues

Vitreoretinal adhesion and traction

Full-thickness tear of the neurosensory retina

Dense and partially detached area of the neurosensory retina

Shallow neurosensory detachment at the tear margins

Areas of dense pigment epithelium within the chorioretinal lesion

Hyporeflective area at the operculum level

Thinned and dense neurosensory retina

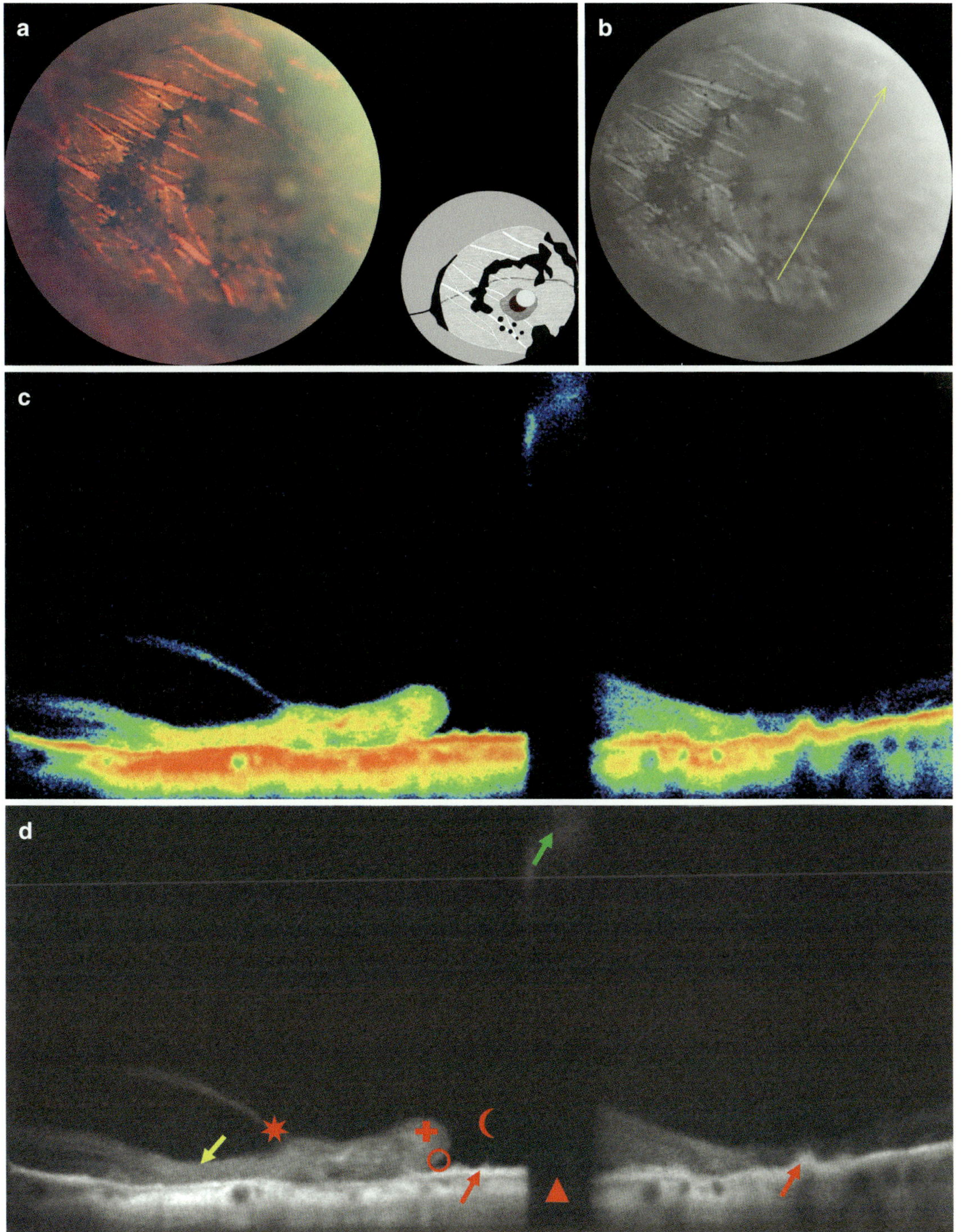

Fig. 5.52 (**a**) Chorioretinitis with an operculated retinal tear in the center. (**b**) *Line* indicates OCT-scanning direction. (**c, d**) OCT-scanning results according to the *line* direction in (**b**)

Case 53. Peripheral Retinal Tear with Honeycomb Degeneration

An asymptomatic 70-year-old female patient with low hyperopia and early-stage cortical cataract. The degeneration was found during routine examination.

Ophthalmoscopic Findings (Fig. 5.53a, b)

Multiple pigment clumps of various forms and sizes corresponding to the honeycomb degeneration are observed in the mid-periphery of the temporal quadrant of the right eye. A gray area of retinal elevation with blurred borders is visible along a retinal vessel further in the far-periphery. Due to cortical cataract, ocular media are not enough transparent and retinal layers are poorly distinguished.

OCT Scan Description (Fig. 5.53c, d)

The neurosensory retina is detached and has a full-thickness tear at the apex with considerable vitreoretinal adhesion and traction. There is a shadow effect (decrease in reflectivity) in the underlying tissues at the level of adhesion. There are areas of dense pigment epithelium within the detachment.

OCT Scan Details (Fig. 5.53c, d)

✴ Vitreoretinal adhesion and traction

☾ Full-thickness tear of the neurosensory retina

↗ The detached margin of the neurosensory retina with vitreous traction

✚ The detached margin of the neurosensory retina without traction

○ Hyporeflective space under the retinal detachment

↗ Locally dense pigment epithelium

▲ Decreased choroidal reflectivity in the area of the vitreoretinal adhesion

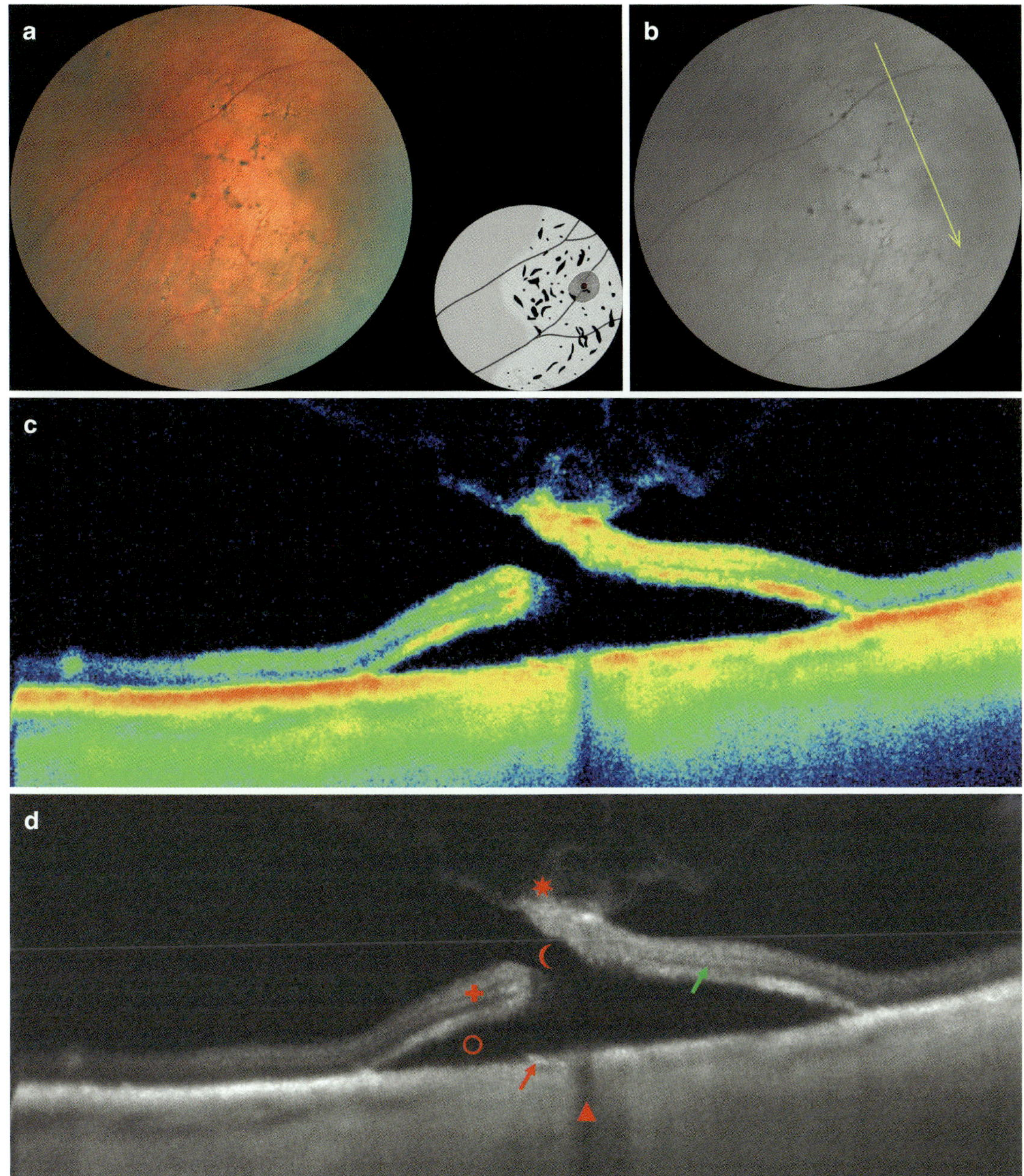

Fig. 5.53 (**a**) Retinal tear with honeycomb degeneration. (**b**) *Line* indicates OCT-scanning direction. (**c, d**) OCT-scanning results according to the *line* direction in (**b**)

Case 54. Tractional Retinal Tear in the Center of Atrophic Lesion

A 47-year-old emmetropic female patient with no symptomatic complaints came to have her reading glasses prescribed. Routine fundus examination revealed a clearly outlined atrophic lesion.

Ophthalmoscopic Findings (Fig. 5.54a, b)

An isolated oval area of pigment epithelium atrophy is observed in the mid-periphery of the inferior quadrant of the right eye. The lesion has clear borders, with pigment clumps along them. The choroid pattern is visible through the lesion. There is a retinal vessel in the nasal part of the lesion. The vitreous over the degenerative lesion is opaque.

OCT Scan Description (Fig. 5.54c)

Scans 1 and 3 Scans were performed through the upper (central) and lower (peripheral) segments of degeneration (lines 1 and 3, respectively). The retinal surface is irregular. The neurosensory retina is considerably thinned, has multiple intraretinal cavities. The pigment epithelium and photoreceptor layer are atrophic. The reflectivity of the retinal layers is increased because of atrophic changes in the pigment epithelium.

Scan 2 A full-thickness tear with vitreous traction is observed in the center of the atrophic area. Pigment epithelium and photoreceptor layer are destructed and the choroid is hyperreflective.

OCT Scan Details (Fig. 5.54c)

✳ Marked vitreoretinal adhesion and traction

✚ Multiple intraretinal cavities with hyporeflective content

➚ Pigment epithelium and photoreceptor layer destruction

◆ Increased choroidal reflectivity in the area of pigment epithelium destruction

☾ Full-thickness tear within the atrophic retina

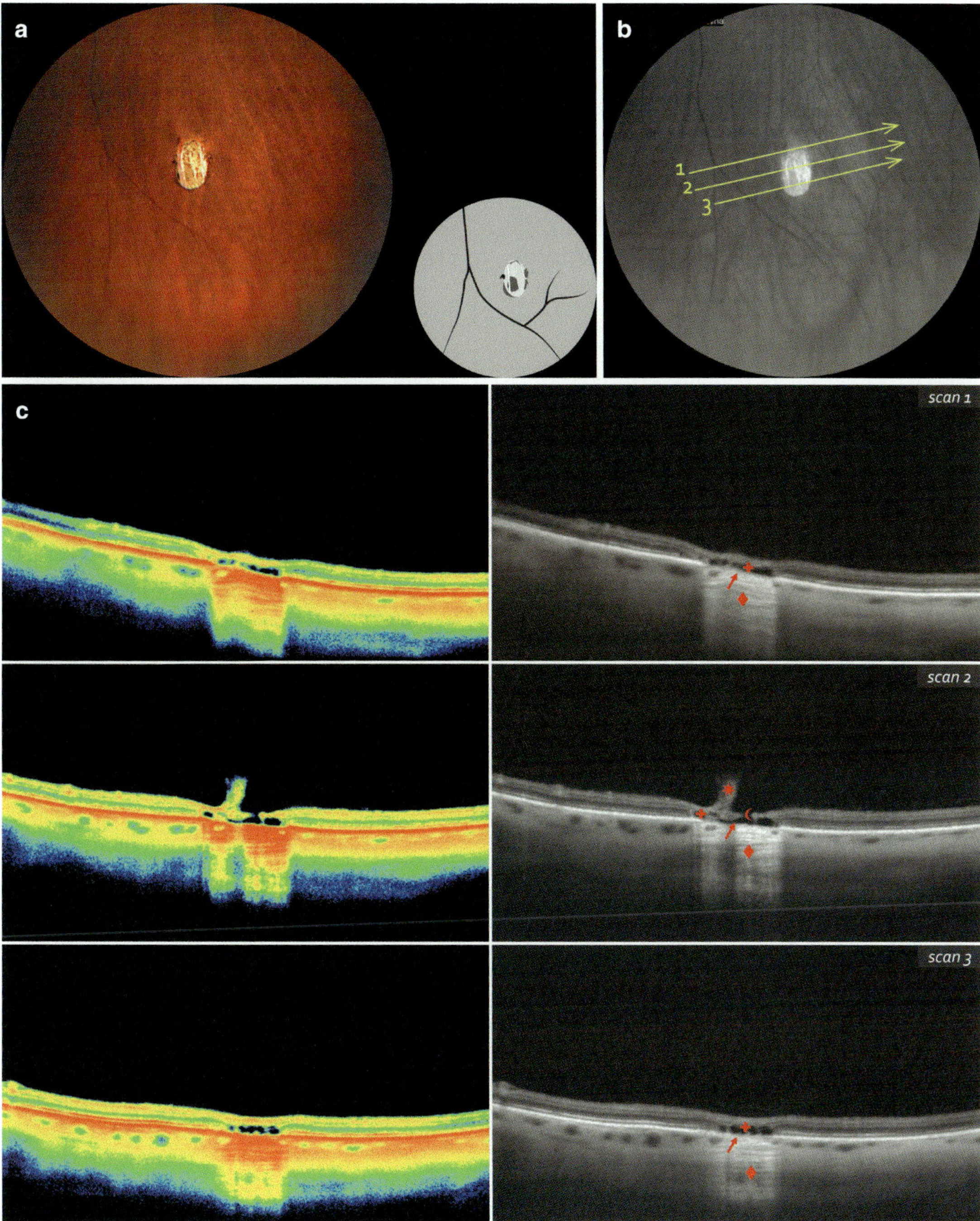

Fig. 5.54 (**a**) Tractional tear in the center of the pigment epithelium atrophy. (**b**) *Lines* indicate OCT-scanning direction. (**c**) OCT-scanning results according to the *lines* direction in (**b**)

Case 55. Operculated Retinal Tear Against Multiple Drusen

A 59-year-old female patient with partial posterior vitreous detachment presented with a 3-day history of floaters affecting her right eye.

Ophthalmoscopic Findings (Fig. 5.55a, b)

Multiple whitish hyperpigmented retinal drusen are seen in the mid- and far-periphery of the temporal quadrant of the right eye. In the mid-periphery, a bright-red full-thickness tear of the neurosensory retina is seen against the multiple peripheral drusen near the retinal vessel (at 8:30 o'clock position). A shallow (subclinical) retinal detachment is at the edges of the tear. Medially there is a gray operculum in the vitreous and a small area of retinal haemorrhage on the retinal surface.

OCT Scan Description (Fig. 5.55c, d)

A full-thickness operculated tear with shallow neurosensory detachment at the edges is observed. An operculum in the vitreous over the tear casts a hyporeflective shadow over the choroid. Pigment epithelium is partially dense and elevated.

OCT Scan Details (Fig. 5.55c, d)

↗ Free-floating operculum in the vitreous over the tear (the neurosensory retina tissue with vitreoretinal adhesion)

(Full-thickness tear of the neurosensory retina

+ Dense and detached neurosensory retina at the edges of the tear

○ Shallow neurosensory detachment at the edges of the tear

↗ Dense and elevated pigment epithelium at the edges of the shallow detachment

▲ Hyporeflective shadow of the operculum over the choroid

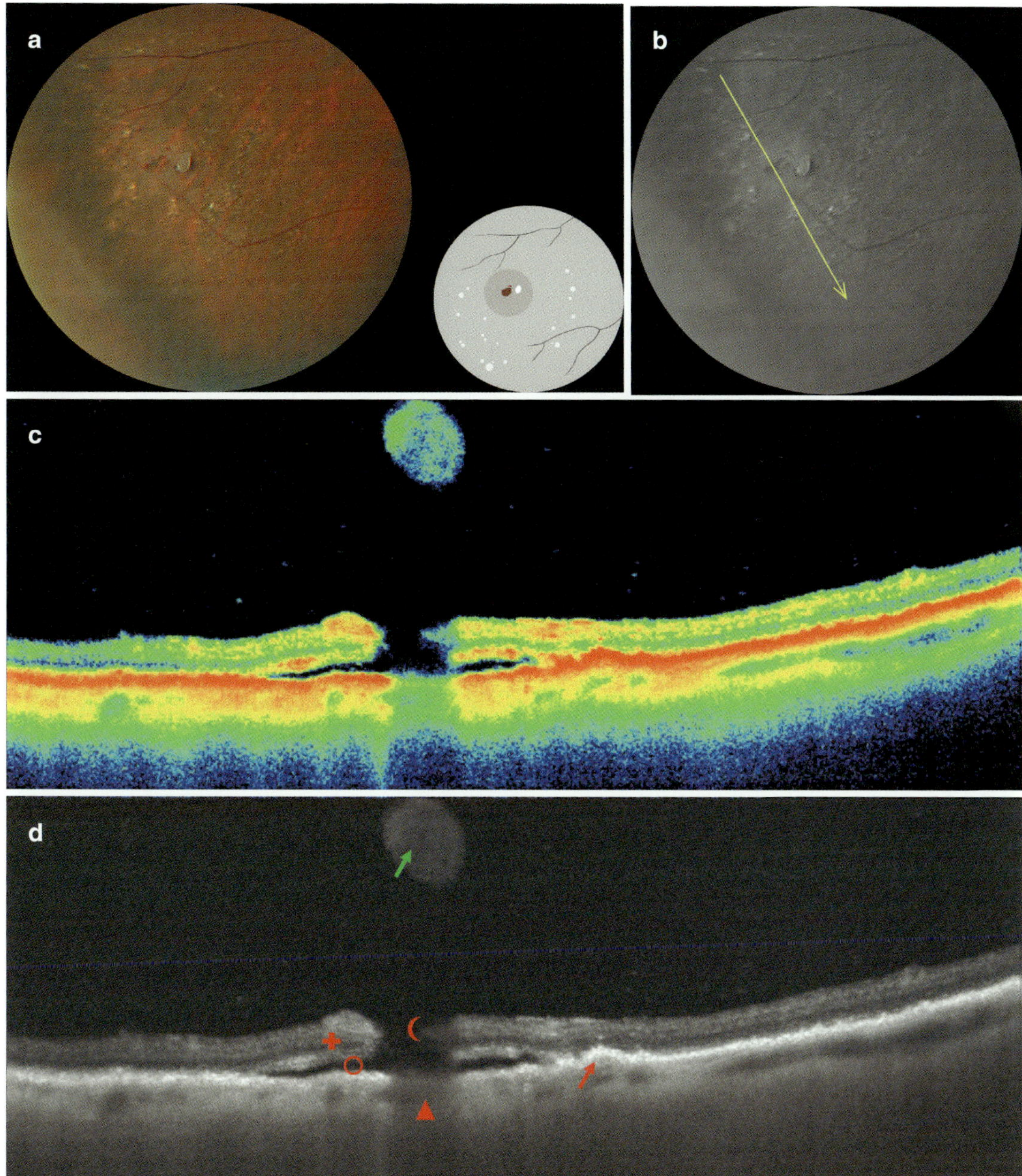

Fig. 5.55 (**a**) Operculated retinal tear against drusen. (**b**) *Line* indicates OCT-scanning direction. (**c, d**) OCT-scanning results according to the *line* direction in (**b**)

Case 56. Flap Tear

A 45-year-old emmetropic male patient with partial posterior vitreous detachment presented with complaints of sudden floaters affecting his right eye for 2 days.

Ophthalmoscopic Findings (Fig. 5.56a, b)

A full-thickness flap tear (horseshoe tear) with sharp borders is visible in the mid-periphery of the superotemporal quadrant of the right eye. The flap is light gray and slightly elevated. The retina along the tear margins is spongy and gray. There are isolated haemorrhage areas next to the tear along the retinal vessel.

OCT Scan Description (Fig. 5.56c, d)

A full-thickness flap tear makes the retinal profile irregular. The neurosensory flap is dense and elevated. The choroid is hyporeflective because of the shadow effect of the flap.

OCT Scan Details (Fig. 5.56c, d)

↗ Dense and elevated neurosensory retina (retinal flap)

☾ Full-thickness tear of the neurosensory retina

▲ Decreased reflectivity of the choroid at the level of the retinal tear

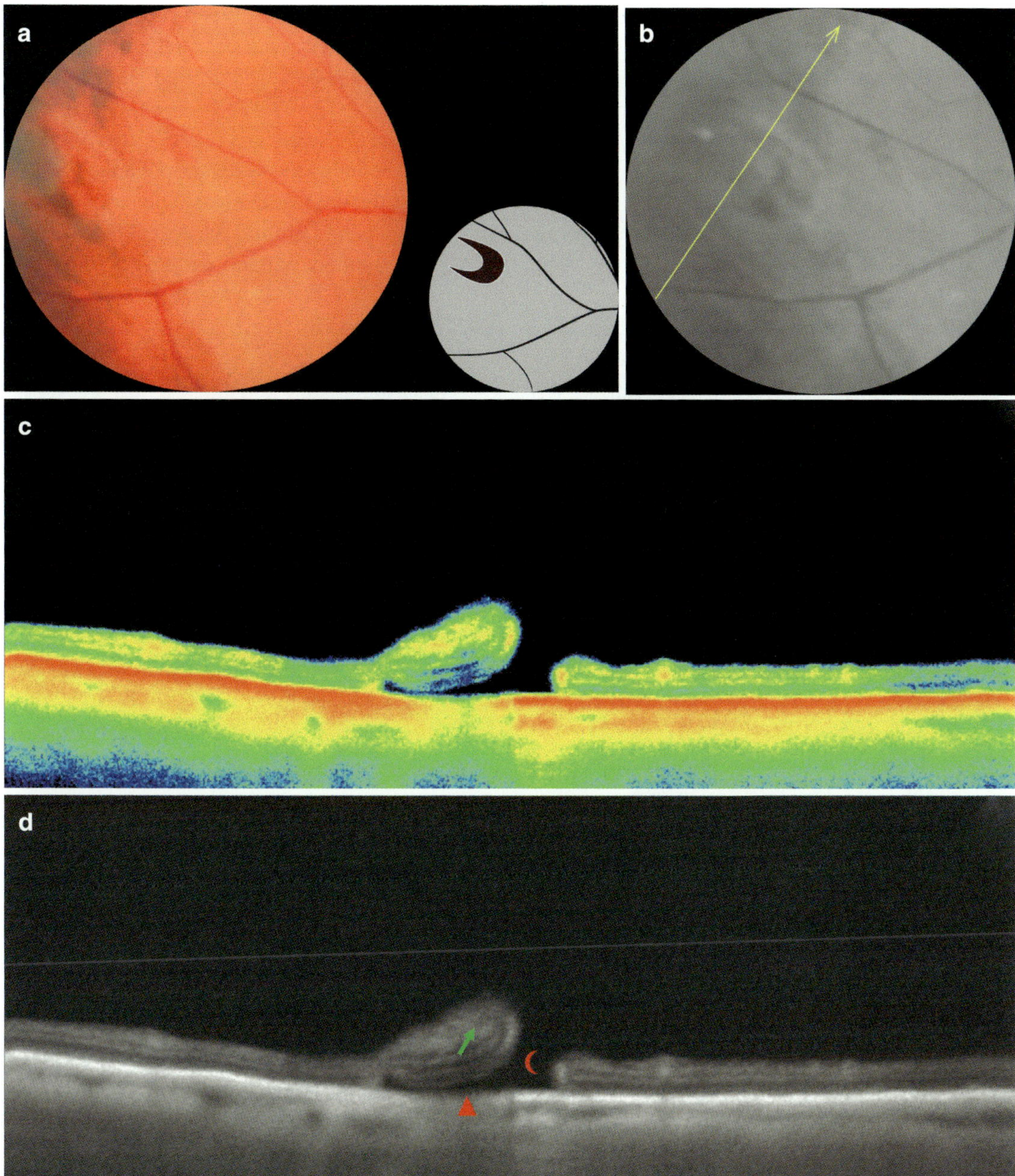

Fig. 5.56 (**a**) Flap tear. (**b**) *Line* indicates OCT-scanning direction. (**c, d**) OCT-scanning results according to the *line* direction in (**b**)

Case 57. Flap Tear with Vitreous Traction and Multiple Haemorrhages

A 58-year-old female patient with severe myopia and partial posterior vitreous detachment presented with sudden vision deterioration, flashes of light and blurry vision affecting her right eye after physical exercises.

Ophthalmoscopic Findings (Fig. 5.57a, b)

An extensive, well-outlined flap tear (horseshoe tear) and associated ruptured retinal vessel are observed in the mid-periphery of the superior quadrant of the right eye. A circular grayish area of the dense vitreous with traction is seen at the top of the flap. Multiple red haemorrhages of various size are observed near the ruptured vessel. A clearly outlined area of gray retina is elevated along the tear edges, indicating a subclinical retinal detachment.

OCT Scan Description (Fig. 5.57c)

Scan 1 The scan is made closer to the bottom of the retinal tear. The retinal surface is dome-shaped because of an extensive flap tear. The flap is elevated into the vitreous, with no adhesion or traction observed. A hyperreflective shadow (comet tail) is observed at the tear. The neurosensory retina is detached around the tear.

Scan 2 and 3 Scans are made across the condensed vitreous at the vitreoretinal adhesion and traction at the apex of the tear. The neurosensory retina is detached around the tear. The retina on the flap is thinned, with an atrophic hole in it.

OCT Scan Details (Fig. 5.57c)

✳ Vitreoretinal adhesion and traction

↗ Detached neurosensory retina (retinal flap)

☾ Full-thickness tear of the neurosensory retina

◤ Local retinal thinning of the retinal flap (atrophic hole)

✚ Detached neurosensory retina around the tear

○ Hyporeflective space under the detached retina

▲ Decreased choroidal reflectivity in the area of retinal flap and vitreoretinal adhesion

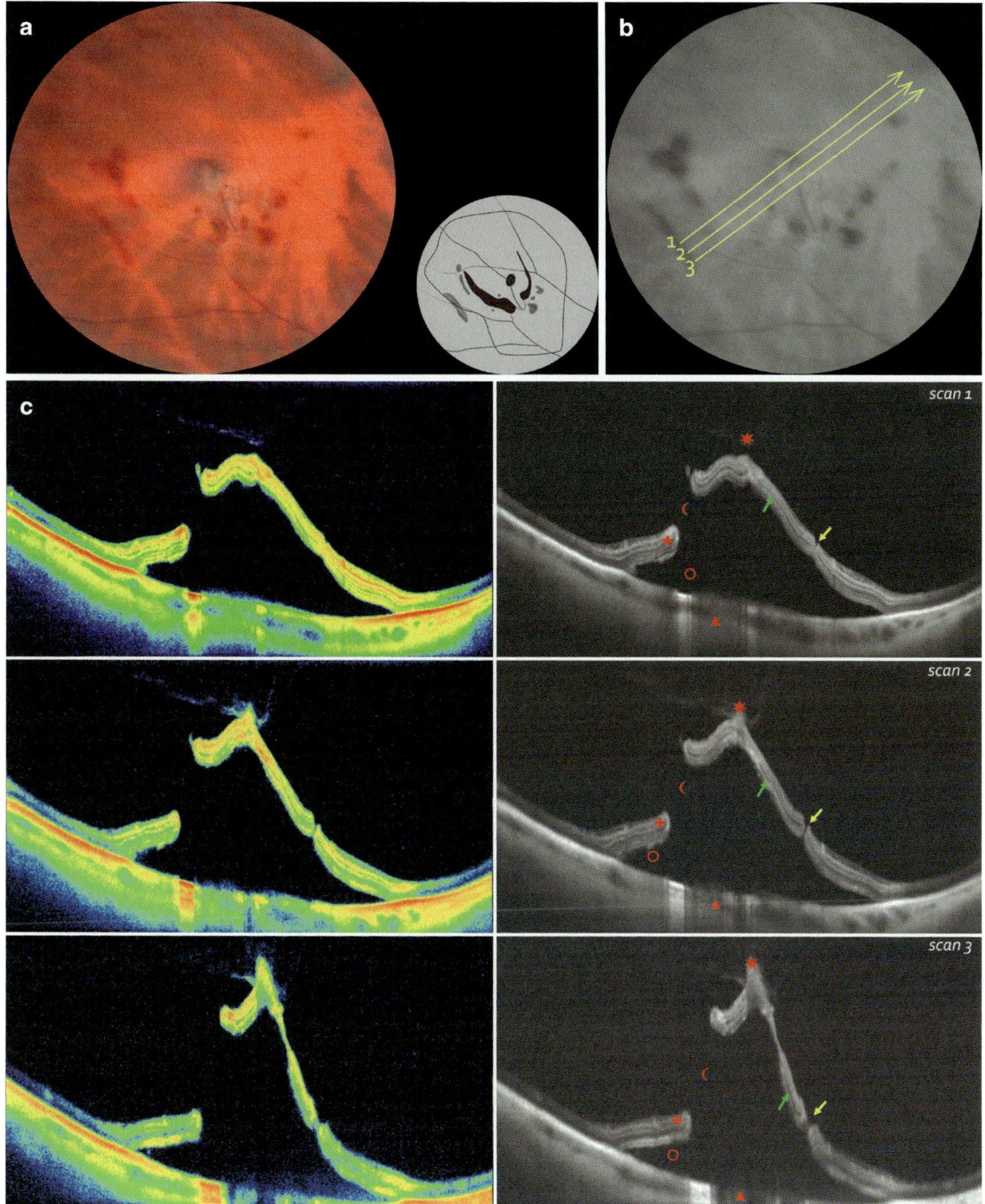

Fig. 5.57 (**a**) Flap tear with traction and multiple haemorrhages. (**b**) *Lines* indicate OCT-scanning direction. (**c**) OCT-scanning results according to the *lines* direction in (**b**)

Case 58. Flap Tear with Haemorrhages

A 57-year-old male patient with moderate myopia and incomplete posterior vitreous detachment presented with a 3-day history of visual deterioration and blurry vision affecting his left eye after a hypertensive episode.

Ophthalmoscopic Findings (Fig. 5.58a, b)

A flap tear is seen in the superotemporal quadrant of the left eye. A retinal vessel is observed passing through the tear and the flap. The flap margins are irregular and deformed, with full-thickness tears. The flap appears to be adherent to the retinal vessel. Isolated haemorrhages are visible at the tear edges.

OCT Scan Description (Fig. 5.58c)

Scan 1 The retinal surface is changed by a large flap tear. The tear edges are dense, with the underlying neurosensory detachment. The choroid is hyporeflective at the level of the tear, with a hyperreflective shadow at the tear edges.

Scan 2 Full-thickness tears are seen at the flap, with its apex elevated towards the vitreous by vitreous traction. The neuroepithelium is detached at the tear edges. The choroid reflectivity in the area of the tear is decreased.

OCT Scan Details (Fig. 5.58c)

↗ Dense and elevated neurosensory retina (cross-section image of retinal flap)

☾ Full-thickness tear of the neurosensory retina

✚ Detached neurosensory retina around the tear

◯ Hyporeflective space under the detached retina

▲ Decreased choroidal reflectivity at the level of the flap

↙ Area of dense neurosensory retina with the retinal vessel inside

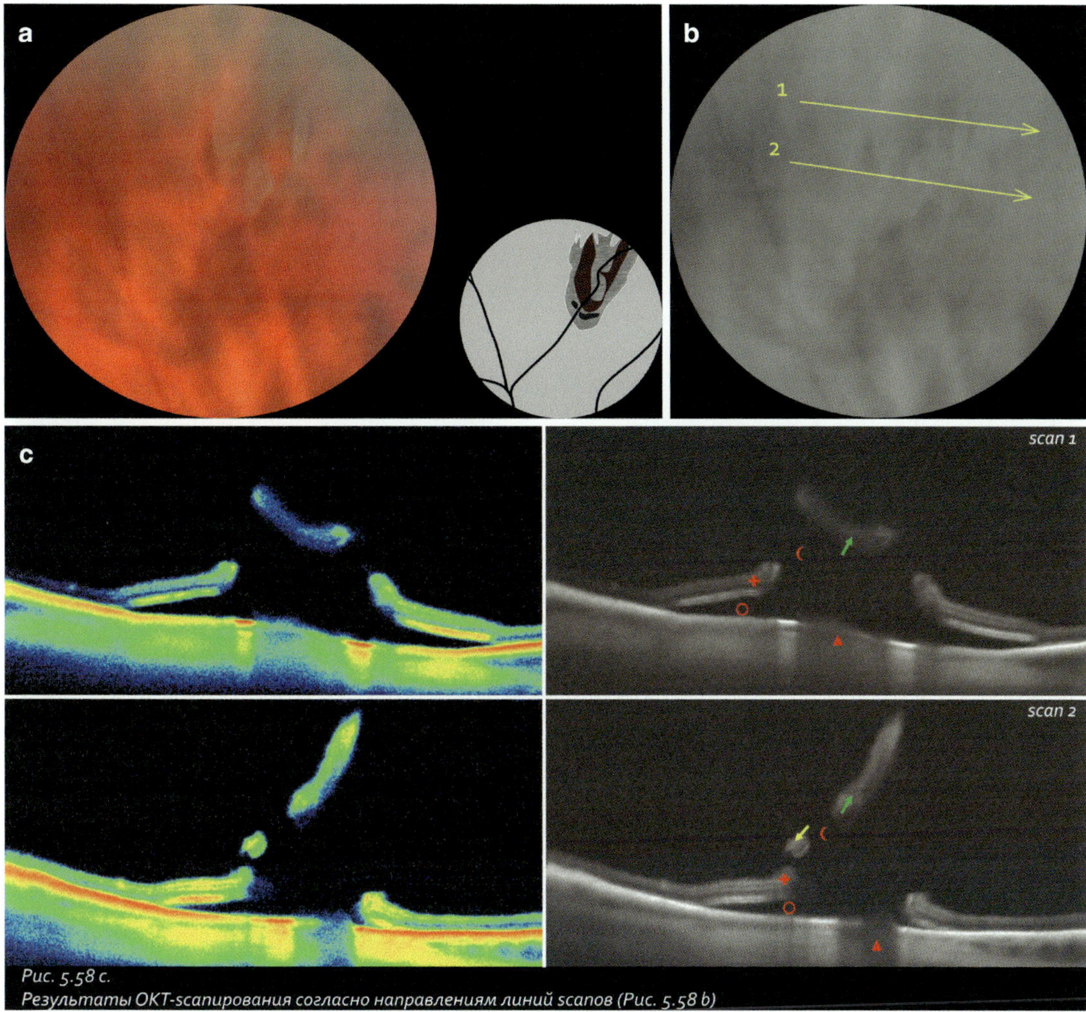

Fig. 5.58 (**a**) Flap tear with haemorrhages. (**b**) *Lines* indicate OCT-scanning direction. (**c**) OCT-scanning results according to the *lines* direction in (**b**)

Case 59. Flap Tear with an Intact Retinal Vessel

A 64-year-old female patient with moderate myopia, early stage cortical cataract, and partial posterior vitreous detachment presented with a 10-day history of floaters affecting her left eye.

Ophthalmoscopic Findings (Fig. 5.59a, b)
A full-thickness U-shaped tear is seen in the far-periphery of the superior quadrant of the left eye. An intact retinal vessel is observed passing through the center of the tear and the flap. The retina around the tear is gray and spongy.

OCT Scan Description (Fig. 5.59c, d)
The retinal surface is irregular because of a large full-thickness tear. In the center of the tear there is an elevated area of neurosensory retina with a vessel. There are areas of hyperpigmentation at the flap along the vessel. Shallow neurosensory detachment is seen at the tear edges.

OCT Scan Details (Fig. 5.59c, d)

↗ Detached neurosensory retina with an intact vessel

☾ Full-thickness tear of the neurosensory retina

✚ Detached neurosensory retina around the tear with tiny intraretinal hyporeflective cavities

○ Hyporeflective space under the shallow neurosensory detachment at the edges of the tear

▲ Decreased choroidal reflectivity at the level of the retinal vessel

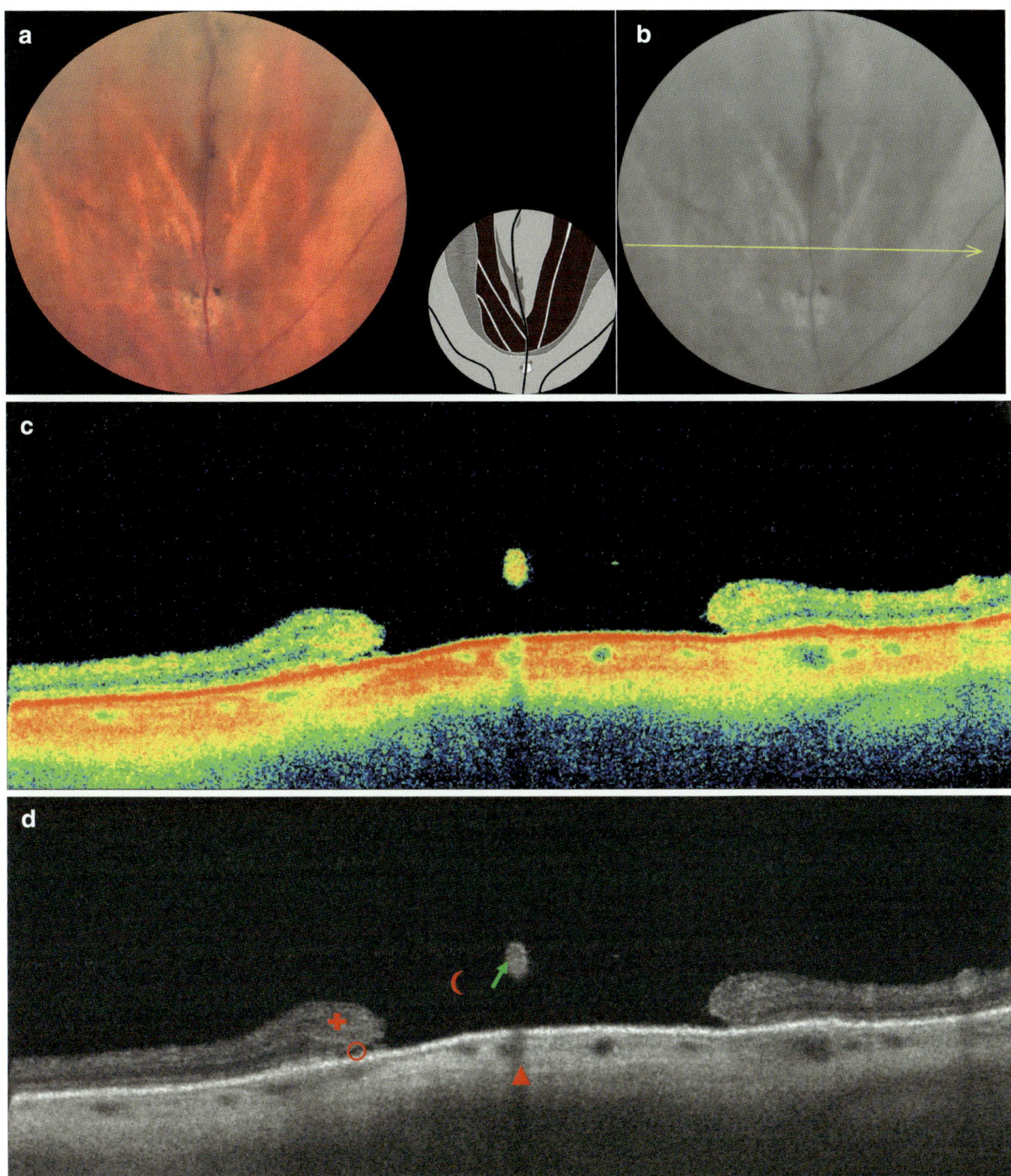

Fig. 5.59 (a) Flap tear with an intact retinal vessel. (b) *Line* indicates OCT-scanning direction. (c, d) OCT-scanning results according to the *line* direction in (b)

Case 60. Flap Tear (U-Shaped)

A 50-year-old male patient presented with complaints of photopsias in his left eye that appear after physical exercises. Examination revealed a flap tear (U-shaped) in the periphery of the left eye.

Ophthalmoscopic Findings (Fig. 5.60a, b)

A full-thickness U-shaped tear is seen at 9 o'clock position in the mid-periphery of the left eye. The neuroepithelial flap is clearly outlined and bright red in color. The retina around the tear is grayish (localized retinal detachment). There is a scarlet haemorrhage on the retinal surface below the tear.

OCT Scan Description (Fig. 5.60c, d)

The retinal surface is irregular because of the full-thickness tear of the neuroepithelium with clear margins and an overhanging hyperreflective flap in the vitreous. There is a shallow neurosensory retinal detachment around the tear margins. The flap causes a hyporeflective effect at the level of the pigment epithelium and the choroid.

OCT Scan Details (Fig. 5.60c, d)

↗ Dense and elevated area of the neurosensory retina (cross-section image of the flap)

☾ Full-thickness tear of the neurosensory retina

✚ Detached neurosensory retina at the tear margin

○ Hyporeflective space under the detached neurosensory retina

↗ Thickened pigment epithelium at the tear margin

▲ Decreased choroidal reflectivity at the level of the pigment epithelium and the flap

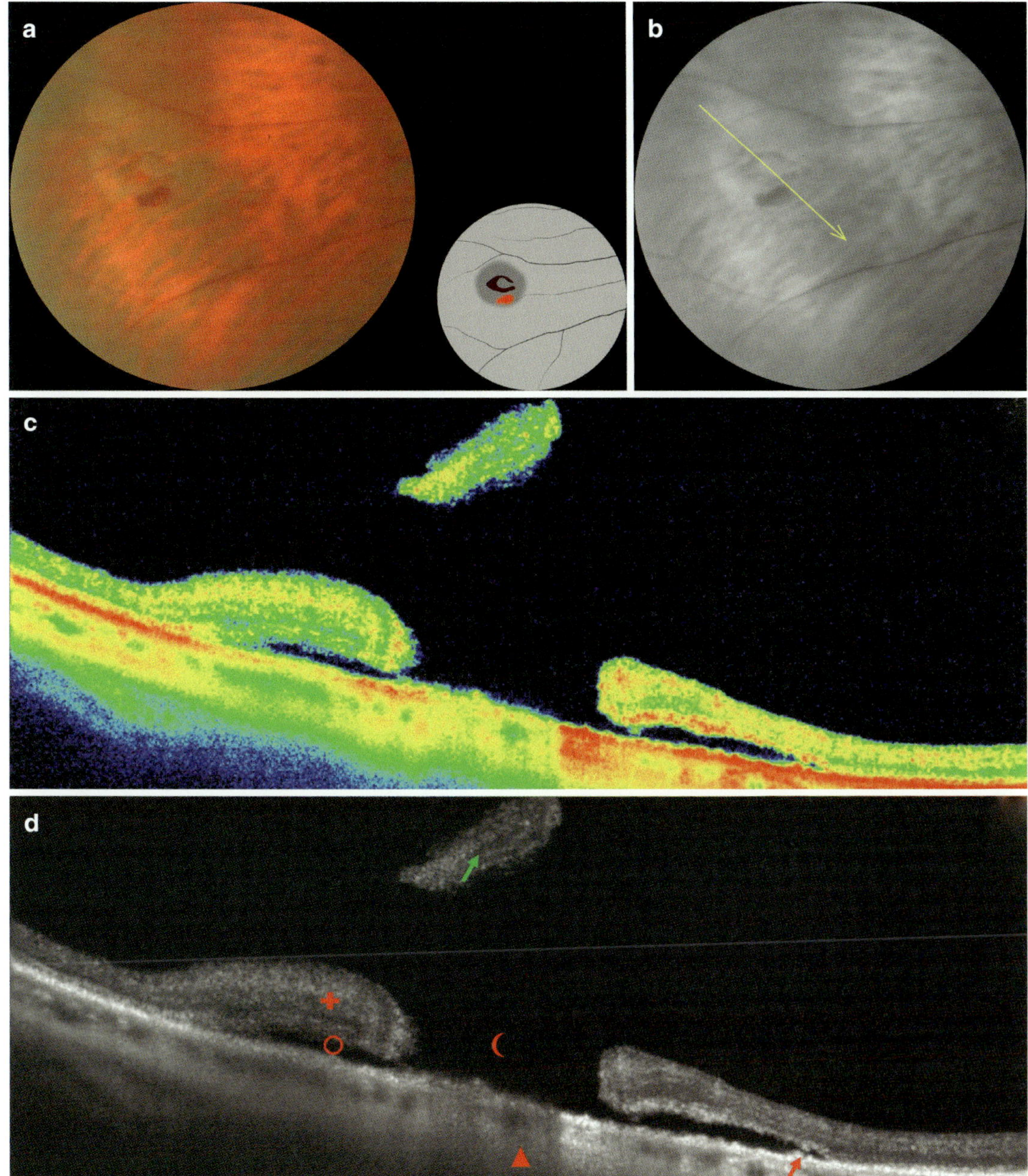

Fig. 5.60 (**a**) Flap tear (U-shaped). (**b**) *Line* indicates OCT-scanning direction. (**c, d**) OCT-scanning results according to the *line* direction in (**b**)

Case 61. Flap Tear with Demarcated Shallow Retinal Detachment

A 65-year-old female patient presented with complaints of floaters affecting her right eye, that intensified in the past 3 days.

Ophthalmoscopic Findings (Fig. 5.61a, b)

A flap retinal tear with shallow detachment demarcated by a pigment line is seen in the temporal quadrant of the right eye. The pigmentation is irregular.

OCT Scan Description (Fig. 5.61c)

Scan 1 The retinal surface is irregular because of a full-thickness tear of the neurosensory retina. There are intraretinal round hyporeflective cavities at the tear margins. Elevated hyperreflective retinal tissue is observed at the vitreous level over the tear, and is adherent to the posterior hyaloid membrane (cross-section image of the retinal flap).

Scan 2 The retinal surface is irregular because of a flap tear. There is a shallow retinal detachment and an intraretinal cystoid oedema at the tear margins. Large hyporeflective cavities are observed at the level of the flap. Vitreoretinal adhesion and traction at the tear margins are caused by the posterior hyaloid membrane.

OCT Scan Details (Fig. 5.61c)

↗ Dense and elevated neurosensory retina (cross-section image of the flap)

✳ Vitreoretinal adhesion at the edge of the flap

✛ Intraretinal hyporeflective cavities in the detached neurosensory retina at the tear edges

☾ Full-thickness tear of the neurosensory retina

○ Shallow neurosensory detachment around the tear

↗ Thickened and dense pigment epithelium around the shallow detachment

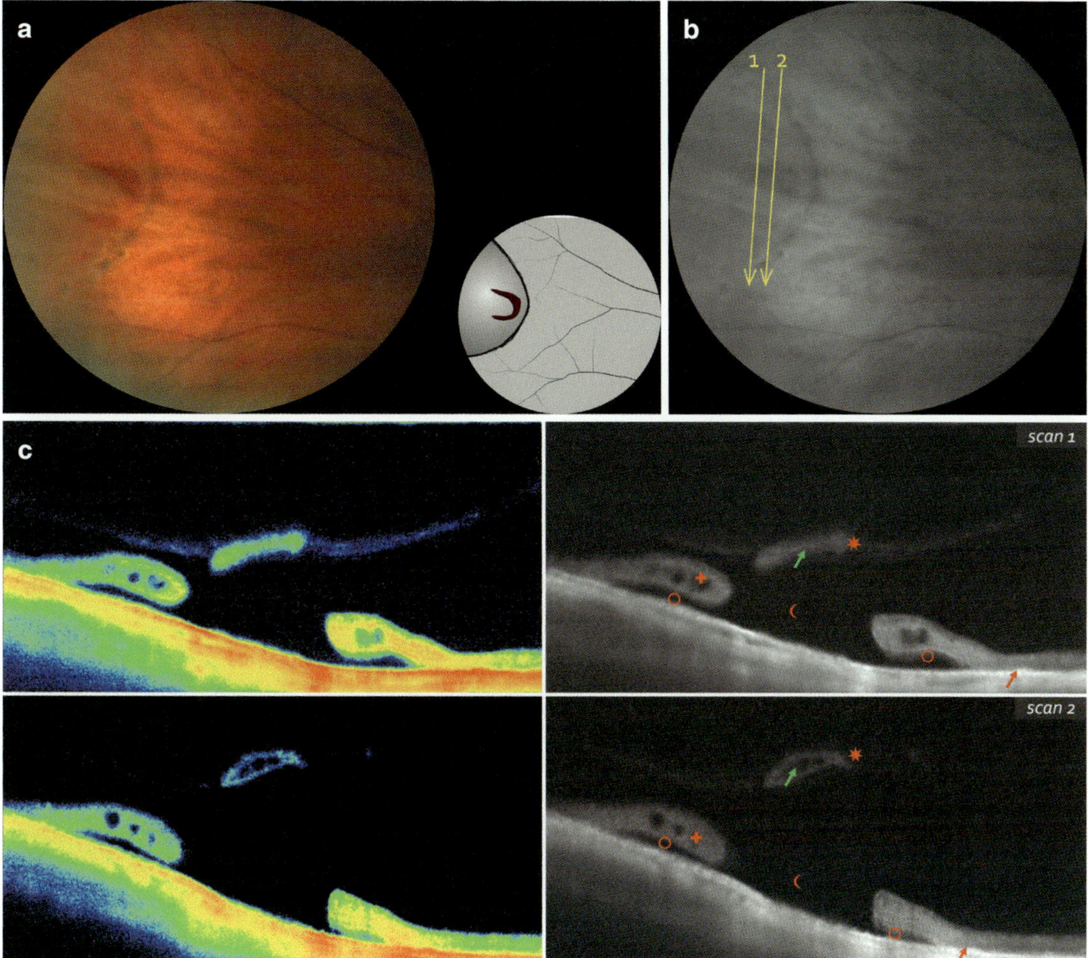

Fig. 5.61 (**a**) Flap tear with demarcated shallow retinal detachment. (**b**) *Lines* indicate OCT-scanning direction. (**c**) OCT-scanning results according to the *lines* direction in (**b**)

References

1. Jones WL et al. Care of the patient with retinal detachment and related peripheral vitreoretinal disease. St. Louis: Mosby; 2004.
2. Jones WL. Peripheral ocular fundus. 3rd ed. St. Louis: Elsevier Butterworth-Heinemann; 2007.
3. Pasechnikova NV. Laser treatment of the eye fundus pathology. Kiev: Naukova Dumka (In Russian); 2007.
4. Aaberg TM, Stevens TR. Snail-track degeneration of the retina. Am J Ophthalmol. 1972;73(3):370–6.
5. Conart JB, Baron D, Berrod JP. Degenerative lesions of the peripheral retina. J Fr Ophtalmol. 2014;37(1):73–80. doi:10.1016/j.jfo.2013.09.001.
6. Brinton DA, Wilkinson CP. Retinal detachment: principles and practice. 3rd ed. Oxford: Oxford University Press; 2009.
7. Graue-Wiechers FA, Verduzco NS. Laser treatment for retinal holes, tears and peripheral degenerations. In: Boyd S, Wilkinson CP, editors. Retinal detachment surgery and laser treatment. Panama: Jaypee Highlights Med Publ; 2009. p. 47–57.
8. Neroev VV, Zaharova GY, Kondratieva YP. Peripheral retinal degenerations in fellow eyes of patients with unilateral retinal detachment. Russ Ophthalmol J. 2014;3:5–10. (In Russian)
9. Shukla M, Ahuja CP. A possible relationship between lattice and snail track degeneration of the retina. Amer J Ophthalmol. 1981; 92(4):482–5. Adrean SD, Elliot D. Prophylaxis for retinal detachment. Rev Ophthalmol. 2005;5(6). http://www.reviewofophthalmology.com/content/d/retinal_insider/i/1314/c/25288/. Accessed 15 Jul 2005.
10. Kothari A, Narendran V, Saravanan VR. In vivo sectional imaging of the retinal periphery using conventional optical coherence tomography systems. Indian J Ophthalmol. 2012;60(3):235–9.
11. Daicker BA. The macular fatty degeneration of the peripheral retina a variety of the snail track degeneration (author's transl). lbrecht Von Graefes Arch Klin Exp Ophthalmol. 1978;205(3):147–55. Article in German
12. Bec P, Malecaze F, Arne JL, et al. Lattice degeneration of the peripheral retina: ultrastructural study. Ophthalmologica. 1985;191(2):107–13. (In French)
13. Kanski D, Bowling B. Clinical ophthalmology: systemic approach. 7th ed. Edinburgh: Elsevier/Saunders; 2011.
14. Shaimova VA, Pozdeeva OG, Shaimov TB, et al. Optical coherence tomography in peripheral retinal tears diagnostics. Vestn Ophthalmol. 2013;6:51–66. (In Russian)
15. Ho A et al. Retina. Color atlas and synopsis of clinical ophthalmology. Wills Eye Series. McGraw-Hill Professional: New York; 2003.
16. Karlin BD, Curtin BJ. Peripheral chorioretinal lesions and axial length of the myopic eye. Am J Ophthalmol. 1976;81(5):625–35.
17. Macaliester G, Sullivan P. Peripheral retinal degenerations. In: OT CET. 2011. http://goo.gl/PzTidM.
18. Boiko EV, Suetov AA, Maltcev DS. Retinal lattice degeneration. Vestn Ophthalmol. 2014;130(2):77–82. (In Russian)
19. Baron D. Atlas périphérie rétinienne et décollements de rétine. Paris: Med'com éditions; 2013.
20. Straatsma BR, Foos RY. Tipical and reticular retinoshisis. Am J Ophthalmol. 1973;75(4):551–75.
21. Straatsma BR, Zeegen PD, Foss RY, et al. Lattice degeneration of the retina. Am J Ophthalmol. 1974; 77(5):619–49.
22. Byer NE. Lattice degeneration of the retina. Surv Ophthalmol. 1979;23(4):213–48.
23. Byer NE. Long-term natural history of lattice degeneration of the retina. Ophthalmology. 1989;96(9): 1396–401.
24. Byer NE. The peripheral retina in profile: a stereoscopic atlas. Torrance: Criterion Press; 1982.
25. Antelava DI et al. Primary retinal detachment. Tbilisi: Sabchota Sakartvelo (In Russian); 1986.
26. Davis MD. The natural history of retinal breaks without detachment. Trans Am Ophthalmol Soc. 1973;71:343–72.
27. Mitry D, Singh J, Yorston D, et al. The fellow eye in retinal detachment: findings from the Scottish Retinal Detachment Study. Br J Ophthalmol. 2012;96(1): 110–3.
28. Lewis H. Peripheral retinal degenerations and the risk of retinal detachment. Am J Ophthalmol. 2003; 136(1):155–60.
29. Adrean SD, Elliot D. Prophylaxis for retinal detachment. Rev Ophthalmol. 2005;12(7):82–7.
30. Wilkinson CP. Interventions for asymptomatic retinal breaks and lattice degeneration for preventing retinal detachment. Cochrane Database Syst Rev. 2014;9:CD003170. doi:10.1002/14651858.CD003170.pub4.
31. Ehlers JP, Shah CP, editors. Wills Eye Institute The Wills Eye Manual: Office and Emergency Room Diagnosis and Treatment of Eye Disease, 5th edn. Lippincott Williams and Wilkins. Russian edition: Ehlers JP, Shah CP, editors (2012) Ophthalmology: guide (trans: Y. S. Astakhov). MEDpress-inform, Moscow; 2010.
32. Byer NE. Cystic retinal tufts and their relationship to retinal detachment. Arch Ophthalmol. 1981;99:1788–90.
33. Foos RY, Allen RA. Retinal tears and lesser lesions of the peripheral retina in autopsy eyes. Am J Ophthalmol. 1967;64(3):643–55.
34. Foos RY. Zonular traction tufts of the peripheral retina in cadaver eyes. Arch Ophthalmol. 1969;82(5):620–32.
35. Murakami-Nagasako F, Ohba N. Phakic retinal detachment associated with cystic retinal tuft. Graefes Arch Clin Exp Ophthalmol. 1982;219(4):88–92.
36. Robertson DM, Norton EW. Long term follow – up of treated retinal breaks. Am J Ophthalmol. 1973;75(3):395–404.

37. Williams KM, Dogramaci M, Williamson TN. Retrospective study of rhegmatogenous retinal detachments secondary to round retinal holes. Eur J Ophthalmol. 2012;22(4):635–40.
38. Silva RA, Blumenkranz MS. Prophylaxis for retinal detachments. 2013. http://www.aao.org/munnerlyn-laser-surgery-center/prophylaxis-retinal-detachments. Accessed 29 Oct 2013.
39. Bol'shunov AV, editor. Laser ophthalmology problems. Moscow: Aprel' (In Russian); 2013.
40. Coffee RE, Westfall AC, Davis GH, et al. Symptomatic posterior vitreous detachment and the incidence of delayed retinal breaks: case series and meta-analysis. Am J Ophthalmol. 2007;144(3): 409–13.
41. Conart JB, Barron D, Berrod JP. Lessions degeneratives de la peripherie retinienne. EMC Ophthalmol. 2013;10(1):1–12.
42. Bloom SM, Brucker J. Laser surgery of the posterior segment. Philadelphia: Lippincot Raven; 1997.
43. Peyman GA et al. Principles and practice of ophthalmology. Philadelphia: W.B. Saunders Company; 1987.
44. Isola V, Spinelli G, Misefari W. Transpupillary retinopexy of chorioretinal lesions predisposing to retinal detachment with the use of diode (810 nm) microlaser. Retina. 2001;21(5):453–9.
45. Saurabh J, Newsom RSB, McHugh DA. Treatment of retinal breaks with large-spot diode laser photocoagulation. Ophthalmic Surg Lasers Imaging. 2005;36(6): 514–6.

Chorioretinal Degenerations

6

Third Group of Peripheral Retinal Degenerations

Alexey Y. Galin and Tatiana A. Shaimova

A.Y. Galin • T.A. Shaimova (✉)
Center Zreniya Medical Clinic, LLC,
Chelyabinsk, Russian Federation
e-mail: tanya.shaimova@gmail.com

© Springer International Publishing AG 2017
V.A. Shaimova (ed.), *Peripheral Retinal Degenerations*, DOI 10.1007/978-3-319-48995-7_6

Peripheral Chorioretinal Atrophy of the Retinal Pigment Epithelium

Peripheral chorioretinal atrophy (Table 6.1) appears as either multiple lesions known as paving-stone degeneration, or individual areas of pigment epithelium atrophy (one or two lesions). This degeneration is characterized by atrophic changes in the outer retinal layers, pigment epithelium, and choriocapillaris, with no changes in the vitreous [1, 2]. Paving-stone degeneration is usually found between equator and ora serrata. In early stages, it appears as separated round or oval rose-colored lesions of 0.5–1 PD. In advanced stages, the lesions tend to coalesce and become whitish with irregular hyperpigmentation [3, 4].

Paving-stone changes can be congenital and are not considered degenerative by some experts [5]. Paving-stone degeneration is present in 4.4–28.4 % of general population [2, 4, 6].

Although this degeneration can resemble retinal holes, this is an outer retina defect; the inner neurosensory layers are intact, and retinal breaks do not occur [5]. Majority of clinicians consider this degeneration benign with low risk of retinal detachment. Paving-stone degeneration has been reported to have a protective effect against the progression of rhegmatogenous retinal detachment [1].

Many authors consider chorioretinal atrophy of the pigment epithelium as bearing no risk of retinal detachment and not indicated for prophylactic laser treatment [5–7]. However, some authors report 11.1 % frequency of retinal breaks associated with marked stages of chorioretinal degeneration [3].

Table 6.1 Diagram of peripheral retinal degenerations

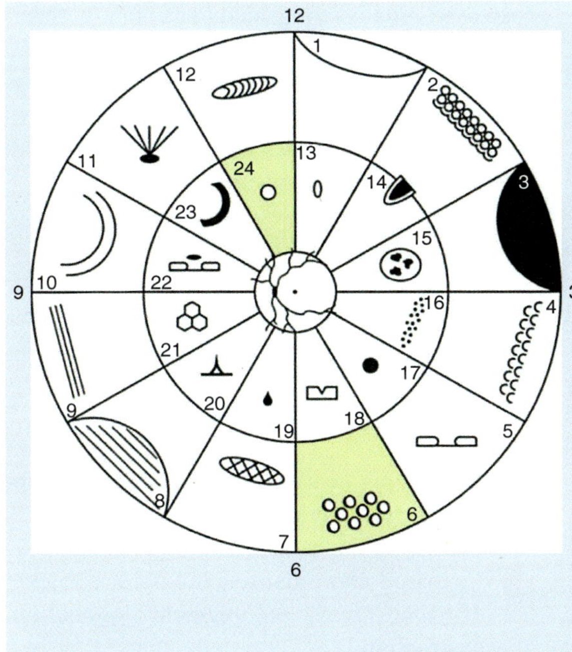

1. Retinal dialysis
2. Peripheral cystoid degeneration
3. Retinal detachment
4. Retinal drusen
5. Full-thickness tear
6. Paving-stone degeneration
7. Lattice degeneration
8. Bullous retinoschisis
9. Flat retinoschisis
10. White-without-pressure
11. Retinal tuft
12. Snail-track degeneration
13. Pearl degeneration
14. Flap tear
15. Grouped congenital hypertrophy of the retinal pigment epithelium ("bear tracks")
16. Snowflake degeneration
17. Unifocal hypertrophy of the retinal pigment epithelium
18. Atrophic retinal hole
19. Haemorrhage
20. Preretinal fibrosis
21. Honeycomb degeneration
22. Operculated retinal tear
23. Dark-without-pressure
24. Unifocal atrophy of the retinal pigment epithelium

Paving-stone degeneration in sector 6 and unifocal atrophy of the retinal pigment epithelium in sector 24 are highlighted in yellow

Case 62. Paving-Stone Degeneration

A 56-year-old female patient with mild myopia and no symptomatic complains was referred for fundus examination because of arterial hypertension.

Ophthalmoscopic Findings (Fig. 6.62a, b)

Multiple atrophic lesions in the pigment epithelium of various forms and sizes are seen in the far-periphery of the inferior quadrant of the right eye. Some lesions merge, others are isolated. Pigment clumps of various forms and intensity are located within and between the chorioretinal atrophy lesions. There is a clearly seen choroidal pattern in the atrophic areas.

OCT Scan Description (Fig. 6.62c, d)

The retinal surface is irregular and wavy. Multiple areas of pigment epithelium destruction are observed. The reflectivity in the neurosensory retina layers is increased. Neurosensory retina is thinned at the level of the pigment epithelium destruction, and hyperreflective shadows are observed at the choroidal level because of increased retinal echogenicity and light permeability. The ellipsoid zone is not seen. Choroid hyperreflectivity correlates with the areas of pigment epithelium destruction. Multiple hyperreflective deposits are present in the vitreous, there is no evidence of vitreous traction.

OCT Scan Details (Fig. 6.62c, d)

- Pre-retinal consolidation of the vitreous with multiple hyperreflective deposits

- Areas of dense pigment epithelium

- Areas of pigment epithelium and photoreceptor layer destruction

- Increased choroidal reflectivity at the level of the areas of pigment epithelium destruction

- Decreased choroidal reflectivity at the level of the areas of dense pigment epithelium

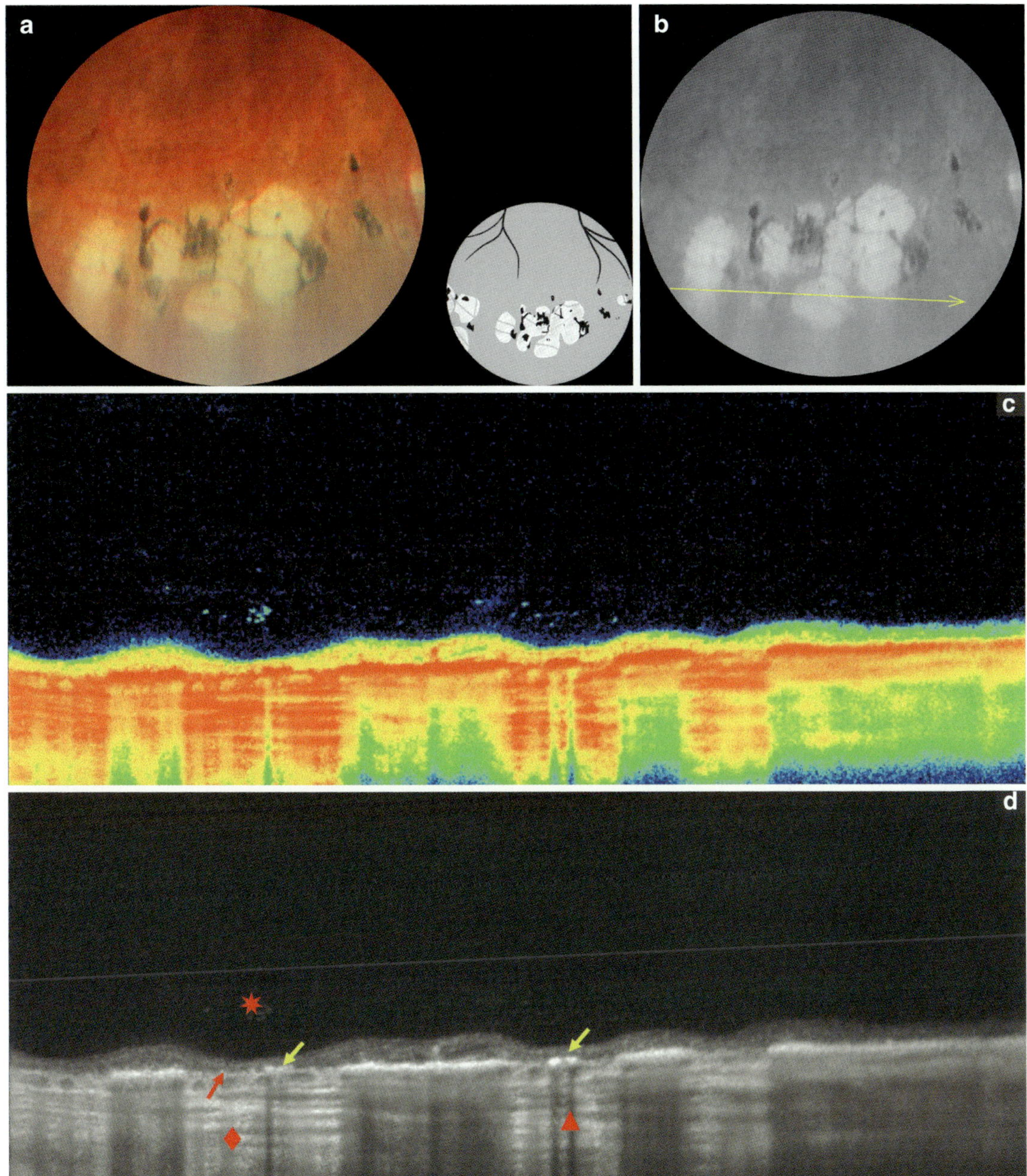

Fig. 6.62 (**a**) Paving-stone degeneration. (**b**) *Line* indicates OCT-scanning direction. (**c, d**) OCT-scanning results according to the line direction in (**b**)

Case 63. Focal Pigment Epithelium Atrophy

An asymptomatic 40-year-old female patient with mild myopia came to have distance glasses prescribed. Fundus examination revealed an atrophic lesion with sharp borders in the infero-temporal quadrant of her left eye. No signs of traction were noted.

Ophthalmoscopic Findings (Fig. 6.63a, b)

A round-shaped area of atrophic pigment epithelium with clearly outlined borders is seen at the 7 o'clock position in the mid-periphery of the inferonasal quadrant of the left eye. Pigment clumps are observed around the borders.

OCT Scan Description (Fig. 6.63c, d)

The retinal profile is deformed, the structure of all layers is altered. Neurosensory retina is thinned, neuroepithelial surface is slopy on one side of the lesion and excavated on the other side. The pigment epithelium is hyporeflective and atrophic. The ellipsoid zone is not distinguishable. Choroidal reflectivity and light transmittance in the atrophic area is considerably increased.

OCT Scan Details (Fig. 6.63c, d)

 Neurosensory retina thinning

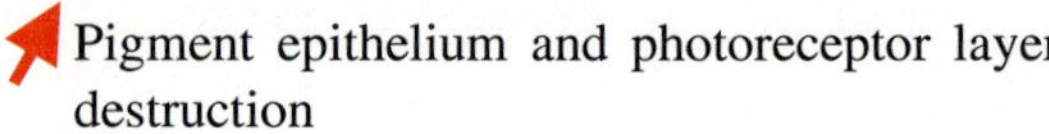 Pigment epithelium and photoreceptor layer destruction

 Increased choroidal reflectivity at the level of the pigment epithelium destruction

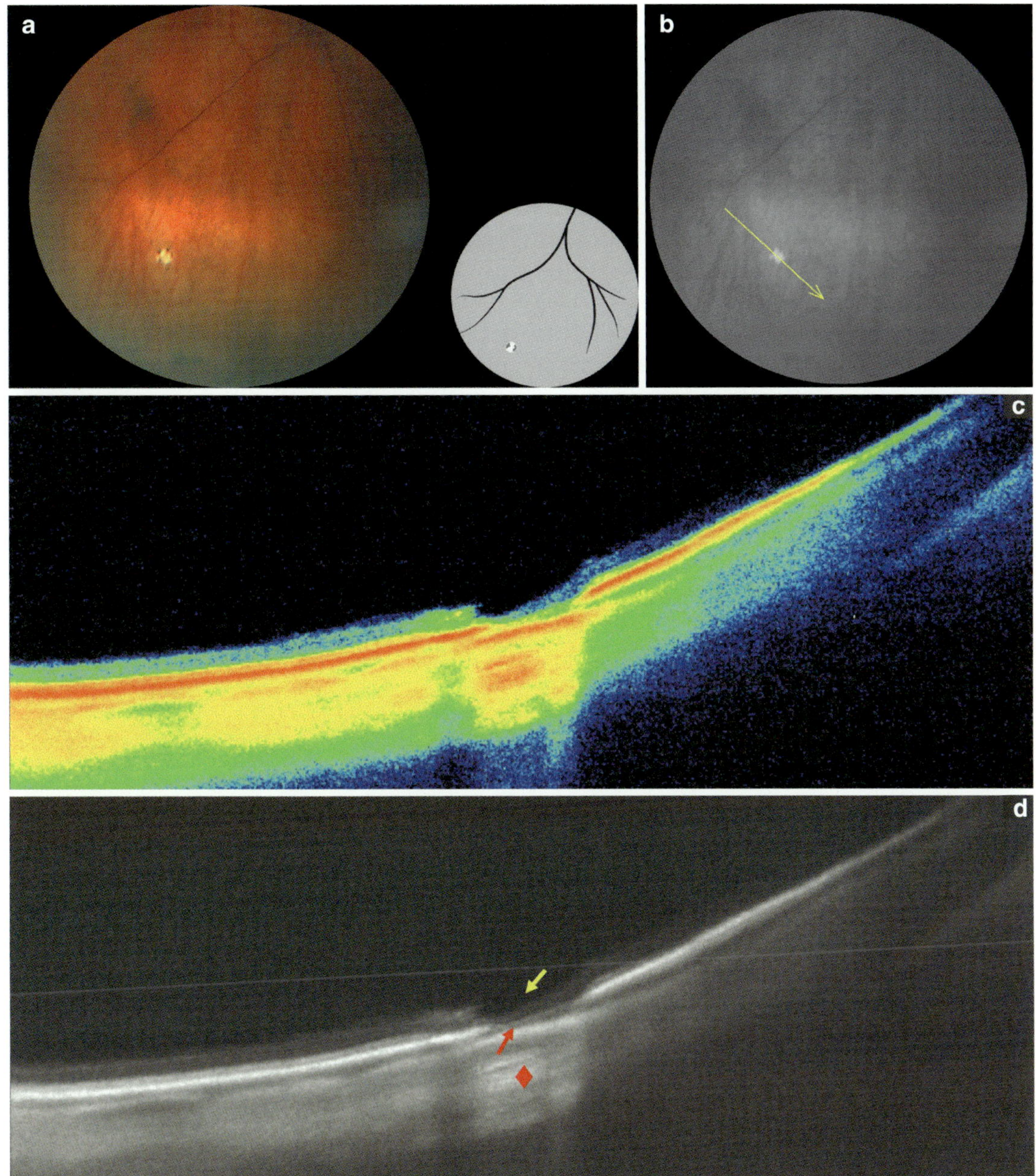

Fig. 6.63 (**a**) Focal pigment epithelium atrophy. (**b**) *Line* indicates OCT-scanning direction. (**c, d**) OCT-scanning results according to the line direction in (**b**)

Congenital Hypertrophy of the Retinal Pigment Epithelium

Congenital hypertrophy of the retinal pigment epithelium (CHRPE) is a common benign retinal condition [6]. According to some authors, CHRPE is characterized by pigment deposits found along the ora serrata, which may extend as far as equator. In early stages pigment spots and clumps reach 1/8 PD, and in advanced stages the lesion occupies 1/4–1.0 PD [3]. Other authors claim that CHRPE can be unifocal or multifocal (Table 6.2). Unifocal CHRPE is a round or oval flat lesion, 1–2 PD in size, with well-defined borders, that can be deep gray or black. The lesion can be surrounded by a hypopigmented halo. Multifocal CHRPE appears as grouped pigmented deep gray or black spots of various sizes, that resemble animal tracks ("bear tracks") [5].

Histological studies have established CHRPE to be a result of pigment redistribution [2, 3]. Patients with multifocal CHRPE (bear tracks) should be evaluated for familial adenomatous polyposis of colon and rectum, which may lead to colorectal cancer after 50 years of age [5, 6].

As reported by many authors, CHRPE is not usually associated with vitreous traction, changes in the vitreoretinal interface, or risk of retinal detachment. However, there have been reports of retinal tears in 11.9 % of cases of advanced CHRPE [3]. Nonetheless, prophylactic laser treatment for this condition is not indicated [5].

Table 6.2 Diagram of peripheral retinal degenerations

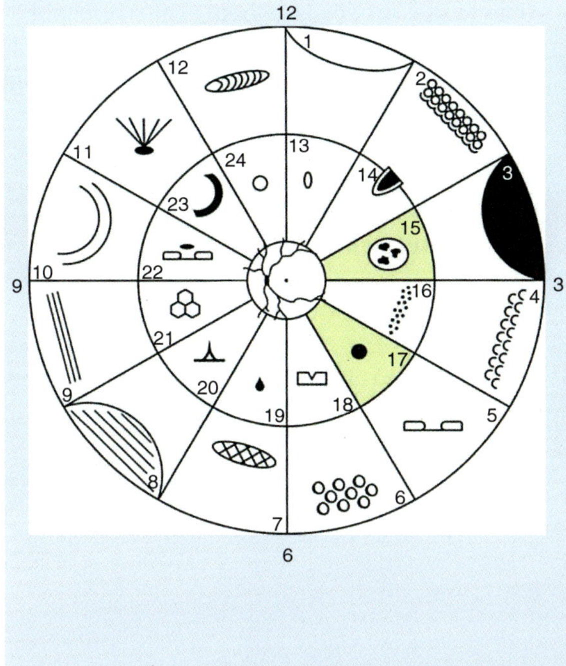

1. Retinal dialysis
2. Peripheral cystoid degeneration
3. Retinal detachment
4. Retinal drusen
5. Full-thickness tear
6. Paving-stone degeneration
7. Lattice degeneration
8. Bullous retinoschisis
9. Flat retinoschisis
10. White-without-pressure
11. Retinal tuft
12. Snail-track degeneration
13. Pearl degeneration
14. Flap tear
15. Grouped congenital hypertrophy of the retinal pigment epithelium ("bear tracks")
16. Snowflake degeneration
17. Unifocal hypertrophy of the retinal pigment epithelium
18. Atrophic retinal hole
19. Haemorrhage
20. Preretinal fibrosis
21. Honeycomb degeneration
22. Operculated retinal tear
23. Dark-without-pressure
24. Unifocal atrophy of the retinal pigment epithelium

Multifocal hypertrophy of the retinal pigment epithelium (bear tracks) in sector 15 and unifocal hypertrophy of the retinal pigment epithelium in sector 17 are highlighted in yellow

Case 64. Unifocal Congenital Hypertrophy of the Pigment Epithelium

An asymptomatic 29-year-old emmetropic female patient was found to have a hyperpigmented lesion in her left eye during a routine examination.

Ophthalmoscopic Findings (Fig. 6.64a, b)

A round area of hyperpigmented pigment epithelium is seen in the mid-periphery of the superior quadrant of the left eye. The lesion has distinct borders. The adjacent retinal vessel is intact. No vitreoretinal traction is observed.

OCT Scan Description (Fig. 6.64c, d)

The retinal surface is smooth. The neuroepithelial thickness is normal. An area of pigment epithelium hyperplasia shadows the underlying tissues because the light transmittance decreases. The choroid thickness is unaltered. No vitreoretinal adhesions or tractions are observed.

OCT Scan Details (Fig. 6.64c, d)

➤ Area of the dense pigment epithelium

▲ Decreased choroidal reflectivity at the hyperreflective pigment epithelium level

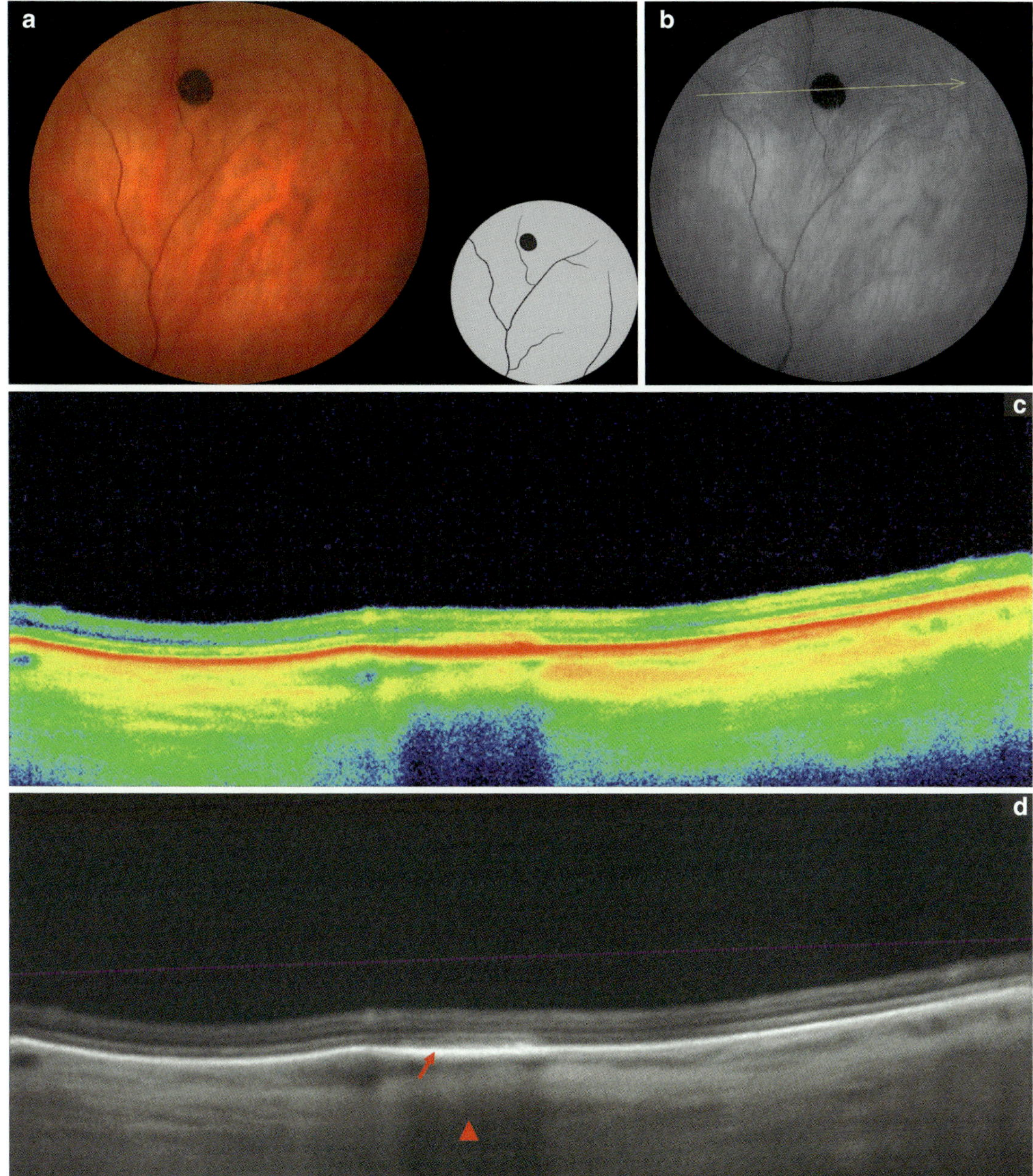

Fig. 6.64 (**a**) Unifocal congenital hypertrophy of the pigment epithelium. (**b**) *Line* indicates OCT-scanning direction. (**c, d**) OCT-scanning results according to the line direction in (**b**)

Case 65. Multifocal Hypertrophy of the Pigment Epithelium (Bear Tracks)

An asymptomatic 23-year-old female patient with mild myopia was found to have retinal degeneration during routine examination.

Ophthalmoscopic Findings (Fig. 6.65a, b)

Multiple hyperpigmented areas of irregular forms and various sizes are observed from the equatorial up to the far-peripheral retina in the inferotemporal quadrant of the left eye. Lesions are seen along the vessel arcades, and their contours resemble bear tracks. The vitreous is unchanged, with no vitreoretinal traction identified.

OCT Scan Description (Fig. 6.65c, d)

The retinal surface is smooth. Neuroepithelial structure in the area of degeneration is unchanged, and its thickness is retained. The ellipsoid zone integrity is reduced within the lesion, and the dense area of pigment epithelium casts a hyporeflective shadow over the choroid. The vitreoretinal interface is unchanged.

OCT Scan Details (Fig. 6.65c, d)

 Photoreceptor layer destruction

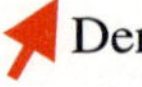 Dense pigment epithelium

 Decreased choroidal reflectivity at the level of dense pigment epithelium

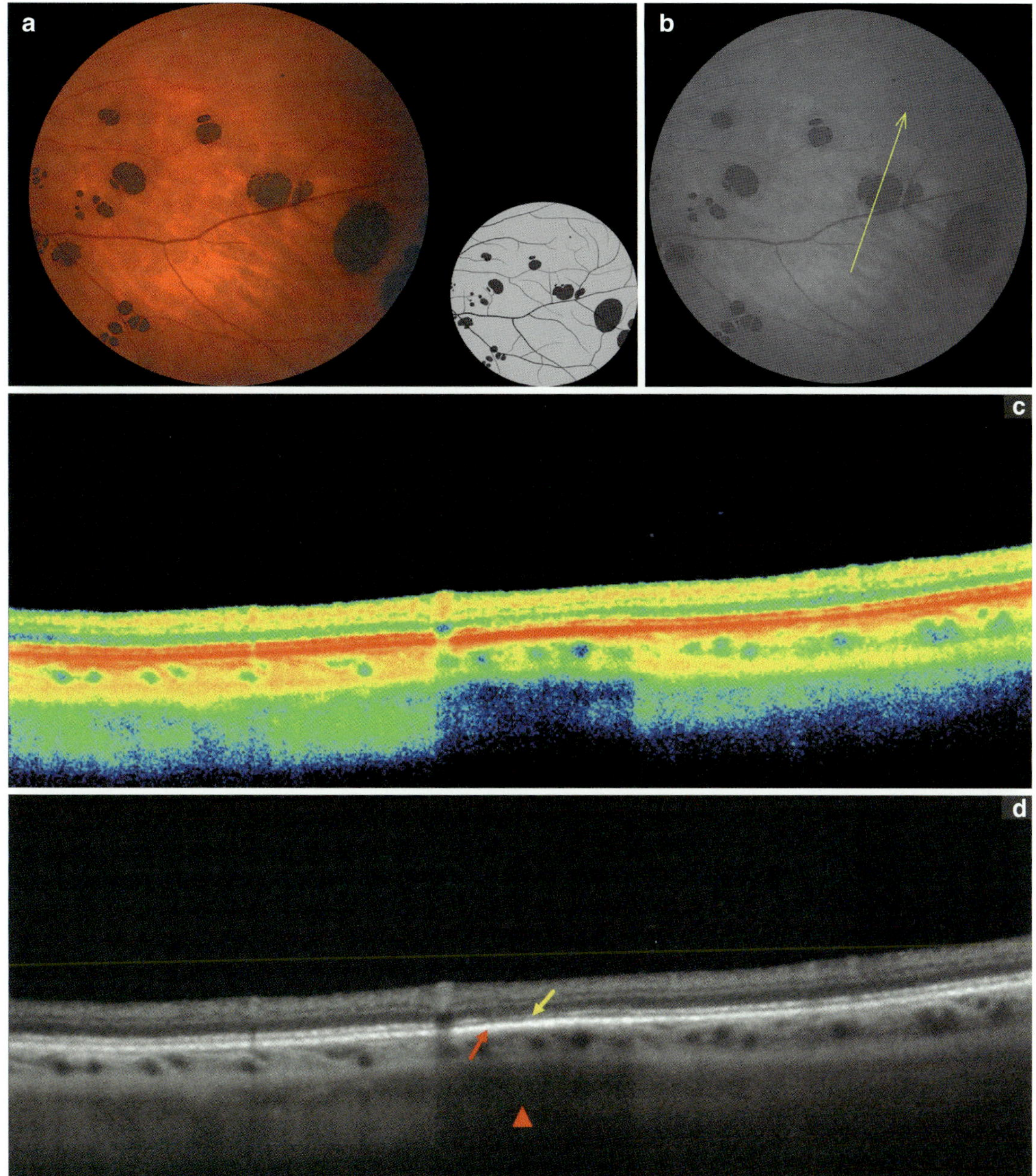

Fig. 6.65 (**a**) Multifocal congenital hypertrophy of the pigment epithelium (bear tracks). (**b**) *Line* indicates OCT-scanning direction. (**c, d**) OCT-scanning results according to the line direction in (**b**)

Honeycomb Degeneration

Honeycomb (reticular) degeneration is an age-related retinal degeneration characterized by hyperpigmented net, that can extend up to equator [6]. The etiology and pathogenesis of honeycomb degeneration remain unclear. Its clinical manifestations include hyperpigmented honeycomb (lace) pattern; the lesion is found in individuals of 46–90 years of age (mean age, 69.2 ± 8.54 years). Less than 10 % of patients are less than 55 years of age. Both sexes are almost equally affected [8].

According to some experts, honeycomb degeneration is usually bilateral and most commonly located at the equator. It is characterized by hyperpigmentation of pigment epithelium and linear hyperpigmented hexagons [9]. The loss of pigment is attributed to the degenerative process in pigment epithelium cells, and its geometrical, reticular appearance – to thinning, shrinking, and reactive hyperplasia of the pigment epithelium cells.

Honeycomb degeneration (Table 6.3) is reported to be most frequently found in advanced age and considered a benign condition, that does not cause retinal detachment; thus, prophylactic laser treatment is not indicated [5].

Table 6.3 Diagram of peripheral retinal degenerations

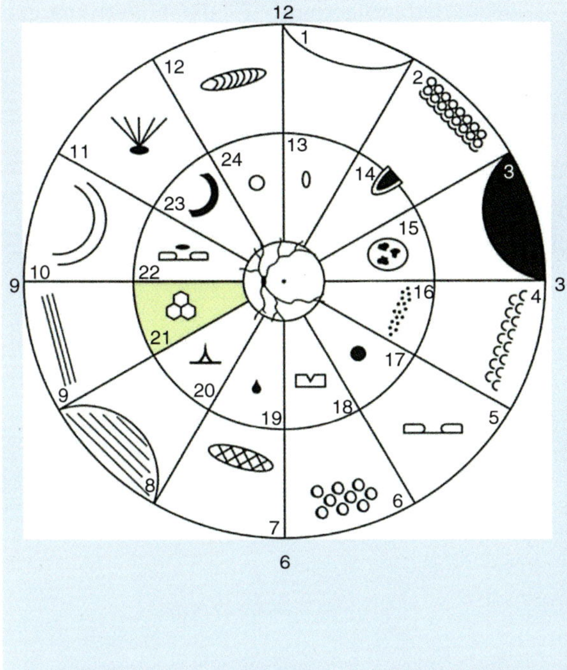

1. Retinal dialysis
2. Peripheral cystoid degeneration
3. Retinal detachment
4. Retinal drusen
5. Full-thickness tear
6. Paving-stone degeneration
7. Lattice degeneration
8. Bullous retinoschisis
9. Flat retinoschisis
10. White-without-pressure
11. Retinal tuft
12. Snail-track degeneration
13. Pearl degeneration
14. Flap tear
15. Grouped congenital hypertrophy of the retinal pigment epithelium ("bear tracks")
16. Snowflake degeneration
17. Unifocal hypertrophy of the retinal pigment epithelium
18. Atrophic retinal hole
19. Haemorrhage
20. Preretinal fibrosis
21. Honeycomb degeneration
22. Operculated retinal tear
23. Dark-without-pressure
24. Unifocal atrophy of the retinal pigment epithelium

Honeycomb degeneration in sector 21 is highlighted in yellow

Case 66. Honeycomb Degeneration

A 76-year-old female patient with moderate hyperopia and early stage cortical cataract presented with complaints of decreased vision.

Ophthalmoscopic Findings (Fig. 6.66a, b)
Multiple pigment clumps of various forms and sizes, with a honeycomb appearance are observed in the mid-periphery of the temporal quadrant of the left eye.

OCT Scan Description (Fig. 6.66c, d)
The retinal surface is smooth with no vitreoretinal adhesion or traction. The retina contains hyperreflective deposits causing a shadow effect (decreased reflectivity) in the underlying tissues. Areas of dense pigment epithelium are seen.

OCT Scan Details (Fig. 6.66c, d)

Intraretinal hyperreflective deposits

Areas of dense pigment epithelium

Decreased reflectivity of the pigment epithelium and the choroid at the level of intraretinal deposits

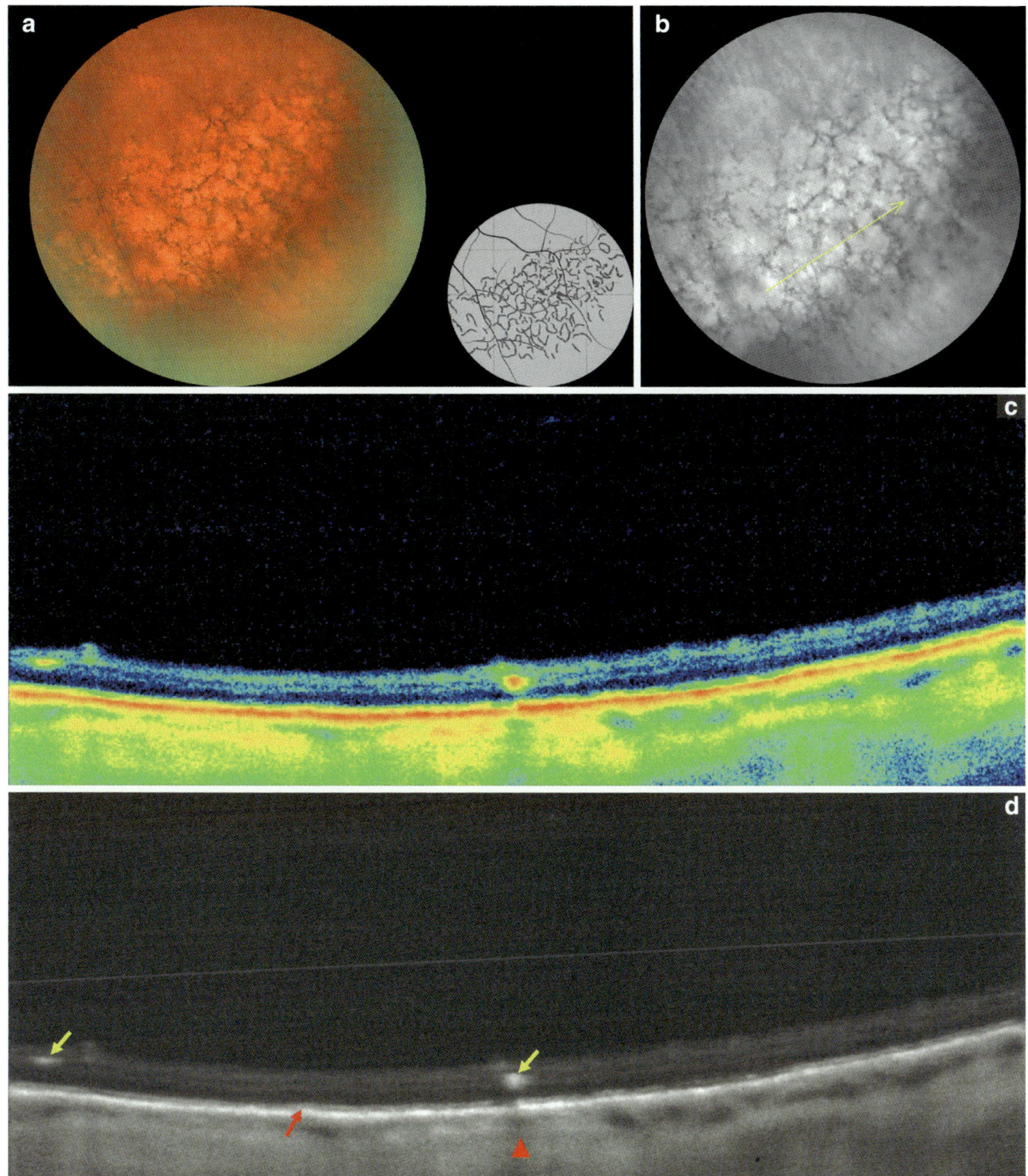

Fig. 6.66 (**a**) Honeycomb degeneration. (**b**) *Line* indicates OCT-scanning direction. (**c, d**) OCT-scanning results according to the line direction in (**b**)

Case 67. Honeycomb Degeneration with an Atrophic Lesion of the Pigment Epithelium

A 76-year-old male patient with mild hyperopia and early stage cataract presented with complaints of decreased vision. Examination revealed honeycomb degeneration with an atrophic lesion of the pigment epithelium.

Ophthalmoscopic Findings (Fig. 6.67a, b)

Multiple pigment clumps of various forms and sizes, with a honeycomb appearance are observed in the mid- and far periphery of the inferior quadrant of the left eye. An atrophic lesion of the pigment epithelium with sharp borders is seen at 7 o'clock position. A choroidal pattern is noticeable in the center of atrophic area.

OCT Scan Description (Fig. 6.67c, d)

The retinal surface is irregular because of local thinning, neuroepithelium atrophy and pigment epithelium destruction with a hyperreflective shadow in the choroid (comet tail). There are multiple areas of pigment epithelium elevation and hypertrophy at the lesion margins. Choroid is hyporeflective because the light transmittance decreases.

OCT Scan Details (Fig. 6.67c, d)

Area of retinal thinning at the level of the atrophic lesion

Area of pigment epithelium destruction

Dense pigment epithelium

Increased choroidal reflectivity at the level of the pigment epithelium destruction

Decreased reflectivity of the choroid at the level of the dense pigment epithelium

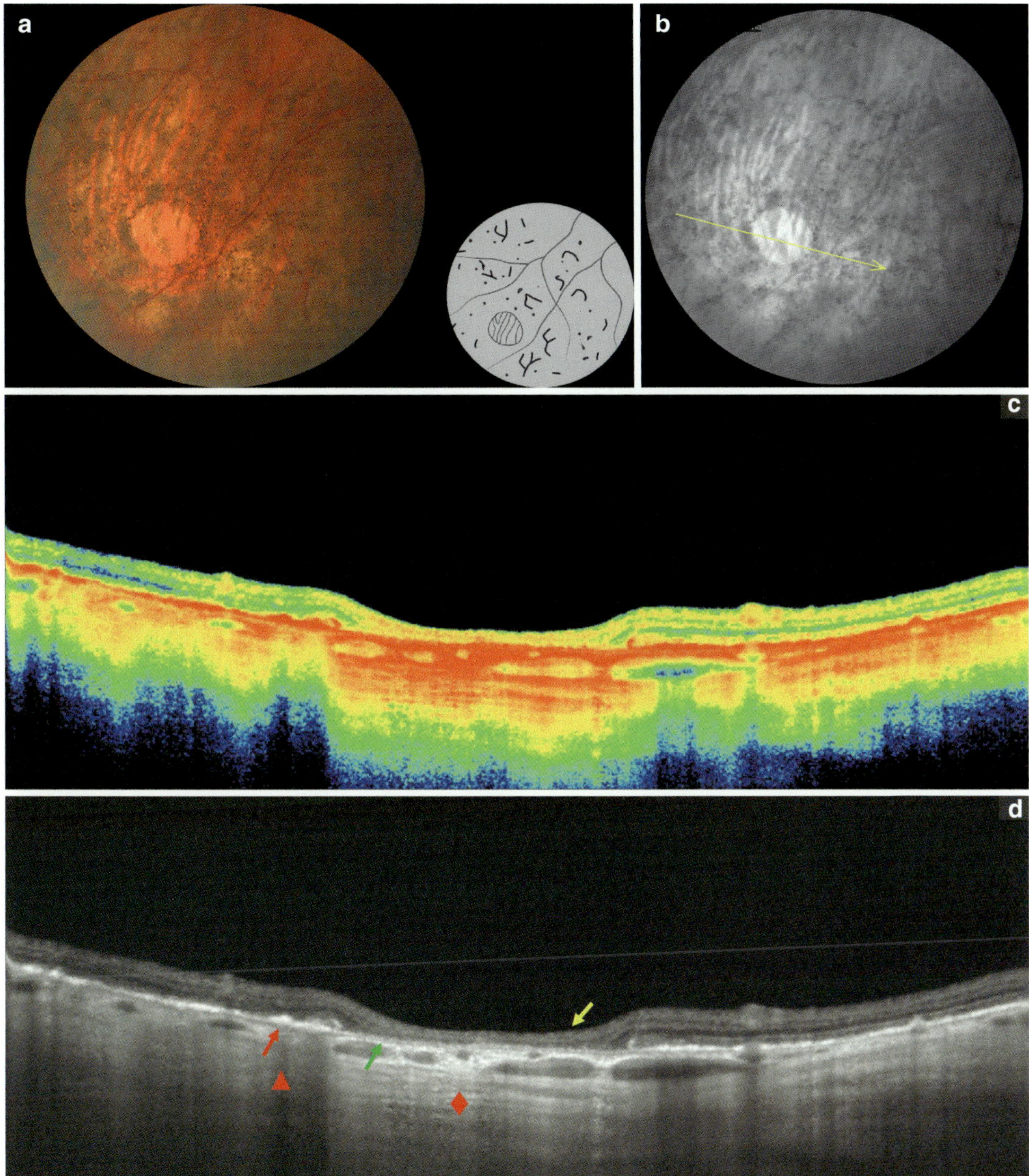

Fig. 6.67 (**a**) Honeycomb degeneration with an atrophic lesion of the pigment epithelium. (**b**) *Line* indicates OCT-scanning direction. (**c, d**) OCT-scanning results according to the line direction in (**b**)

Peripheral Retinal Drusen

Peripheral retinal drusen are extracellular deposits of proteins and fatty unstructured material between the basement membrane of the pigment epithelium and the inner collagenous layer of Bruch's membrane [10]. Retinal drusen appear as glistening crystals, and the term itself refers to a German word meaning "stone nodule or geode" [12]. Drusen are reported to result from the degeneration of pigment epithelial cells, which accumulate metabolic waste products and exude them in the inner layers of Bruch's membrane in the form of small dome-shaped lesions [11, 12].

The universal classification of drusen has not yet been established. Drusen have been described as hard, soft, mixed, complex, and diffuse (laminar or cuticular) [12, 13].

"Hard" drusen are usually found in the peripheral retina. They consist of solid, hyaloid, homogenous material and are usually small (mean diameter, 47.3 nm) [12]. Retinal drusen have different forms and sizes but are most commonly small, round- or dome-shaped, and clearly outlined in front of the healthy retina. This degeneration is commonly age related and bilateral and reported to be found in individuals >40 years of age. During fluorescein angiography, "hard" drusen demonstrate hyperfluorescent spots during choroidal flush (window effect) with subsequent gradual hypofluoresence [10, 13]. There has been a report of spontaneous resolution of drusen [14]. Different patterns of pigment epithelium hyperplasia result in pigment-ringed drusen [11] or small multifocal hyperpigmented lesions [14].

In addition to retinal drusen, reticular pseudo-drusen, also known as subretinal drusenoid deposits, are described. Reticular pseudo-drusen form yellow deposits arranged in a network, which are located between the pigment epithelium and photoreceptor layer in the superior quadrant of the retina [15]. Pseudo-drusen are best visualized during ophthalmoscopy or fundus photography in blue light but are not seen during fluorescein angiography [14].

Peripheral retinal drusen (Table 6.4) are considered to be a benign degeneration, which most commonly occurs with increasing age and is rarely associated with clinically significant consequences. Prophylactic laser treatment is not indicated [5, 11].

Table 6.4 Diagram of peripheral retinal degenerations

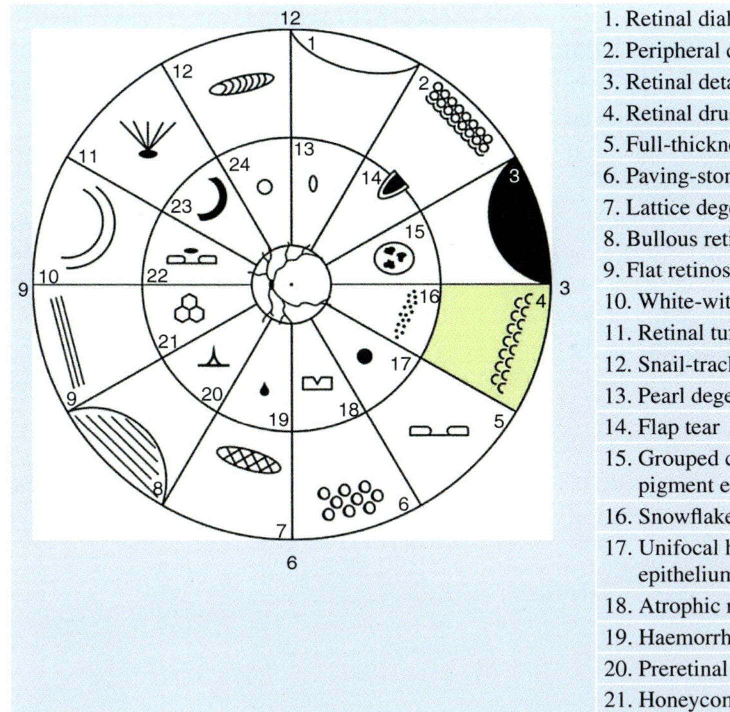

1. Retinal dialysis
2. Peripheral cystoid degeneration
3. Retinal detachment
4. Retinal drusen
5. Full-thickness tear
6. Paving-stone degeneration
7. Lattice degeneration
8. Bullous retinoschisis
9. Flat retinoschisis
10. White-without-pressure
11. Retinal tuft
12. Snail-track degeneration
13. Pearl degeneration
14. Flap tear
15. Grouped congenital hypertrophy of the retinal pigment epithelium ("bear tracks")
16. Snowflake degeneration
17. Unifocal hypertrophy of the retinal pigment epithelium
18. Atrophic retinal hole
19. Haemorrhage
20. Preretinal fibrosis
21. Honeycomb degeneration
22. Operculated retinal tear
23. Dark-without-pressure
24. Unifocal atrophy of the retinal pigment epithelium

Retinal drusen in sector 4 are highlighted in yellow

Case 68. Peripheral Retinal Drusen

A 48-year-old female patient presented with complaints of reduced vision in her right eye. Examination revealed low hyperopia, early stage cataract and multiple drusen in the equatorial zone and in the retinal periphery of her right eye.

Ophthalmoscopic Findings (Fig. 6.68a)

Multiple circular, spot-like whitish lesions are seen in the equatorial and peripheral retina of the right eye. The retina around the lesions is unaltered.

OCT Scan Description (Fig. 6.68c, d)

The retinal surface is smooth. Multiple regions of pigment epithelium elevation and areas of increased density are observed. Signs of ellipsoid zone destruction are evident. Hyperreflective inclusions are seen in the vitreous. No vitreous traction is present.

OCT Scan Details (Fig. 6.68c, d)

Multiple pigment epithelium elevations and dense areas with moderately reflective content

Areas of ellipsoid layer destruction

Decreased choroidal reflectivity at the level of the dense areas of pigment epithelium

Multiple hyperreflective deposits in the vitreous

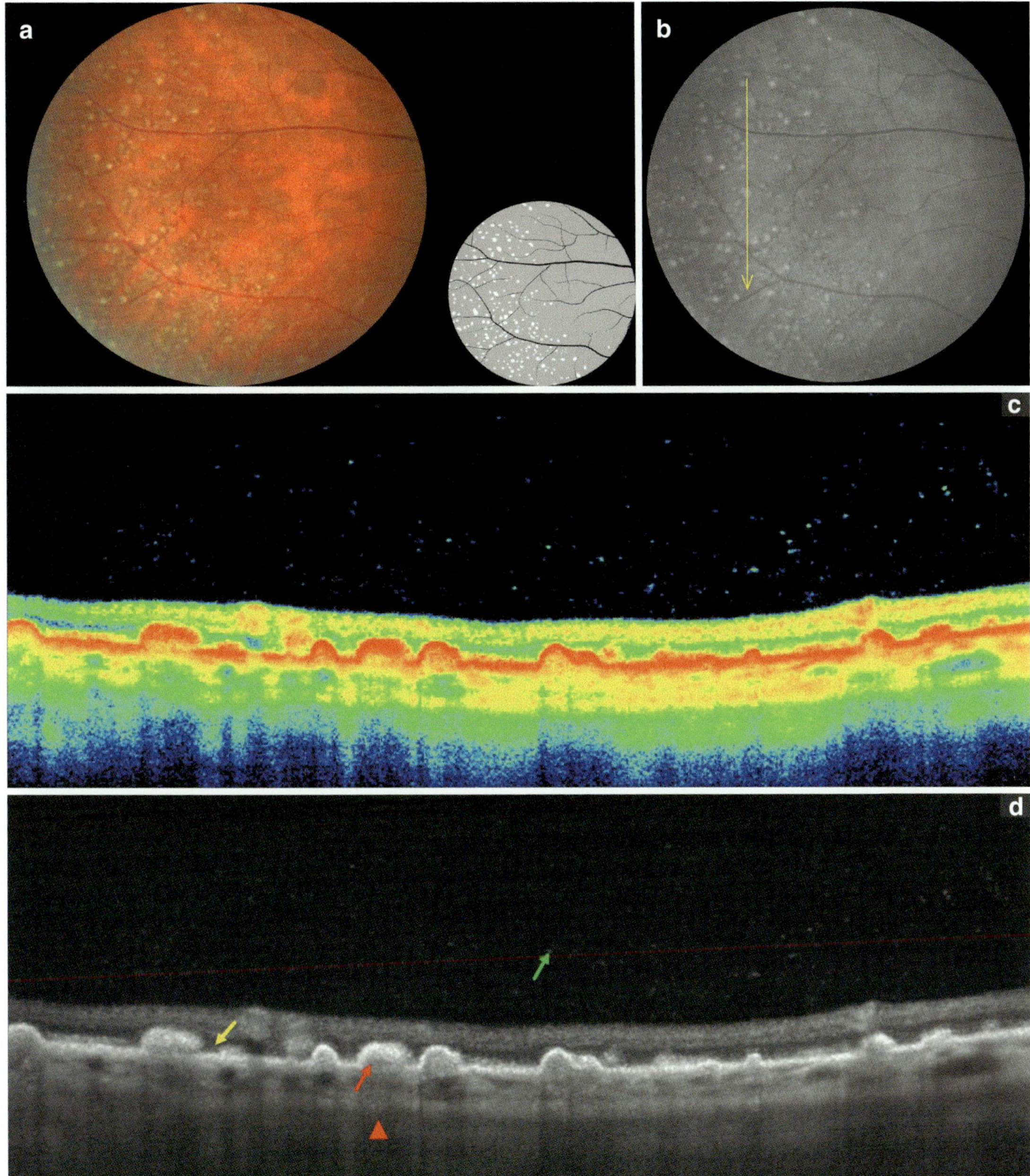

Fig. 6.68 (**a**) Peripheral retinal drusen. (**b**) *Line* indicates OCT-scanning direction. (**c, d**) OCT-scanning results according to the line direction in (**b**)

References

1. Ho A, et al. Retina. Color atlas and synopsis of clinical ophthalmology. Wills Eye Series. McGraw-Hill Professional; 2003.
2. Pasechnikova NV. Laser treatment of the eye fundus pathology. Kiev: Naukova Dumka (In Russian); 2007.
3. Franchuk AA. Prophylactic retinal laser photocoagulation in peripheral retinal degeneration in fellow eyes after unilateral retinal detachment. Dissertation, Odessa research Institute of eye diseases and tissue therapy (In Russian); 1981.
4. Rutnin U, Schepens CL. Fundus appearance in normal eyes. IV. Retinal breaks and other finding. Am J Ophthalmol. 1967;64(6):1040–1.
5. Macalister G, Sullivan P. Peripheral retinal degenerations. In: OT CET. 2011. http://www.metropolia.fi/fileadmin/user_upload/Liiketoimintapalvelut/Sosiaali-_ja_terveysala/Optikoiden_DG-koulutuksen_materiaalit/Peripheral_retinal_degenerations.pdf. Accessed 24 June 2011.
6. Kanski D, Bowling B. Clinical ophthalmology: systemic approach. 7th ed. Edinburgh: Elsevier/Saunders; 2011.
7. Morhat MV, Marchenko LN, Morhat VI. Prophylactic laser photocoagulation in peripheral retina irregularities (literature review). Ophthalmol East Eur. 2011;4(11):85–92.
8. Humphrey WT, Carlson RE, Valone Jr JA. Senile reticular pigmentary degeneration. Am J Ophthalmol. 1984;98(6):717–22.
9. Lewis H, Straatsma BR, Foos RY, et al. Reticular degeneration of the pigment epithelium. Ophthalmology. 1985;92(11):1485–95.
10. Heimann H, Kelner U, Forster M. Atlas of fundus angiography. Stuttgart: Thieme; 2006.
11. Jones WL. Peripheral ocular fundus. 3rd ed. St. Louis: Elsevier; 2007.
12. Rudolf M, Clark ME, Chimento MF, et al. Prevalence and morphology of druse types in the macula and periphery of eyes with age-related maculopathy. Invest Ophthalmol Vis Sci. 2008;49(3):1200–9.
13. Ditmar S, Holz FG. Fluorescent angiography in ophthalmology. Heidelberg: Springer; 2008.
14. Yannuzzi L. The retinal atlas. Amsterdam: Elsevier Science; 2010.
15. Van der Schaft TL, de Bruijn WC, Mooy CM, et al. Basal laminar deposit in the aging peripheral human retina. Graef's Arch Clin Exp Ophthalmol. 1993; 231(8):470–5.

Retinal Laser Photocoagulation in Peripheral Retinal Degenerations

Venera A. Shaimova, Ernest V. Boyko, and Olga G. Pozdeeva

Indications for Retinal Laser Photocoagulation in Peripheral Retinal Degenerations

Peripheral vitreochorioretinal degenerations represent a risk factor for rhegmatogenous retinal detachment (RRD) [1–4]. RRD prevalence is 1 case per 10,000 of population, and it is bilateral in 1.18–10 % of patients according to different authors [5–8].

While retinal tears that originate from vitreoretinal degenerations during posterior vitreous

V.A. Shaimova (✉)
Chelyabinsk State Laser Surgery Institute,
Chelyabinsk, Russian Federation

Center Zreniya Medical Clinic, LLC,
Chelyabinsk, Russian Federation
e-mail: shaimova.v@mail.ru

E.V. Boyko
St. Petersburg Branch of S. Fyodorov Eye
Microsurgery Federal State Institution,
St. Petersburg, Russian Federation

Department of Ophthalmology, Mechnikov
North-West State Medical University,
St. Petersburg, Russian Federation

Department of Ophthalmology, S.M. Kirov Military
Medical Academy, St. Petersburg, Russian Federation

O.G. Pozdeeva
Municipal City Clinical Hospital No 2,
Chelyabinsk, Russian Federation

Eye Diseases Department, South Ural State Medical
University, Chelyabinsk, Russian Federation

detachment are the main cause of RRD, many authors consider it necessary to prevent retinal detachment creating chorioretinal adhesions around the retinal tears and/or its precursors by means of laser photocoagulation or cryotherapy [8–11].

Degenerative changes of the peripheral retina may be divided into two categories: predisposing or not predisposing to the RRD. Preventive retinopexy may be indicated in cases of retinal degenerations of the first category among mentioned above [1]. However, there is no consensus at present time, which peripheral degenerations are really predisposing (rhegmatogenous). Therefore, prophylactic treatment of retinal detachment is still debated, because it is not clear which type of the lesion should be treated and which therapeutic method should be used [12].

According to some authors [13], prophylactic treatment of peripheral retinal degenerations remains clinical and economic problem in which more profound evidence is needed. According to other authors' data [9], preventive laser treatment or cryopexy is an effective method to prevent retinal detachment.

Retinal laser photocoagulation (LPC) is considered more preferable, while cryopexy should be used in cases when media opacities prevent laser treatment [2]. Laser retinopexy is based on obtaining the effect of tissue coagulation followed with scar adhesions formation between the choroid and the retina, which prevents neurosensory retinal detachment from the pigment epithe-

© Springer International Publishing AG 2017
V.A. Shaimova (ed.), *Peripheral Retinal Degenerations*, DOI 10.1007/978-3-319-48995-7_7

lium and blocks the flow of the liquefied vitreous into the subretinal space [11, 14, 15].

After photocoagulators had become widely available, retinopexy has been performed in almost all clinical forms of peripheral retinal degenerations [11]. However, in the 1960s there already had been studies showing that retinal tears following degenerative changes of the peripheral retina occur in 13.7 % of the population, but not all of them lead to RRD; therefore, it was recommended to perform preventive laser treatment only when indicated [11, 16–18]. To determine the indications, RRD risk factors were identified: flap tears, PVD (partial), RRD on the fellow eye, aphakia, pseudophakia; symptomatic manifestation as photopsias, floaters and blurred vision; subclinical retinal detachment around the tear, family history (RRD in relatives), and systemic diseases: Marfan syndrome, Stickler syndrome, and Ehler-Danlos syndrome [8, 19].

There are a lot of controversial and sometimes conflicting publications on indications for prophylactic LPC in peripheral retinal degenerations [7, 20–24]. Despite the large number of publications, there had been no randomized trials of the preventive treatment effectiveness in different clinical types of peripheral retinal degenerations, and therefore, there is still no clear consensus on the indications for laser intervention [23, 25, 26]. This makes laser surgeons "solve the problem relying mainly on their own experience" [11].

According to some authors, preventive retinal LPC in peripheral vitreoretinal degenerations should be performed preferably in the presence of symptomatic PVD [7, 20, 21, 27], symptomatic flap tear [22]; or all types of symptomatic tears [24, 28]. However, there is an alternative view, and according to other authors, laser retinopexy is indicated "in all cases of vitreoretinal degeneration" [10], or "at the slightest sign of vitreoretinal traction" in peripheral retinal degeneration [23].

Of interest is the monograph by Bolshunov AV (2013) where he presented indications for preventive retinal LPC in the following types of peripheral degenerations:

1. All symptomatic retinal tears
2. Asymptomatic retinal tears occurring in:
   (a) Myopia
   (b) Aphakia
   (c) Before cataract surgery
   (d) Fellow eye in unilateral retinal detachment
   (e) Hereditary predisposition
3. Chorioretinal degenerations with "malignant" course:
   (a) "lattice"
   (b) "snail track"
   (c) "snowflake"
   (d) Other degeneration types with vitreoretinal tractions
4. All kinds of chorioretinal degenerations with "malignant" course and retinal tears in the fellow eye before refractive surgery
5. Progressive retinoschisis

Lacking consensus on the indications for prophylactic retinal LPC in patients with peripheral retinal degenerations it is advisable to take into account the Preferred Practice Patterns for treatment (Table 7.1) and follow-up (Table 7.2) recommended by the American Academy of Ophthalmology in 2014 [29].

Therapeutic efficacy of LPC as a preventive method in different types of peripheral vitreochorioretinal degenerations is 75–100 % according to literature data [30, 31]. The need for retinal LPC in peripheral vitreoretinal degenerations is supported by many publications: the risk of retinal detachment with deferred symptomatic tears' treatment may reach 30–50 % [32]. The risk of retinal tear and retinal detachment in patients with lattice degeneration and retinal detachment in the fellow eye without preventive laser treatment was 2.5 times higher than in same patients after retinopexy (5.1 % vs 1.8 %, $p = 0.0125$) [33]. Preventive retinal LPC in aphakic patients with vitreoretinal degeneration reduced the incidence of retinal detachment to 0.33 % of the cases compared to

Table 7.1 Management options in peripheral retinal degenerations

Type of lesion	Treatment[a]
Acute symptomatic horseshoe tears	Treat promptly
Acute symptomatic operculated holes	Treatment may not be necessary
Acute symptomatic dialyses	Treat promptly
Traumatic retinal breaks	Usually treated
Asymptomatic horseshoe tears (without subclinical retinal detachment)	Often can be followed without treatment
Asymptomatic operculated tears	Treatment is rarely recommended
Asymptomatic atrophic round holes	Treatment is rarely recommended
Asymptomatic lattice degeneration without holes	Not treated unless PVD causes a horseshoe tear
Asymptomatic lattice degeneration with holes	Usually does not require treatment
Asymptomatic dialyses	No consensus on treatment and insufficient evidence to guide management
Eyes with atrophic holes, lattice degeneration, or asymptomatic horseshoe tears where the fellow eye has had a retinal detachment	No consensus on treatment and insufficient evidence to guide management

Reprinted with permission of American Academy of Ophthalmology Retina/Vitreous Panel. Preferred Practice Pattern®Guidelines. *Posterior Vitreous Detachment, Retinal Breaks, and Lattice Degeneration.* San Francisco, CA: American Academy of Ophthalmology; 2014. Available at: www.aao.org/ppp
[a]There is insufficient evidence to recommend prophylaxis of asymptomatic retinal breaks for patients undergoing cataract surgery

Table 7.2 Follow-up guidelines in peripheral retinal degenerations

Type of lesion	Follow-up interval
Symptomatic PVD with no retinal break	Depending on symptoms, risk factors, and clinical findings, patients may be followed in 1–8 weeks, then 6–12 months
Acute symptomatic horseshoe tears	1–2 weeks after treatment, then 4–6 weeks, then 3–6 months, then annually
Acute symptomatic operculated holes	2–4 weeks, then 1–3 months, then 6–12 months, then annually
Acute symptomatic dialyses	1–2 weeks after treatment, then 4–6 weeks, then 3–6 months, then annually
Traumatic retinal breaks	1–2 weeks after treatment, then 4–6 weeks, then 3–6 months, then annually
Asymptomatic horseshoe tears (without subclinical retinal detachment)	1–4 weeks, then 2–4 months, then 6–12 months, then annually
Asymptomatic operculated tears	1–4 months, then 6–12 months, then annually
Asymptomatic atrophic round holes	1–2 years
Asymptomatic lattice degeneration without holes	Annually
Asymptomatic lattice degeneration with holes	Annually
Asymptomatic dialyses	If untreated, 1 month, then 3 months, then 6 months, then every 6 months
	If treated, 1–2 weeks after treatment, then 4–6 weeks, then 3–6 months, then annually
Eyes with atrophic holes, lattice degeneration, or asymptomatic horseshoe tears where the fellow eye has had a retinal detachment	Every 6–12 months

Reprinted with permission of American Academy of Ophthalmology Retina/Vitreous Panel. Preferred Practice Pattern® Guidelines. *Posterior Vitreous Detachment, Retinal Breaks, and Lattice Degeneration.* San Francisco, CA: American Academy of Ophthalmology; 2014. Available at: www.aao.org/ppp

2 % in the control group [34]. Ora secunda cerclage effectively protects against RRD [26]. LPC and cryotherapy are considered effective methods to prevent retinal detachment [9]. Prophylactic LPC significantly reduces the risk of retinal detachment [10], and many authors consider laser treatment an easy-to-use and convenient treatment method [35].

However, there is an alternative viewpoint, that laser treatment performed in the visible areas of degeneration may increase the invisible vitreoretinal traction and cause new tears and retinal detachment in unsuspected areas, and sometimes the treatment itself should be recognized as a risk factor for RRD [18, 36].

According to most of the foreign and national authors, one should carefully examine each patient and take into account all risk factors before performing a prophylactic treatment in peripheral degenerations. These risk factors include: the presence of symptoms, vitreoretinal traction, tear, and subretinal fluid around the break; localization of lesions, family history of retinal detachment, the state of the fellow eye, refraction, age, gender, patient's profession; special circumstances, such as aphakia or pseudophakia, posterior capsulotomy due to the secondary cataract, planned refractive surgery. Laser is a useful treatment tool, and it must be used wisely [11, 14].

Performing optical coherence tomography of the retinal periphery may be of great help in determining the risk of RRD, necessity and timing (promptness) of preventive LPC (see Figs. 7.1, 7.2, and 7.3), and in assessing the state of the retina and laser burns in the postoperative period (see Figs. 7.4 and 7.5). OCT in the retinal periphery makes it possible to determine the morphometric parameters (length and height) of the vitreoretinal traction and its changes over time, that allows to refine the indications for retinal LPC. Analysis of OCT data in different clinical types of retinal tears allowed to identify three risk levels according to the probability of RRD development: retinal tears with high risk of RRD, retinal tears with moderate risk of RRD, and retinal tears with low risk of RRD. Below we present examples of three clinical cases, corresponding to different levels of RRD risk.

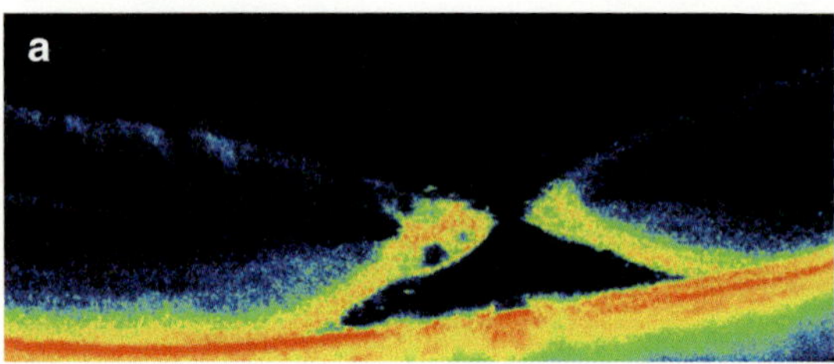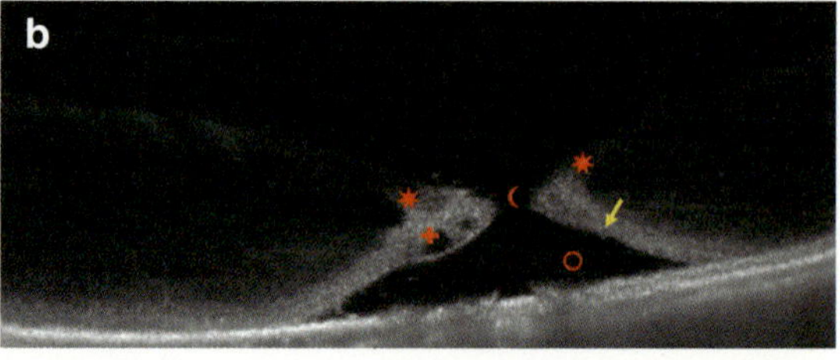

Fig. 7.1 Spectral Domain OCT scan (6 mm) in the area of the retinal tear with neurosensory retinal detachment. (**a**) Color image, (**b**) Black and white image. Full-thickness retinal tear (*crescent*) with neurosensory retinal detachment (*circle*) is seen with its edges thickened (*yellow arrow*) and containing hyporeflective cavities (*crisscross*), and vitreoretinal traction (*asterisk*) at the edges of the tear

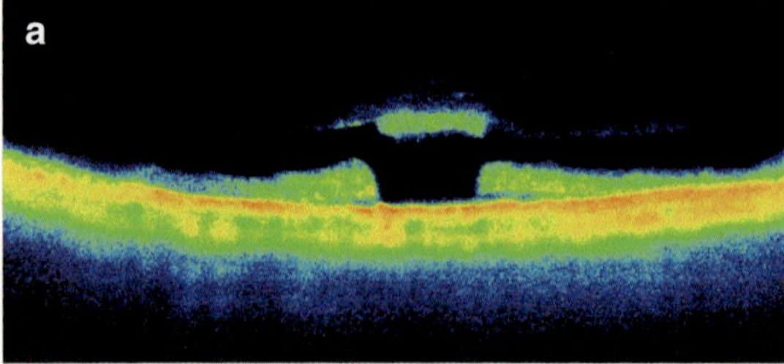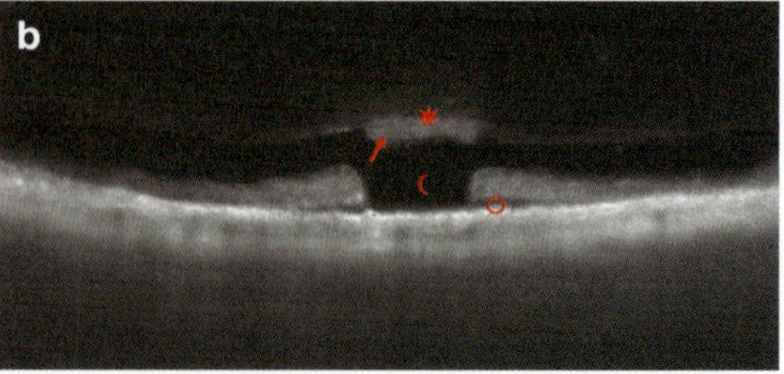

Fig. 7.2 Spectral Domain OCT scan (6 mm) in the area of the retinal tear with operculum and shallow retinal detachment. (**a**) Color image, (**b**) Black and white image. Full-thickness retinal tear (*crescent*) with flat (*slit*-like) neurosensory retinal detachment (*circle*) is seen with hyperreflective operculum (*arrow*) on the outer surface of the detached vitreous (*asterisk*); no vitreoretinal traction is seen in the tear area

First case A 29-year-old male patient complained of intermittent lightnings and floaters affecting his right eye for 1 week. Ophthalmoscopic exam revealed a tractional tear in the upper-temporal segment of the peripheral retina. OCT scan showed a full-thickness retinal tear with a shallow neurosensory retina detachment and severe vitreoretinal traction (Fig. 7.1a, b). This case represents a high level of RRD risk and is an absolute indication for urgent delimiting retinal LPC on the right eye.

Second case A 45-year-old male patient came to the ophthalmologist to have glasses prescribed, as he complained of blurred vision while reading. Ophthalmoscopic exam revealed an isolated tear with an operculum floating in the vitreous over the tear in the peripheral retina lower segment of the left eye. OCT scanning showed the full-thickness retinal tear with shallow neurosensory retinal detachment and hyperreflective operculum on the outer surface of the detached vitreous. Vitreoretinal traction is absent (see Fig. 7.2a, b).

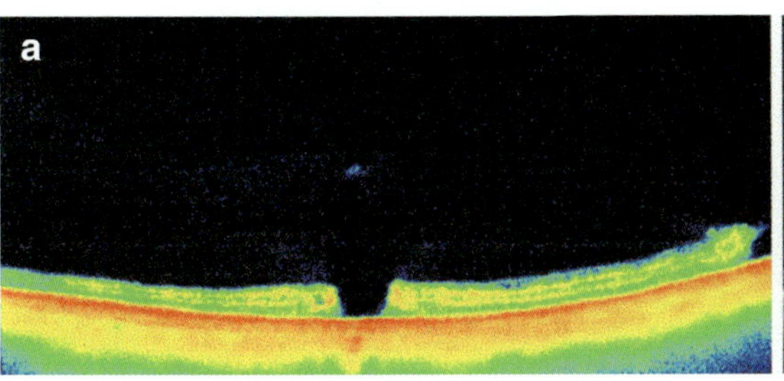
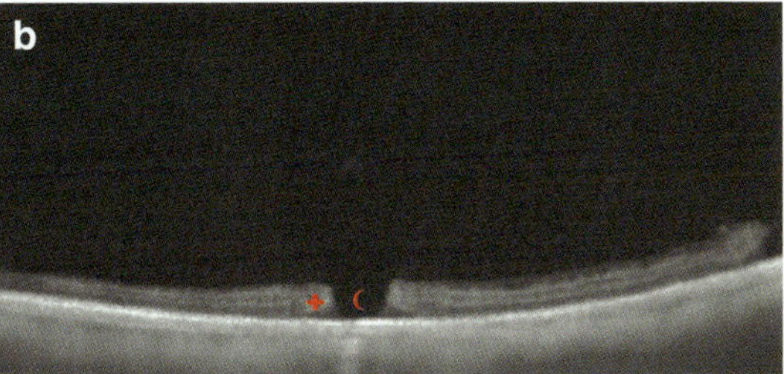

Fig. 7.3 Spectral Domain OCT scan (6 mm) in the area of the full-thickness retinal tear. (**a**) Color image, (**b**) *Black* and *white* image. Full-thickness retinal tear (*crescent*) is seen with surrounding neurosensory retina (*crisscross*) attached to the retinal pigment epithelium; no vitreoretinal traction is seen

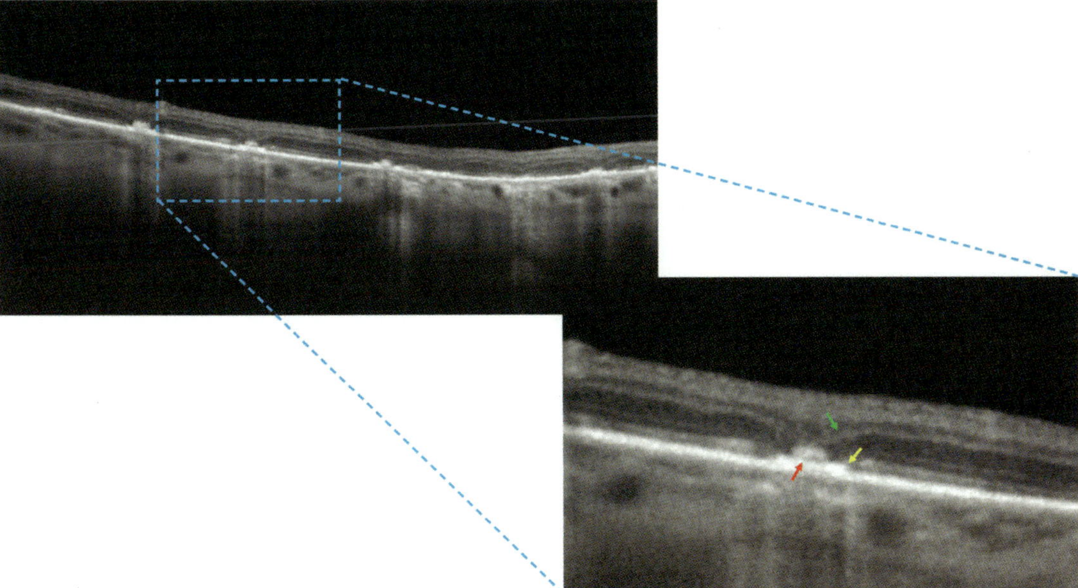

Fig. 7.4 Retinal OCT scan 2 weeks after retinal laser photocoagulation. Localized hyperreflective areas at the level of the pigment epithelium and outer nuclear layer of the neurosensory retina (*red arrow* pointing at RPE thickening) are seen at laser burns, with photoreceptors and RPE destruction at the edges of these lesions (*yellow arrow*). The outer plexiform and inner nuclear layers became funnel-shaped (green arrow) in the direction of the retinal pigment epithelium

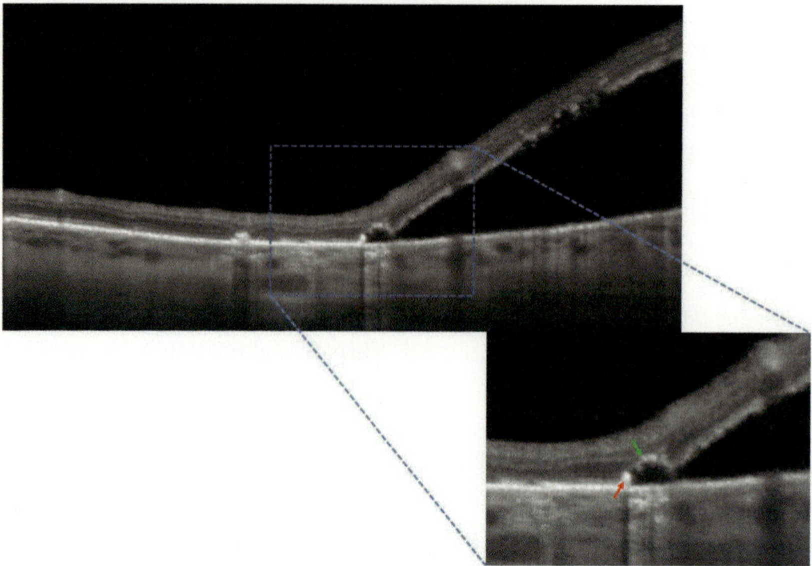

Fig. 7.5 OCT image of retinal detachment occurring after the delimiting LPC. Neurosensory retinal detachment reaches laser burns (RPE thickening, *red arrow*), and its outer layers' arcuate deformation (*green arrow*) is formed

Taking into account both clinical data (absence of symptomatic complaints) and OCT results, this case illustrates a moderate RRD risk and is a relative indication for retinal LPC. It is recommended to follow changes over time.

Third case A 59-year-old female patient complained of blurred vision in her right eye for six months. Ophthalmoscopic exam revealed mild cortical cataract and isolated tear in the lower-temporal segment of the retinal periphery. OCT (see Fig. 7.3a, b) revealed the full-thickness neurosensory retinal tear with its edges completely attached to RPE, no subretinal fluid and vitreo-retinal traction. This case can be attributed to the third group with a low level RRD risk. There are no indications for urgent preventive LPC, but the patient should be instructed to visit an ophthalmologist in case of any visual symptom. It is recommended to follow changes over time.

Methods of Retinal Laser Photocoagulation

Characteristics of laser radiation are unique: it is highly coherent in time (monochromaticity) and in space (small beam divergence), which allows to focus the light energy on the small diameter spot. Simply said, the mechanism of laser action in the fundus tissues is to convert light energy into heat, and to perform the primary coagulative damage of the pigment epithelium, choriocapillaris and photoreceptors' outer layers. In long-term prospective, these necrotic masses are replaced by the reparative tissue rich in pigment cells, and the chorioretinal scar is formed [37]. Furthermore, retina should be fully attached in the LPC area, which is an obligatory condition for a strong chorioretinal adhesion. The direct clinical effect is produced if the desired intensity of the retinal burns is achieved [38].

Optical coherence tomography in vivo reveals the destructive changes in the pigment epithelium during preventive retinopexy and the redistribution of pigment epithelium at the burn's borders. Cells are destructed and deformed during LPC, as a result, pigment epithelium is proliferated and chorioretinal adhesions are formed in 1 or 2 weeks after the operation (see Figs. 7.4 and 7.5).

Lasers with the wavelength of visible (yellow, green, red, etc.) or near-infrared range (approximately to 1 μm) may be used for retinopexy. Exposure varies from tenths of seconds to seconds. Selection of power begins with the minimum value [11, 15, 39] which then is gradually increased until the 1 degree burn is achieved. For more severe burns one should continue to increase the output power to meet the coagulation step. Burns of greater intensity may also be obtained by increasing the exposure without increasing the power.

When performing retinal LPC with the argon laser (blue-green part of the spectrum: 488–514 nm) or the solid-state YAG laser with doubled frequency (wavelength of the green part of the spectrum: 532 nm), it is necessary to achieve 2–3 degree burns, and 1–2 degree burns when using the diode (infrared: 810 nm) laser.

Burn degree is more homogeneous when using lasers with a wavelength of the visible spectrum, and may differ slightly between burns when using infrared lasers, which is determined, as a rule, by the inhomogeneity of the fundus pigmentation. Burn's degree and size are influenced by optical media opacities, and the denser is optical haze, the larger may be the laser spot diameter on the fundus and the lower burn's degree. In the presence of optical media opacities, infrared lasers provide obvious advantage for fundus coagulation, but infrared laser retinopexy weaknesses include the lack of visual control of the tissue response to laser irradiation.

Depending on the extent of degenerative process, its localization and the "malignancy" of its course, that may lead to retinal tear and detachment, there are different methods of LPC: barrier, delimiting, and circular. Several different types of the preventive laser retinopexy have been proposed in the literature: two rows of confluent laser burns [8]; two to three rows of staggered burns with the distance of ≤1 burn diameter between them [11, 39]; three to four rows of adjoined burns along the lesion edge [14].

The most possible attenuated coagulation modes should be used for preventive LPC of peripheral tears and rhegmatogenous retinal degenerations. When performing retinal LPC with an argon laser or a solid-state YAG laser with doubled frequency the continuous mode is used with spot diameter of 300–500 μm and exposure of 0.2 s, the power is adjusted individually depending on the fundus pigmentation and optical media transparency (2–3 degree burn is considered the best). In cases when a diode laser (infrared: 810 nm) is used, burn diameter is 200–300 μm, exposure is 0.1–0.2 s, and the power that is required to achieve 1–2 degree laser burns. The results of treatment are evaluated after 2 weeks after retinal LPC.

A constant follow-up is recommended after retinal LPC: first in 1–2 weeks, then after 3–6 months, and then annually [22]. Additional retinal LPC should be performed in cases of new degenerative foci or progressive and complicated course of retinal lesion [11].

Many authors have warned about the possible complications after retinal LPC, including maculopathy, macular epiretinal membranes, new tears, RRD, exudative retinal detachment, and intraretinal and preretinal haemorrhages [8, 22, 23, 40]. According to several authors, some changes in macular area were observed in 1.7 % of cases after prophylactic laser treatment, vitreous haemorrhage – in 3.7 % of cases, new retinal tears in the early postoperative period – in 5.5 % of cases, and in the late postoperative period – in 8.3 % of cases [41]. Generally, serious adverse events after peripheral LPC are uncommon and usually are associated with different violations of the LPC basic principles: excess of radiation power [40, 42], inadequate or incomplete treatment due to lack of retinopexy along the tear's anterior margin [41] or obviously excessive overtreatment of large retinal areas [8].

We carried out the follow-up monitoring of the laser burns state using OCT scan in the following periods: the day of the retinal LPC (after 1 h), 2 weeks and 4 weeks after LPC (Case 69, Fig. 7.69); before treatment and 2 weeks after retinal LPC in case of the operculated tear with subclinical flat retinal detachment (Case 70, Fig. 7.70). Parameters used: solid-state YAG laser with doubled frequency, continuous mode, spot diameter of 200 μm, exposure of 0.1 sec, power of 80–100 mW depending on the fundus pigmentation until the 2–3 degree burn according to L'Esperance classification.

Here we present photographically and OCT-documented cases of complications after prophylactic laser treatment: post-LPC atrophy of the pigment epithelium (Case 71, Fig. 7.71), and post-LPC flap retinal tear (Case 72, Fig. 7.72).

Thus, layer-by-layer OCT scanning of peripheral degenerative lesions provides a better identification of vitreochorioretinal structures' pathological relationships compared to other diagnostic techniques and comes to the fore in the diagnosis and clarifying the nature of vitreoretinal tractions, adhesions, and retinal tears, allowing to determine the indications for prophylactic retinal LPC and to evaluate the treatment effectiveness.

Case 69. OCT Monitoring of Prophylactic Laser Photocoagulation for Lattice Degeneration

A 35-year-old male patient with severe myopia and partial posterior vitreous detachment presented with a 7-day history of floaters and flashes of light affecting his right eye.

Ophthalmoscopic Findings

Lattice degeneration with both full-thickness and atrophic tears, and considerable vitreous traction at the margins of the lesion is visible in the superotemporal quadrant of the right eye. Prophylactic laser photocoagulation was performed. The surgery was performed using a diode-pumped Oculight GL/GLx laser (532 nm) (IRIDEX, USA). The following parameters were used: laser spot diameter, 200 µm; pulse duration, 0.1 s; and pulse power, 80–90 mW. OCT monitoring was performed 1 h after surgery and during postoperative weeks 2 and 4.

Fundus Photographs and OCT Scans
(Fig. 7.69a–c)

1. **At 1 h postoperatively** (Fig. 7.69a)
   Fundus photo of lattice degeneration with laser burns at 1 h postoperatively is shown in Fig. 7.69a. The laser spots are light gray and clearly outlined. OCT scan shows areas of increased reflectivity in the neuroepithelium and dense areas of the pigment epithelium corresponding to the photocoagulation spots.
2. **At 2 and 4 weeks postoperatively**
   (Fig. 7.69b, c)
   Fundus photo of lattice degeneration with laser spots at 2 weeks (Fig. 7.69b) and 4 weeks (Fig. 7.69c) postoperatively. The laser spots are dark, their margins – distinct. OCT scans show areas of dense neuroepithelium with chorioretinal adhesions corresponding to the laser spots.

OCT Scans Details (Fig. 7.69a–c)

Dense areas of pigment epithelium

Increased reflectivity of all retinal layers (laser burn spots)

Increased reflectivity of the choroid at the level of the pigment epithelium destruction

Areas of dense pigment epithelium with chorioretinal adhesions (laser burn spots)

Decreased reflectivity of the choroid at the level of the dense pigment epithelium

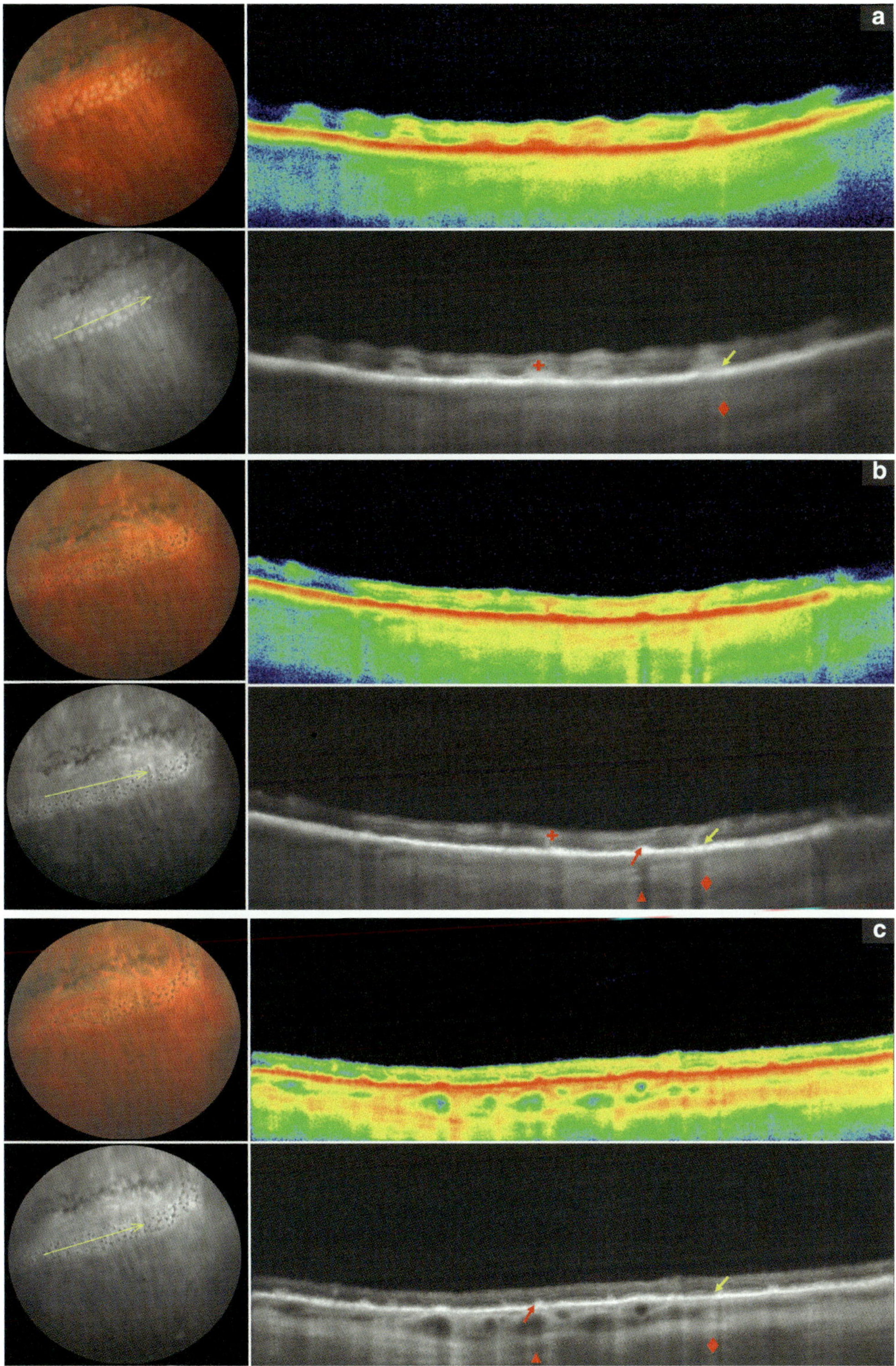

Fig. 7.69 (**a**) Fundus photographs and OCT scans of lattice degeneration with laser spots at 1 h postoperatively. (**b**) Fundus photographs and OCT scans of lattice degenera- tion with laser spots at 2 weeks postoperatively. (**c**) Fundus photographs and OCT scans of lattice degeneration with laser spots at 4 weeks postoperatively

Case 70. OCT Monitoring of Laser Photocoagulation of a Forming Retinal Tear

A 20-year-old male patient presented with 7-day history of photopsias in his right eye.

Ophthalmoscopic Findings

A small round area of hyperpigmentation with blurred borders and vitreoretinal traction is seen in the mid-peripheral retina of the inferior quadrant of the right eye. The retinal vessels are intact. The OCT-scanning revealed a forming flap tear. Prophylactic laser photocoagulation was performed with OCT-monitoring at 1 h and 2 weeks postoperatively.

Fundus Photographs and OCT Scans (Fig. 7.70a–c)

1. **Prior to the laser surgery** (Fig. 7.70a)
   Fundus photo of the forming tear before the surgery shows a small round area of hyperpigmentation with blurred borders. The OCT scan shows irregular retinal surface with multiple epiretinal folds. A large intraretinal cavity with hyporeflective content and clear borders is evident within the neuroepithelium.
2. **At 1 h postoperatively** (Fig. 7.70b)

Fundus photo shows well-defined white laser spots placed in two to three rows around and in the center of the tear. The OCT-scan shows that the size of the hyporeflective cavity has significantly decreased. Pigment epithelium in the center and at the margins of the tear is thickened, which corresponds to the laser burns.

3. **At 2 weeks postoperatively** (Fig. 7.70c)
   Fundus photo shows laser burns in two to three rows around and in the center of the tear, they are pigmented and have distinct irregular margins. The OCT scan shows that the retinal surface is smooth, with areas of thickened pigment epithelium (laser burns). The hyporeflective intraretinal cavity is no longer seen.

OCT Scans Details (Fig. 7.70a–c)

Isolated irregular intraretinal cavity

Increased reflectivity of all neurosensory retina layers (laser spots)

Areas of dense pigment epithelium (laser spots)

Destructive changes around the dense areas of pigment epithelium

Increased reflectivity of the choroid at the level of the pigment epithelium destruction

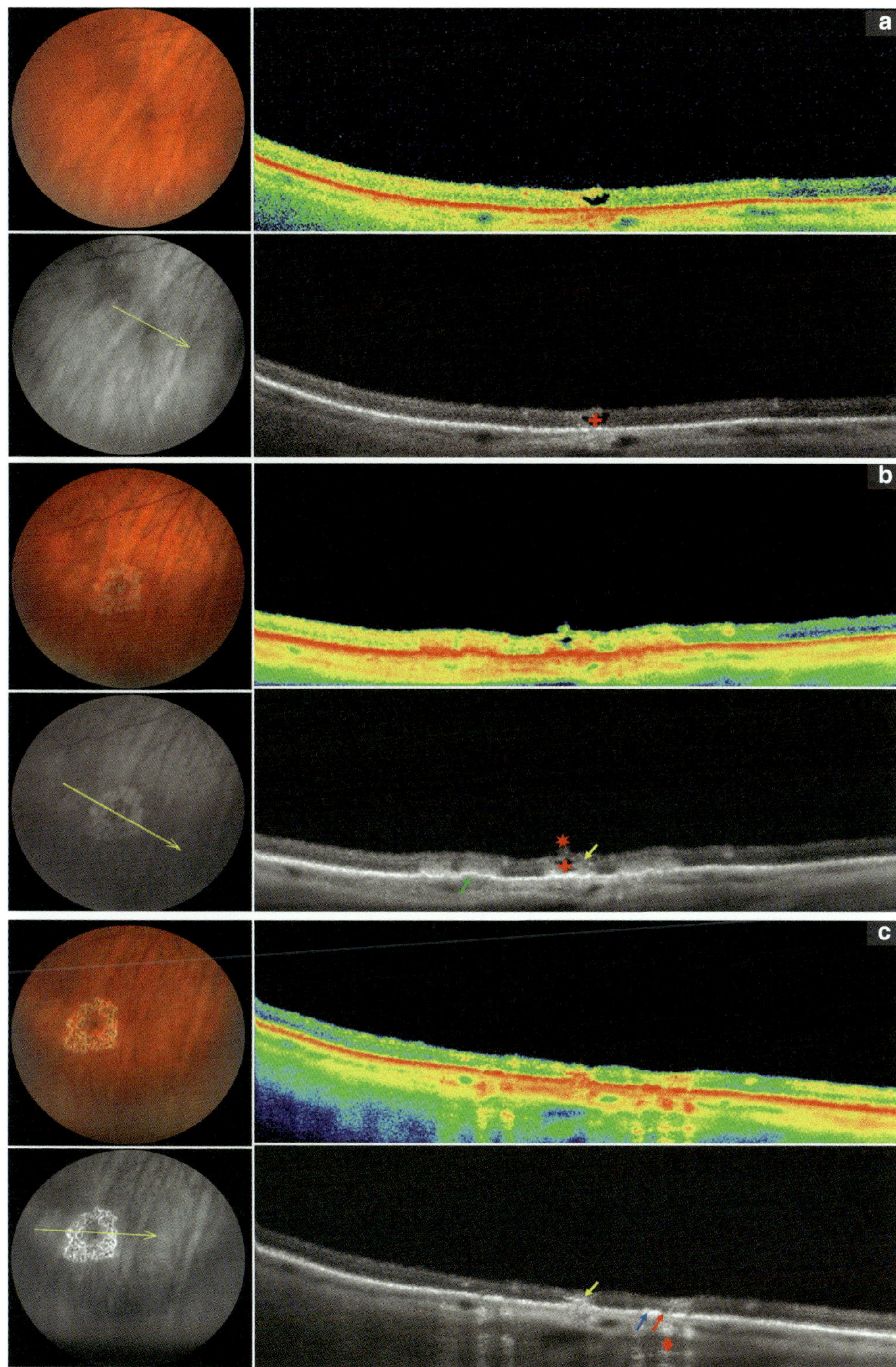

Fig. 7.70 (**a**) Fundus photograph and OCT scan of the forming flap tear prior to the surgery. (**b**) Fundus photograph and OCT scan of the forming flap tear at 1 h postoperatively. (**c**) Fundus photograph and OCT scan of the forming flap tear at 2 weeks postoperatively

Case 71. OCT Monitoring of Laser Photocoagulation of a Full-Thickness Operculated Tear with Shallow Retinal Detachment and Associated Honeycomb Degeneration

A 25-year-old female patient presented with flashes of light and floaters affecting her right eye.

Ophthalmoscopic Findings

A full-thickness operculated neurosensory tear is seen in the mid-peripheral retina of the infero-temporal quadrant of the right eye. The tear is bright red and irregular. There is a small haemorrhage on the retina surface next to the tear. There is a shallow (subclinical) retinal detachment around the tear margins.

The prophylactic laser photocoagulation was performed using a solid-state YAG laser with doubled frequency (532 nm green). The following parameters were used: laser spot diameter, 200 μm; pulse duration, 0.2 s; and pulse power, 80–90 mW.

Fundus Photographs and OCT Scans (Fig. 7.71a–c)

1. **Prior to the laser surgery** (Fig. 7.71a)
   The fundus photo shows the full-thickness operculated tear of the neurosensory retina associated with honeycomb degeneration. The tear is bright red and irregular.
2. **Prior to the laser surgery** (Fig. 7.71b)
   Fundus photo of the full-thickness operculated tear before the surgery. OCT scan shows the full-thickness tear (inner diameter, 367 μm; outer diameter, 513 μm) with shallow neurosensory detachment around the edges (length, 1.48 mm). There is an operculum in

the vitreous over the tear, shadowing the choroid, and areas of dense and elevated pigment epithelium.

3. **At 2 weeks postoperatively** (Fig. 7.71c)
   Fundus photo of the full-thickness operculated tear 2 weeks after the surgery. The laser spots are clearly seen, pigmented and have distinct irregular margins. The detached retina has re-attached. The haemorrhage has resolved. OCT scan shows the full-thickness retinal tear (inner diameter, 361 μm; outer diameter, 336 μm). Shallow retinal detachment is adherent. The retinal margins are thickened with chorioretinal adhesions secondary to laser photocoagulation.

OCT Scan Details (Fig. 7.71a–c)

Hyperreflective operculum in the vitreous at the level of the full-thickness neurosensory tear

Full-thickness tear of the neurosensory retina

Detached neurosensory retina around the tear

Cavity formed by the shallow detachment

Hyporeflectivity at the level of the pigment epithelium and the choroid at the level of the hyperreflective operculum

Areas of dense pigment epithelium (honeycomb degeneration)

Adherent neurosensory retina around the full-thickness tear

Areas of dense pigment epithelium with chorioretinal adhesions at the level of the laser burns

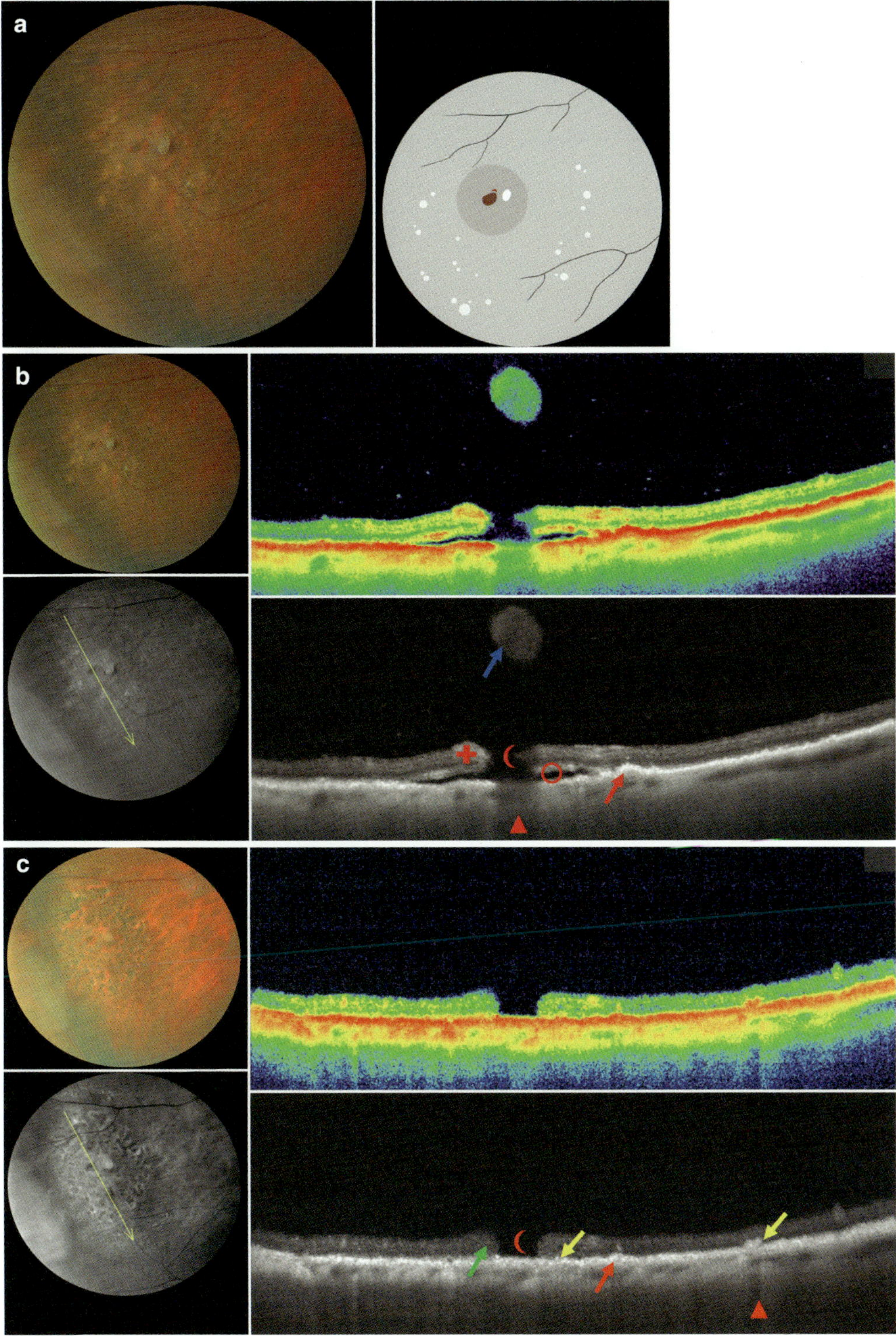

Fig. 7.71 (**a**) Operculated tear with shallow retinal detachment and honeycomb degeneration prior to the surgery. (**b**) Fundus photograph and OCT scan prior to the surgery. (**c**) Fundus photograph and OCT scan at 2 weeks postoperatively

Case 72. Pigment Epithelium Atrophy Secondary to Laser Photocoagulation

An asymptomatic 48-year-old female patient came for a routine fundus examination. According to the patient, she had a laser photocoagulation 5 years before.

Ophthalmoscopic Findings
(Fig. 7.72a, b)

Laser spots are seen in the inferior quadrant with atrophic changes of the pigment epithelium around some of them.

OCT Scan Description (Fig. 7.72c, d)

The retinal surface is irregular with areas of thinning at the level of the atrophic changes. Some areas of pigment epithelium are totally destructed and some are dense.

OCT Scan Details

Areas of pigment epithelium destruction (laser spots)

Increased reflectivity of the choroid at the level of the pigment epithelium destruction.

Areas of dense pigment epithelium

Decreased reflectivity of the choroid at the level of the dense pigment epithelium

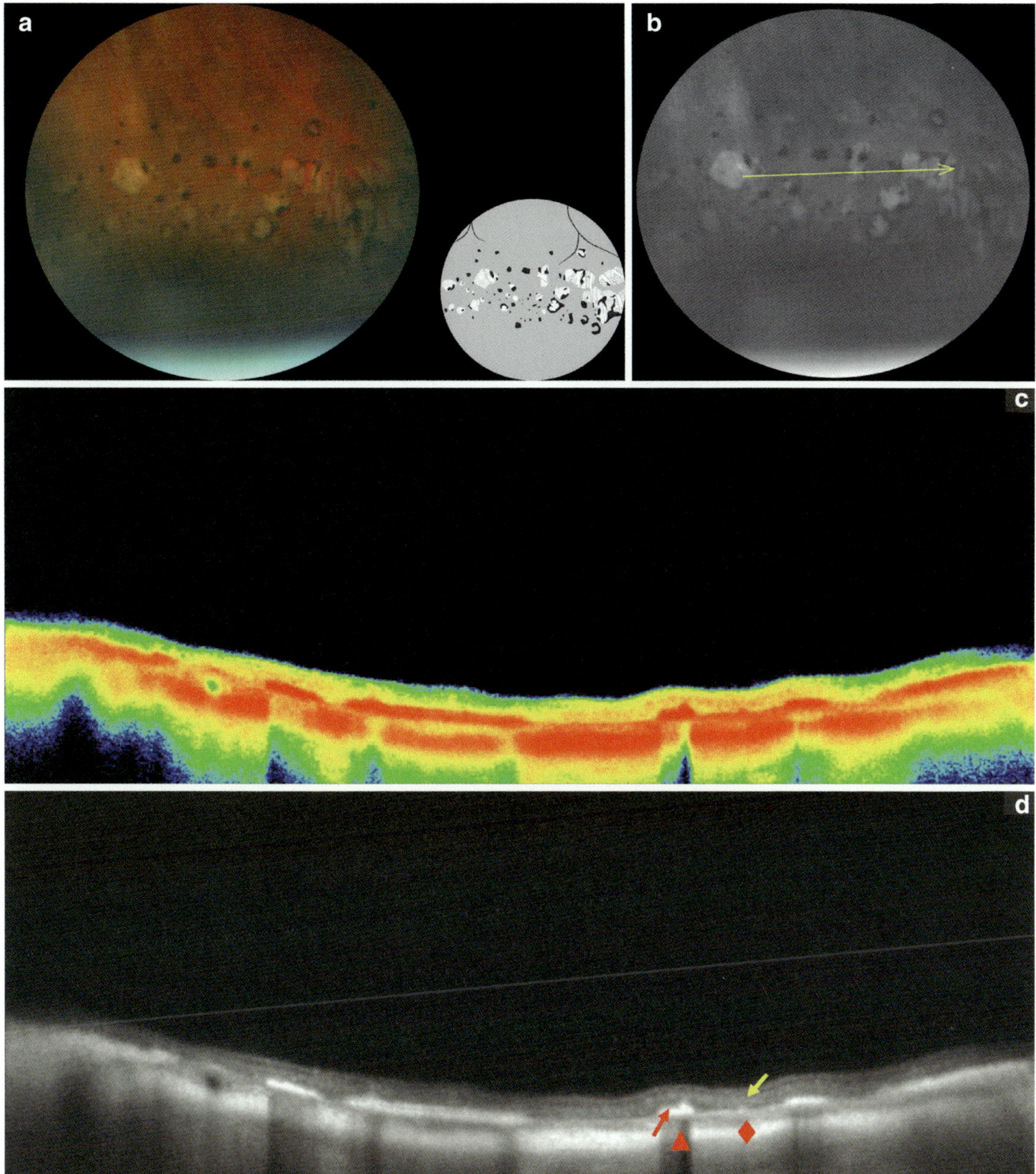

Fig. 7.72 (**a**) Pigment epithelium atrophy secondary to laser photocoagulation. (**b**) *Line* indicates OCT-scanning direction. (**c**, **d**) OCT scans of atrophic areas of pigment epithelium after the surgery

Case 73. Long-Term Post-Laser Flap Tear

A 53-year-old male patient presented with a 7 day-history of flashes of light and floaters disturbing him after physical exercise. According to the patient, he had had laser photocoagulation for peripheral retinal degeneration 1 year earlier. The patient was found to have moderate myopia and incomplete posterior vitreous detachment.

Ophthalmoscopic Findings (Fig. 7.73a, b)

Several rows of laser spots are seen in the far periphery of the inferior quadrant of the right eye. Laser burns are pigmented, some of them are surrounded by atrophic pigment epithelium. Two retinal tears are seen at the level of the laser spots: the U-shaped flap tear at 8 o'clock and the oval full-thickness tear with an operculum in the vitreous at 7 o'clock position.

OCT Scan Description (Fig. 7.73c)

Scan 1 The retinal surface is irregular, with marked vitreoretinal adhesion, traction, shallow retinal detachment and pigment epithelium destruction on the left and a full-thickness retinal tear and areas of dense pigment epithelium on the right. The retina over the tear is elevated and adherent to the posterior hyaloid membrane (cross-section image of the flap).

Scan 2 There are two full-thickness retinal tears in the neuroepithelium. The pigment epithelium at the tear edges is partially destroyed.

The retinal operculum, adherent to the posterior hyaloid membrane, is seen above the tear on the right.

OCT Scan Details (Fig. 7.73c)

Vitreoretinal adhesion and traction. Layers of moderate reflectivity in the vitreous

Cross-section image of the flap in the vitreous, with several hyporeflective cavities

An operculum floating in the vitreous over the tear (neurosensory tissue with vitreoretinal adhesion)

Full-thickness tear of the neurosensory retina

Area of dense neurosensory retina at the tear edges

Destruction of the pigment epithelium at the level of the vitreoretinal adhesion and traction

Hyporeflective space of the shallow neurosensory detachment

Area of dense pigment epithelium at the edge of the flap tear (laser spot)

Increased reflectivity of the choroid at the level of the pigment epithelium destruction

Decreased reflectivity of the choroid at the level of the dense retina under the vitreoretinal adhesion

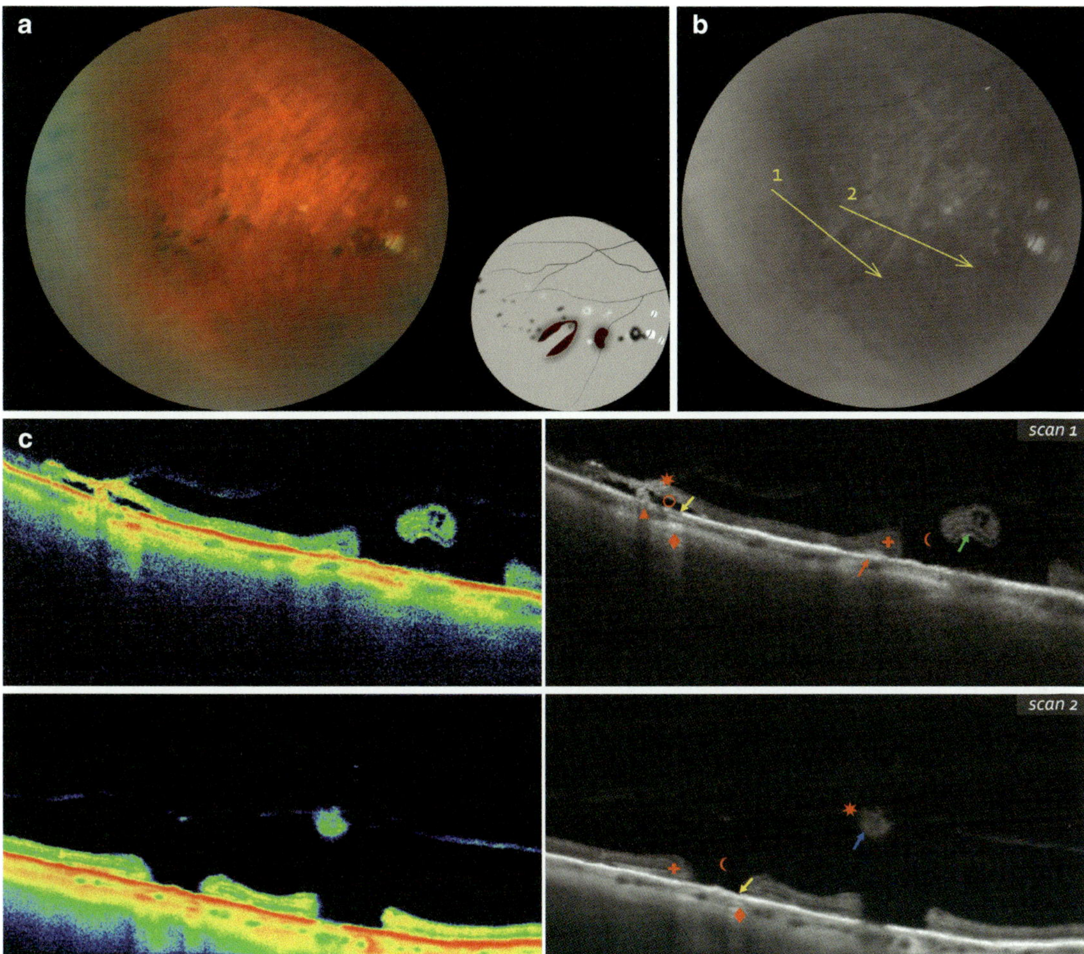

Fig. 7.73 (**a**) Post-laser flap tear. (**b**) *Line* indicates OCT-scanning direction. (**c**) OCT-scanning results according to the *line* direction in (**b**)

References

1. Conart JB, Baron D, Berrod JP. Degenerative lesions of the peripheral retina. J Fr Ophtalmol. 2014;37(1):73–80. doi:10.1016/j.jfo.2013.09.001. (In French)
2. Adrean SD, Elliot D. Prophylaxis for retinal detachment. Rev Ophthalmol. 2005;12(7):82–7.
3. Saksonova EO, Petropavlovskaja GA, Nesterov SA. Retinoschizis and retinal cysts. Ophthalmol J. 1991;30(3):173–6. (In Russian)
4. Kolenko OV, Sorokin EL, Egorov VV. Relationship between constitutional type of systemic hemodynamics and formation of peripheral vitreo-chorioretinal dystrophies during pregnancy. Vestn oftalmol. 2002;118(3):20–3. (In Russian)
5. Krohn J, Seland JH. Simultaneous, bilateral rhegmatogenous retinal detachment. Acta Ophthalmol Scand. 2000;78(3):354–8.
6. Bodanowitz S, Hesse L, Kroll P. Simultaneous bilateral rhegmatogenous retinal detachment. Klin Monatsbl Augenheilkd. 1995;206(3):148–51.
7. Lewis H. Peripheral retinal degenerations and the risk of retinal detachment. Am J Ophthalmol. 2003;136(1):155–60.
8. Kanski J. Clinical ophthalmology: a systemic approach. 5th ed. London: Butterworth Heinemann; 2003.
9. Soni M, Kirkby G. Prophylaxis of retinal detachment. 2005. http://www.medscape.com/viewarticle/513229_6.
10. Franchuk AA. The clinical characteristics of different types of peripheral retinal degeneration and their relationship to retinal breaks and detachment. Oftalmol Zh. 1989;8:451–4.
11. Bol'shunov AV, editor. Laser ophthalmology problems. Moscow: Aprel' (In Russian); 2013.
12. Mastropasqua L, Carpineto P, Ciancaglini M, et al. Treatment of retinal tears and lattice degenerations in fellow eyes in high risk patients suffering retinal detachment: a prospective study. Br J Ophthalmol. 1999;83(9):1046–9.
13. Kreis AJ, Aylward GW, Wolfensberger TJ. Prophilaxis for retinal detachment. Evidence or eminence based? Retina. 2007;27(4):468–72.
14. Graue-Wiechers FA, Verduzco NS. Laser treatment for retinal holes, tears and peripheral. In: Boyd S, Wilkinson CP, editors. Retinal detachment surgery and laser treatment. Panama: Jaypee Highlights Med Publ; 2009. p. 47–57.
15. Boiko EV. Lasers in ophthalmologic surgery: theoretical and practical basis. St.-Petersburg: Voen Med Acad (In Russian); 2004.
16. Straatsma BR, Foos RY. Typical and reticular retinoshisis. Am J Ophthalmol. 1973;75(4):551–75.
17. Straatsma BR, Zeegen PD, Foss RY, et al. Lattice degeneration of the retina. Am J Ophthalmol. 1974;77(5):619–49.
18. Byer NE. Long-term natural history of lattice degeneration of the retina. Ophthalmology. 1989;96(9):1396–401.
19. Feltgen N, Walter P. Rhegmatogenous retinal detachment – an ophthalmologic emergency. Dtsch Arztebl Int. 2014;111(1–2):12–21.
20. Kain HL. Chorioretinal adhesion after argon laser photocoagulation. Arch Ophthalmol. 1984;102(4):612–5.
21. Byer NE. Can rhegmatogenous retinal detachment be prevented? Reflections on the history of "prophylactic" treatment of retinal detachment. Ophthalmologe. 2000;97(10):696–702.
22. Morhat MV, Marchenko LN, Morhat VI. Prophylactic laser photocoagulation in peripheral retina irregularities (literature review). Ophthalmol East Eur. 2011;4(11):85–92. (In Russian)
23. Pasechnikova NV. Laser treatment of the eye fundus pathology. Kiev: Naukova Dumka (In Russian); 2007.
24. Bloom SM, Brucker J. Laser surgery of the posterior segment. Philadelphia: Lippincot Raven; 1997.
25. Wilkinson CP. Interventions for asymptomatic retinal breaks and lattice degeneration for preventing retinal detachment. Cochrane Database Syst Rev. 2014;9:CD003170. doi:10.1002/14651858.CD003170.pub4.
26. Morris R, Witherspoon CD, Kuhn F, et al. Retinal detachment laser prophylaxis. Ora secunda cerclage (OSC): creating a secondora. Retina Today. 2008;March/April:63–67.
27. Chauhan DS, Downie JA, Eckstein M, et al. Failure of prophylactic retinopexy in fellow eyes without a posterior vitreous detachment. Arch Ophthalmol. 2006;124(7):968–71.
28. Peyman GA, Sanders DR, Goldberg MF. Principles and practice of ophthalmology. Philadelphia: WB Saunders Company; 1987.
29. Garrant S, editor. Posterior vitreous detachment, retinal breaks and lattice degeneration. San Francisco: American Academy of Ophthalmology; 2014.
30. Francois J, Gamble E. Argon laser slitlamp photocoagulation. Indications and results. Ophthalmologica. 1974;169(5):362–70.
31. Bonnet MP, Camean F. Rhegmatogenous retina detachment after prophylactic argon laser photocoagulation. Graefe's Arch Clin Ophthalmol. 1987;225(1):5–8.
32. Davis MD. The natural history of retinal breaks without detachment. Trans Am Ophthalmol Soc. 1973;71:343–72.
33. Folk JC, Arrindell EL, Klugman MR. The fellow eye of patients with phakic lattice retinal detachment. Ophthalmology. 1989;96(1):72–9.
34. Saracco JB, Estachy GM, Gastaud P. Maymard Prophylactic treatment of aphakic retinal detachment by argon laser photocoagulation. Ophthalmologica. 1980;181(3–4):142–8.

35. Pollak A, Oliver M. Argonlaser photocoagulation of symptomatic flap tears and retinal breaks of fellow eyes. Br J Ophthalmol. 1981;65(7):469–72.

36. Byer NE. Rethinking prophylactic therapy of retinal detachment. In: Stirpe M, editor. Advances in vitreoretinal surgery. New York: Ophthalmic Communications Society; 1992. p. 399–411.

37. Balashevich LI, Izmailov AS. Diabetic ophthalmopathy. St.- Petersburg: Chelovek (In Russian); 2012.

38. L'Esperance FA. Ophthalmic lasers. Photocoagulation, photoradiation and surgery. St. Louis: Mosby; 1989.

39. Krasnoshchekova EE, Pankrushova TG, Boĭko EV. Peripheral vitreochorioretinal dystrophies and retinal detachment in pregnant women: diagnosis, treatment, and choice of a delivery procedure. Vestn Oftalmol. 2009;125(2):40–2. (In Russian).

40. Mester U, Volker B, Kroll P, et al. Complications of prophylactic argon laser treatment of retinal breaks and degenerations in 2,000 eyes. Ophthalmol Surg. 1988;19(7):482–4.

41. Robertson DM, Norton EW. Long term follow–up of treated retinal breaks. Am J Ophthalmol. 1973;75(3):395–404.

42. Quezada C, Pieramici DJ, Martsue R, et al. Demarcation laser photocoagulation induced retinal necrosis and rupture resulting in large retinal tear formation. Photodiagn Photodyn Ther. 2015;12(2):314–6. doi:10.1016/j.pdpdt.2015.02.006.

Printed by Printforce, the Netherlands

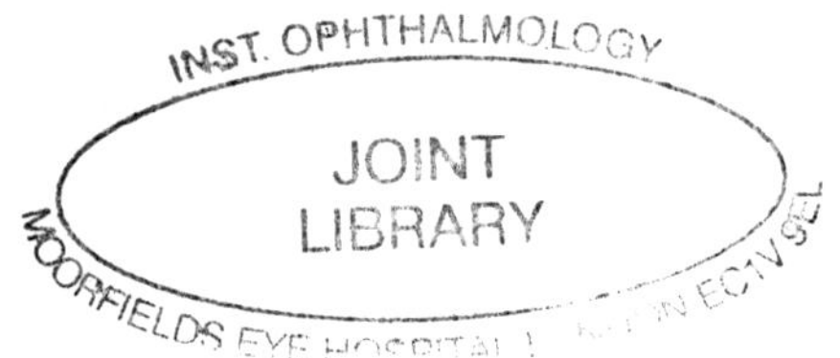